Global Burden and Challenges
of Melioidosis

Global Burden and Challenges of Melioidosis

Special Issue Editors

Direk Limmathurotsakul
David AB Dance

MDPI • Basel • Beijing • Wuhan • Barcelona • Belgrade

MDPI

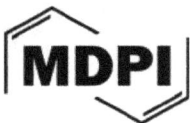

Special Issue Editors
Direk Limmathurotsakul   David AB Dance
Mahidol University   Lao-Oxford-Mahosot Hospital-Wellcome Trust
Thailand   Research Unit (LOMWRU)
                                Laos

Editorial Office
MDPI
St. Alban-Anlage 66
4052 Basel, Switzerland

This is a reprint of articles from the Special Issue published online in the open access journal *Tropical Medicine and Infectious Disease* (ISSN 2414-6366) from 2018 to 2019 (available at: https://www.mdpi.com/journal/tropicalmed/special_issues/melioidosis).

For citation purposes, cite each article independently as indicated on the article page online and as indicated below:

LastName, A.A.; LastName, B.B.; LastName, C.C. Article Title. *Journal Name* **Year**, *Article Number*, Page Range.

ISBN 978-3-03897-742-1 (Pbk)
ISBN 978-3-03897-743-8 (PDF)

Cover image courtesy of Stephen Rudgard.

Contents

About the Special Issue Editors

Direk Limmathurotsakul (Associate Professor, Mahidol University) studied medicine at Chulalongkorn University, Thailand. He obtained a PhD in Life and Biomolecular sciences from the Open University, UK, in 2008, and an MSc in Medical Statistics at the London School of Hygiene and Tropical Medicine in 2009. Since 2004, he has been working at the Mahidol-Oxford Tropical Medicine Research Unit (MORU), Mahidol University, mainly on melioidosis. He also works on sepsis and antimicrobial resistance. From 2012–present (2019), Direk has also run a Wellcome Trust-funded Intermediate Fellowship programme on melioidosis. He is also chair of the International Melioidosis Society (http://www.melioidosis.info) and the Melioidosis Threat Reduction Network (Melioidosis TRN). Direk has convened and contributed to a number of meetings about melioidosis between researchers and policy makers in multiple countries, including Thailand, Vietnam, Malaysia, Cambodia, Indonesia, India, Sri Lanka, and Brazil. These have helped to attract the attention of public health officials and policy makers, with the result that at last actions are being taken to improve diagnosis, treatment, and prevention of melioidosis in many tropical countries.

David Dance (Honorary Visiting Research Fellow, University of Oxford; Honorary Professor, London School of Hygiene and Tropical Medicine) studied medicine at the University of Bristol. He then trained in microbiology with the Public Health Laboratory Service (PHLS) in Southampton and London, completing an MSc in Medical Microbiology at the London School of Hygiene and Tropical Medicine in 1984 and Membership of the Royal College of Pathologists in 1986. From 1986 to 1990 he helped to establish clinical, microbiological, and epidemiological studies on melioidosis in northeast Thailand, which continue to this day. He returned to England for 20 years, working for the PHLS in Plymouth and the Health Protection Agency, and serving on the Councils of the Royal College of Pathologists and the British Infection Society and the Executive Committee of the Association of Medical Microbiologists. He returned to Asia in 2010, working at the Lao-Oxford-Mahosot Hospital-Welcome Trust Research Unit. Melioidosis has been his main research interest for the past 33 years, although he has also published on a wide range of other bacterial infections.

Preface to "Global Burden and Challenges of Melioidosis"

Melioidosis is one of the most neglected tropical diseases (NTDs), so much so that it is not even included in the WHO list of NTDs. Yet modeling suggests that it kills more people worldwide every year than diseases that are much better known, such as leptospirosis and dengue. The reasons for this under-recognition are numerous, including the fact that it mainly affects the disadvantaged rural poor in areas that are poorly supplied with the diagnostic capability to make the diagnosis. Furthermore, as it is strongly associated with diabetes, melioidosis is likely to become more common in the years to come as the prevalence of diabetes increases, and rising global travel will mean that it could be encountered anywhere in the world. Unless treated appropriately, many of those affected by this disease will die. We are passionate about increasing the profile of melioidosis in the hope that this will save some of those lives.

The articles in this book were commissioned from authors around the world in order to provide as complete a picture as possible of the current status (in 2018) of melioidosis in the respective countries or regions, and the challenges faced in relation to the disease. The articles were published online as they were completed, but are now gathered here in one book to form a definitive reference for researchers, healthcare workers, and policy makers. We hope that this will encourage others to study this fascinating infection, and go some way towards securing it the attention it deserves.

Direk Limmathurotsakul, David AB Dance
Special Issue Editors

Tropical Medicine and Infectious Disease

MDPI

Editorial

Global Burden and Challenges of Melioidosis

David AB Dance [1,2,3,*] and Direk Limmathurotsakul [2,4,5,*]

1 Lao-Oxford-Mahosot Hospital-Wellcome Trust Research Unit (LOMWRU), Vientiane, Laos
2 Centre for Tropical Medicine & Global Health, University of Oxford, Oxford OX3 7FZ, UK
3 Faculty of Tropical Medicine and Infectious Diseases, London School of Hygiene and Tropical Medicine, London WC1E 7HT, UK
4 Mahidol-Oxford Research Unit (MORU), Bangkok 10400, Thailand
5 Faculty of Tropical Medicine, Mahidol University, Bangkok 10400, Thailand
* Correspondence: David.d@tropmedres.ac (D.A.B.D.); direk@tropmedres.ac (D.L.)

Received: 23 January 2018; Accepted: 24 January 2018; Published: 29 January 2018

Melioidosis, an infectious disease caused by the environmental bacterium *Burkholderia pseudomallei*, has remained in the shadows for far too long. Described over 100 years ago by Alfred Whitmore in Rangoon [1], the disease is so neglected that it is not even on any of the lists of neglected tropical diseases, despite the fact that it probably kills more people each year than diseases that are much better known, such as leptospirosis and dengue [2]. We aim to set the record straight.

In the first few years after its discovery, melioidosis was considered a relatively rare infection confined to areas where colonial medical services had been established, for example by the British in Burma (now Myanmar) [1], Ceylon (now Sri Lanka) [3] and the Federated Malay States (now Malaysia) [4], the French in Indochina (now Cambodia, Laos and Vietnam) [5–7], and the Dutch in the Dutch East Indies (now Indonesia) [8–10]. It was the French in Indochina who proved that the organism was a saprophyte rather than a zoonosis as had originally been suspected [11,12]. It was discovered for the first time in northern Australia in 1949 [13], although it appears that this is really where it actually originated [14]. *B. pseudomallei* appears to have spread from there to southeast Asia, and thence to Africa and the Americas [15,16]. The disease gained brief notoriety as a cause of infection amongst French and American troops serving in Southeast Asia [17–19]. Its unusual ability to remain latent after acquisition and cause a fatal disease many years later has given rise to the nickname 'Vietnam Time Bomb' [20]. *B. pseudomallei* has more recently been categorised as a 'Tier 1 Select Agent' because of its biothreat potential (https://www.ecfr.gov/cgi-bin/retrieveECFR?gp=&SID=8a4be60456973b5ec6bef5dfeaffd49a&r=PART&n=42y1.0.1.6.61).

Undoubtedly, it was the work of the Infectious Disease Association of Thailand that led to the recognition that melioidosis was actually a greatly-underestimated public health problem in some parts of the world. In 1985, they organised a meeting devoted to melioidosis that highlighted 686 cases of the disease occurring in Thailand over a relatively short time period [21]. This heralded a new wave of interest in the disease that has culminated in this current special issue of Tropical Medicine and Infectious Diseases. Writing in 1991, after spending 4 years observing what an important disease melioidosis was in northeast Thailand [22], one of us reviewed existing evidence and suggested that the disease was probably far more common worldwide than was currently appreciated [23]. This was not a new idea, as Fournier had made similar suggestions some 3 decades earlier [24,25]. The reasons for its under-recognition are a lack of diagnostic microbiology laboratories serving the rural poor in the tropics, who are most likely to acquire melioidosis, and a lack of familiarity and awareness amongst medical and laboratory staff, where such laboratories are available. More recently, the prediction has been vindicated by growing numbers of reports of the disease in new places, and increasing recognition within known endemic areas [26,27]. In 2016, the first attempt was made to estimate the global burden of human melioidosis in terms of cases and deaths, the resulting prediction being 165,000 and 89,000 per year, respectively, a mortality burden similar to that of measles [2].

Now, two years on from this modelling study [2], the time is right to take stock of what we have learned since then. In this issue, we have combined articles from countries and regions around the world that summarise the current status, including what is known locally about the burden of melioidosis, and the key challenges facing local clinicians, laboratory staff and public health and policy makers, in relation to this elusive but common and fatal disease. We hope that this will become a key source of information for those who share our concern and are taking actions against this disease.

Conflicts of Interest: The authors declare no conflict of interest.

References

1. Whitmore, A. On the bacteriology of an infective disease occurring in Rangoon. *Br. Med. J.* **1912**, *2*, 1306–1308.
2. Limmathurotsakul, D.; Golding, N.; Dance, D.A.B.; Messina, J.P.; Pigott, D.M.; Moyes, C.L.; Rolim, D.B.; Bertherat, E.; Day, N.P.J.; Peacock, S.J.; et al. Predicted global distribution of *Burkholderia pseudomallei* and burden of melioidosis. *Nat. Microbiol.* **2016**, *1*, 15008. [CrossRef] [PubMed]
3. Denny, C.R.; Nicholls, L. Melioidosis in a European. *Ceylon J. Sci.* **1927**, *2*, 37–40.
4. Stanton, A.T.; Fletcher, W. *Melioidosis: Studies from the Institute for Medical Research, Federated Malay States*; No. 21; John Bale, Sons & Danielson Ltd.: London, UK, 1932.
5. Vielle, A.; Morin, H.G.S.; Massias, C. Un nouveau cas de mélioïdose en Cochinchine. *Bull. Soc. Med. Chir. Indoch.* **1926**, *4*, 459–465.
6. Pons, R.; Advier, M. Melioidosis in Cochin China. *J. Hyg.* **1927**, *26*, 28–30. [CrossRef] [PubMed]
7. Mesnard, J.; Joyeux, B.G. Un cas de mélioïdose au Tonkin. *Bull. Soc. Med. Chir. Indoch.* **1929**, *7*, 32–39.
8. De Moor, C.E.; Soekarnen; van de Walle, N. Melioidosis op Java. *Mededeeling uit het Geneeskundig Laboratorium te Weltevreden* **1932**, *72*, 1618–1635.
9. Hulshoff, A.A. Een geval van melioïdosis. *Geneeskd Tijdschr Ned Indie* **1933**, *73*, 1218–1222.
10. Pet, M.A.; Fossen, A. Melioidosis der inwendige organen (melioidosis of internal organs). *Geneeskd Tijdschr Ned Indie* **1934**, *74*, 976–981.
11. Vaucel, M. Présence probable du bacille de Whitmore dans l'eau de mare au Tonkin. *Bull. Soc. Pathol. Exot.* **1937**, *30*, 10–15.
12. Chambon, L. Isolement du bacille de Whitmore à partir du milieu extérieur. *Ann. Inst. Pasteur* **1955**, *89*, 229–235.
13. Cottew, G.S. Melioidosis in sheep in Queensland; a description of the causal organism. *Aust. J. Exp. Biol. Med. Sci.* **1950**, *28*, 677–683. [CrossRef] [PubMed]
14. Pearson, T.; Giffard, P.; Beckstrom-Sternberg, S.; Auerbach, R.; Hornstra, H.; Tuanyok, A.; Price, E.P.; Glass, M.B.; Leadem, B.; Beckstrom-Sternberg, J.S.; et al. Phylogeographic reconstruction of a bacterial species with high levels of lateral gene transfer. *BMC Biol.* **2009**, *7*, 78. [CrossRef] [PubMed]
15. Sarovich, D.S.; Garin, B.; De Smet, B.; Kaestli, M.; Mayo, M.; Vandamme, P.; Jacobs, J.; Lompo, P.; Tahita, M.C.; Tinto, H.; et al. Phylogenomic analysis reveals an Asian origin for African *Burkholderia pseudomallei* and further supports melioidosis endemicity in Africa. *mSphere* **2016**, *1*. [CrossRef] [PubMed]
16. Chewapreecha, C.; Holden, M.T.; Vehkala, M.; Valimaki, N.; Yang, Z.; Harris, S.R.; Mather, A.E.; Tuanyok, A.; De Smet, B.; Le Hello, S.; et al. Global and regional dissemination and evolution of *Burkholderia pseudomallei*. *Nat. Microbiol.* **2017**, *2*, 16263. [CrossRef] [PubMed]
17. Patterson, M.C.; Darling, C.L.; Blumenthal, J.B. Acute melioidosis in a soldier home from South Vietnam. *J. Am. Med. Assoc.* **1967**, *200*, 447–451. [CrossRef]
18. Brundage, W.G.; Thuss, C.J.J.; Walden, D.C. Four fatal cases of melioidosis in US soldiers in Vietnam. *Am. J. Trop. Med. Hyg.* **1968**, *17*, 183–191. [CrossRef] [PubMed]
19. Weber, D.R.; Douglass, L.E.; Brundage, W.G.; Stallkamp, T.C. Acute varieties of melioidosis occurring in US soldiers in Vietnam. *Am. J. Med.* **1969**, *46*, 234–244. [CrossRef]
20. Anonymous. Viet Nam's "time bomb". *Time* **1967**, *89*, 6.
21. Punyagupta, S. Review of 686 cases and presentation of a new clinical classification. In *Melioidosis*; Punyagupta, S., Sirisanthana, T., Stapatayavong, B., Eds.; Bangkok Medical Publisher: Bangkok, Thailand, 1989; pp. 217–229.

22. Chaowagul, W.; White, N.J.; Dance, D.A.; Wattanagoon, Y.; Naigowit, P.; Davis, T.M.; Looareesuwan, S.; Pitakwatchara, N. Melioidosis: A major cause of community-acquired septicemia in northeastern Thailand. *J. Infect. Dis.* **1989**, *159*, 890–899. [CrossRef] [PubMed]

23. Dance, D.A.B. Melioidosis: The tip of the iceberg? *Clin. Microbiol. Rev.* **1991**, *4*, 52–60. [CrossRef] [PubMed]

24. Fournier, J. A zoonosis gaining ground: Melioidosis. *Med. d'Egypte* **1960**, *9*, 23–54.

25. Fournier, J. La mélioïdose et le b. de Whitmore. Controverses épidémiologiques et taxonomiques. *Bull. Soc. Pathol. Exot. Filiales* **1965**, *58*, 753–765. [PubMed]

26. Currie, B.J.; Dance, D.A.B.; Cheng, A.C. The global distribution of *Burkholderia pseudomallei* and melioidosis: An update. *Trans. R. Soc. Trop. Med. Hyg.* **2008**, *102* (Suppl. S1), S1–S4. [CrossRef]

27. Limmathurotsakul, D.; Wongratanacheewin, S.; Teerawattanasook, N.; Wongsuvan, G.; Chaisuksant, S.; Chetchotisakd, P.; Chaowagul, W.; Day, N.P.; Peacock, S.J. Increasing incidence of human melioidosis in northeast Thailand. *Am. J. Trop. Med. Hyg.* **2010**, *82*, 1113–1117. [CrossRef] [PubMed]

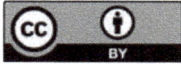

Tropical Medicine and Infectious Disease

MDPI

Review

Melioidosis in Africa: Time to Uncover the True Disease Load

Ivo Steinmetz [1,2,*] , Gabriel E. Wagner [1], Estelle Kanyala [3], Mamadou Sawadogo [3],
Hema Soumeya [4], Mekonnen Teferi [5] , Emawayish Andargie [5], Biruk Yeshitela [5],
Louise Yaba Atsé-Achi [6,7], Moussa Sanogo [6], Bassirou Bonfoh [7], Raphael Rakotozandrindrainy [8],
Célestin Pongombo Shongo [9], Mick Shongoya Pongombo [9], Eric Kasamba Ilunga [9],
Sabine Lichtenegger [1] , Karoline Assig [1,2], Jürgen May [10] , Eric Bertherat [11],
Michael Owusu [12] , Ellis Owusu-Dabo [12,13] and Yaw Adu-Sarkodie [12]

[1] Institute of Hygiene, Microbiology and Environmental Medicine, Medical University of Graz, 8036 Graz,
   Austria; gabriel.wagner-lichtenegger@medunigraz.at (G.E.W.); sabine.lichtenegger@medunigraz.at (S.L.);
   karoline.assig@medunigraz.at (K.A.)
[2] Friedrich Loeffler Institute of Medical Microbiology, University Medicine of Greifswald, KöR,
   17475 Greifswald, Germany
[3] Departement UFR/Science de la Santé, Université d'Ouagadougou, BP 7021, Ouagadougou, Burkina Faso;
   kanyalaestelle@gmail.com (E.K.); elmsawa@yahoo.fr (M.S.)
[4] Centre Muraz, 01 BP 390 Bobo Dioulasso, Burkina Faso; meya_4@yahoo.fr
[5] Armauer Hansen Research Institute, Jimma Road, ALERT Compound, P.O. Box 1005 Addis Ababa, Ethiopia;
   mekonnenteferi@yahoo.com (M.T.); emawaand@gmail.com (E.A.); biruk_23@yahoo.com (B.Y.)
[6] Laboratoire Central Vétérinaire de Bingerville, LANADA, P.O. Box 206 Bingerville, Cote D'Ivoire;
   louisachi@yahoo.fr (L.Y.A.-A.); ssanogomoussas@gmail.com (M.S.)
[7] Centre Suisse de Recherches Scientifiques en Côte d'Ivoire (CSRS), 01 BP 1303 Abidjan, Cote D'Ivoire;
   bassirou.bonfoh@csrs.ci
[8] Department of Microbiology and Parasitology, University of Antananarivo, B.P. 175 Antananarivo,
   Madagascar; rakrapha13@gmail.com
[9] Université de Lubumbashi, 1825 Lubumbashi, Democratic Republic of the Congo;
   pongoshon@gmail.com (C.P.S.); mickshongo@yahoo.fr (M.S.P.); kasambailunga@gmail.com (E.K.I.)
[10] Bernhard Nocht Institute for Tropical Medicine, 20359 Hamburg, Germany; may@bnitm.de
[11] Department of Infectious Hazard Management, World Health Organization, Geneva 27, Switzerland;
   bertherate@who.int
[12] College of Health Sciences, Kwame Nkrumah University of Science and Technology, 00233 Kumasi, Ghana;
   owusumichael-gh@hotmail.com (M.O.); owusudabo@yahoo.com (E.O.-D); yasax@hotmail.co.uk (Y.A.-S.)
[13] Kumasi Centre for Collaborative Research, 00233 Kumasi, Ghana
*   Correspondence: ivo.steinmetz@medunigraz.at; Tel.: +43-316-385-73700

Received: 16 April 2018; Accepted: 1 June 2018; Published: 10 June 2018

Abstract: Melioidosis is an often fatal infectious disease with a protean clinical spectrum, caused by the environmental bacterial pathogen *Burkholderia pseudomallei*. Although the disease has been reported from some African countries in the past, the present epidemiology of melioidosis in Africa is almost entirely unknown. Therefore, the common view that melioidosis is rare in Africa is not evidence-based. A recent study concludes that large parts of Africa are environmentally suitable for *B. pseudomallei*. Twenty-four African countries and three countries in the Middle East were predicted to be endemic, but no cases of melioidosis have been reported yet. In this study, we summarize the present fragmentary knowledge on human and animal melioidosis and environmental *B. pseudomallei* in Africa and the Middle East. We propose that systematic serological studies in man and animals together with environmental investigations on potential *B. pseudomallei* habitats are needed to identify risk areas for melioidosis. This information can subsequently be used to target raising clinical awareness and the implementation of simple laboratory algorithms for the isolation of *B. pseudomallei* from clinical specimens. *B. pseudomallei* was most likely transferred from Asia to the Americas via Africa, which is shown by phylogenetic analyses. More data on the virulence and genomic characteristics of African *B. pseudomallei* isolates will contribute to a better understanding of the global evolution of the pathogen and will also help to assess potential differences in disease prevalence and outcome.

Keywords: melioidosis; Africa; Middle East; *Burkholderia pseudomallei*; genomics; public awareness; environment

1. Introduction

Recently, the global environmental distribution of *B. pseudomallei* and the world-wide incidence and mortality of meliodosis was estimated using a modelling approach. It was predicted that 165,000 melioidosis cases occur per year worldwide, in which 89,000 people die [1]. The estimates suggest not only a massive underreporting in countries known to be endemic but also identified 34 countries in which melioidosis is probably endemic and has never been reported. Among those countries are 24 African countries and three countries in the Middle East. Modelling predicts that 24,000 (95% credible interval 8000–72,000) cases with 15,000 (credible interval 6000–45,000) deaths occur annually in sub-Saharan Africa while less than 1000 annual cases and deaths were predicted for North Africa and the Middle East [1]. Although in some African and Middle East countries sporadic cases of human and animal melioidosis have been reported for many decades [2,3], sound epidemiological data for the disease do not exist for any of those countries. Remarkably, melioidosis has not been classified as a neglected tropical disease. Defining the prevalence of melioidosis in these regions is important for public health. Due to its non-specific clinical presentation, human melioidosis can mimic many common infectious diseases such as malaria or tuberculosis. Due to its severity, misdiagnosis will lead to inappropriate case management and the highest case fatality. Moreover, melioidosis is a differential diagnosis of some epidemic-prone diseases like plague, which means that early diagnosis can be important in a public health perspective. In this paper, we summarize the available information on reported cases of melioidosis in man and animals. Furthermore, we review knowledge on the environmental presence of *B. pseudomallei* in Africa and the Middle East and on the characteristics of African *B. pseudomallei* strains. Lastly, we consider potential strategies to unravel the true burden of the disease in these parts of the world.

2. Melioidosis and Environmental *B. pseudomallei* in Africa and the Middle East

In this section, countries were assigned to sub-regions, according to the United Nations geoscheme. Peer-reviewed published cases of human and animal melioidosis together with reports on environmental *B. pseudomallei* in the various African sub-regions and the Middle East (sub-region Western Asia) were compiled based on journal research and by using the global occurrence database created by Limmathurotsakul et al. [1].

2.1. Northern Africa

Environmental occurrence of *B. pseudomallei* is associated with high amounts of precipitation [1]. It is, therefore, not surprising that most parts of Northern Africa are not considered suitable environments for this pathogen [1]. Neither indigenous nor imported cases of human melioidosis have been reported from this part of Africa. There is, however, a report from Egypt in 1953 describing melioidosis in a horse. This case was identified by a positive reaction to subcutaneous administration of *Burkholderia mallei* antigen (mallein test) while testing horses for glanders. However, because subsequent antigen tests gave inconsistent results, the authors suspected melioidosis. *B. pseudomallei* was isolated from a mesenteric gland after a post-mortem examination and was shown to be virulent in guinea pigs. Metabolic characteristics of the isolate were different from the close relative *Burkholderia mallei*, indicating that the horse suffered from melioidosis but not glanders [4].

2.2. Middle East

The environmental suitability for *B. pseudomallei* seems to vary significantly within the countries of the Middle East [1]. Turkey and parts of the Sinai Peninsula were not predicted to be suitable for *B. pseudomallei*. However, there are regions in Saudi Arabia, Yemen, Iraq, and Oman that seem to be suitable for *B. pseudomallei* [1].

In 1961, a case of pulmonary melioidosis was described in southern Turkey, although the information provided on the bacteriological identification procedure does not allow confirmation of *B. pseudomallei* with certainty [5]. This also applies to a report of *B. pseudomallei* isolation from raw milk samples in different areas of Ankara, Turkey from 1998 [6]. A study from 1997 in Saudi Arabia examined the bacterial flora of the nasal cavity and lungs of healthy and unhealthy sheep and calves. It was reported that *B. pseudomallei* was isolated from the nasal cavity of sheep [7]. Again, the information provided on the bacterial identification procedure does not allow firm conclusions on the identity of the isolated bacteria. In 1997, melioidosis was reported in a camel in Dubai in the United Arab Emirates [8]. Although the clinical signs were suggestive of melioidosis, an inadequate amount of information on microbiological characteristics of the isolated strain was provided [8].

Although large parts of Iran have a relatively dry climate, a subtropical region along the Caspian Sea coast and parts of the south were predicted to be environmentally suitable for *B. pseudomallei* [1]. A report from 1975 described the environmental presence of virulent *B. pseudomallei* in rice fields along the Caspian Sea coast. Out of 157 soil samples, 19 were shown to be positive for *B. pseudomallei* and the virulence of these strains was confirmed in guinea pigs [9]. Furthermore, in 1979, an outbreak of melioidosis among horses and a mule in Iran was reported [10]. The authors isolated motile Gram-negative bacterial strains from abscesses in various organs from the horses and the mule, with biochemical characteristics typical of *B. pseudomallei* but not of *B. mallei* [10]. In 1977, the first case of human pulmonary melioidosis in Iran was published [11]. To our knowledge, there have been no further reports in the international literature of indigenous melioidosis from Iran, except for a case of melioidosis imported from Southeast Asia into Iran [12].

2.3. Western Africa

According to the predicted environmental suitability for *B. pseudomallei*, western sub-Saharan Africa is among the highest risk zones [1]. In line with this forecast, *B. pseudomallei* strains were already isolated between 1967 and 1971 from lesions in pigs in a slaughterhouse in Niamey, Niger [13]. Subsequently, environmental surveys along the route of pig transport revealed the presence of *B. pseudomallei* in the soil of Burkina Faso and Niger [14]. More recently, *B. pseudomallei* was isolated in a blood culture of a 59-year-old man native to and living in Burkina Faso, who presented with a mycotic aneurysm of an iliac artery [15]. Galimand and Dodin reported the isolation of *B. pseudomallei* from the soil of a pig farm in Abidjan, Côte d'Ivoire in 1980. However, identification details were not provided [16]. In 1985, the isolation of *B. pseudomallei* in a 12-year-old girl from Sierra Leone presenting with multiple abscesses was reported in The Gambia [17]. In 2009, a 29-year-old diabetic Gambian man was diagnosed in Spain with bilateral calf abscesses due to *B. pseudomallei* after travelling to The Gambia, Guinea-Bissau, and Senegal [18]. Subsequently, another case of melioidosis was reported in a Caucasian Dutch man after traveling to The Gambia. [19].

Among all African countries, Nigeria is predicted to have by far the highest burden of melioidosis [1]. In sharp contrast to this potential disease load, the only report of melioidosis linked to Nigeria was documented in 2011, in which a case of a diabetic traveler was described who most likely acquired infection during a visit to the country [20]. Taken together, the predicted high disease burden and the low number of documented melioidosis incidences exemplify the urgent need for detailed investigations.

In 2014, 'The African Melioidosis Network' (AMENET), sponsored in the context of the European Union project ERAfrica, was established. The project aims at serological and environmental surveillance and capacity building in the laboratory diagnosis of *B. pseudomallei*. In West Africa,

Burkina Faso, Ghana, and Côte d'Ivoire are among the current target countries. In Côte d'Ivoire, culture screening of lesions in a pig slaughterhouse and some pilot soil sampling did not confirm the presence of *B. pseudomallei* in this country so far [21]. However, a recent report describes cutaneous melioidosis in a 49-year-old man presenting with leg cellulitis and an inguinal abscess after returning from one-year travel in Côte d'Ivoire [22]. Recent environmental qPCR-based direct molecular screening [23] and cultural screening of soil samples in Burkina Faso confirmed the environmental presence of *B. pseudomallei*. The phylogenetic analysis of isolated environmental strains based on whole genome sequencing is under way [24].

2.4. Eastern Africa

The predicted environmental suitability for *B. pseudomallei* in Eastern Africa seems to be scattered and possible risk zones vary in size [1]. Among the first hints of melioidosis in this part of the continent was a case of melioidosis in a traveler reported in 1980, who was diagnosed in Denmark but acquired the infection in Kenya. In this case, *B. pseudomallei* identification from blood, urine, and sputum included biochemical characteristics and virulence in guinea pigs [25]. A subsequent environmental survey testing of 81 soil and 71 water samples from three different provinces, including the possible site of infection of the Danish tourist, failed to isolate *B. pseudomallei* [26]. However, recently five indigenous cases of human melioidosis were uncovered in Kenya, even though the overall incidence in this country seems to be low [27]. The only hint of melioidosis in Uganda is a single serological study from 1982 describing 5.9% seropositivity (25 out of 426 individuals) in healthy adults from different parts of the country using an indirect hemagglutination test titre of 1:40 or greater [28]. In 2011, an indigenous case of melioidosis in a child was described in Malawi [2]. Recently, a case of melioidosis in an Eritrean migrant worker was diagnosed in Israel, which indicated that the disease might exist in the Horn of Africa [29].

Parts of Ethiopia were predicted to be environmentally suitable for *B. pseudomallei*. In the context of AMENET, environmental studies revealed the presence of *B. pseudomallei* in soil samples in various regions of the country using molecular [23] as well as cultural methods. The genomes of isolated environmental Ethiopian *B. pseudomallei* strains are currently being analyzed [24]. Current efforts aim to implement serological studies in humans and animals and capacity building in clinical laboratories.

In contrast to the situation in eastern continental Africa, Madagascar, the second largest island state in the western Indian Ocean, was already recognized as an endemic area in the 1930s [30]. Since there is a comprehensive summary of recent cases of melioidosis in the western Indian Ocean [31], in particular in Madagascar, we will only briefly summarize the current situation. First reports on melioidosis in pigs were published by French scientists in 1936 and a further report on the isolation of *B. pseudomallei* from soil [16] confirmed the presence of this pathogen on the island. It took until 2004 for the first human case to be reported and, in 2017, five more cases were described [32]. However, the epidemiological situation for the indigenous population in Madagascar is unknown. Cases were also described from La Réunion, Mauritius, and Seychelles [33–35]. In the framework of AMENET, environmental qPCR-based molecular and cultural screening of soil samples was performed and the environmental presence of *B. pseudomallei* could be demonstrated in various regions of Madagascar [36].

2.5. Central Africa

B. pseudomallei environmental suitability was predicted for all countries of Central Africa. However, significant regional differences seem to exist [1]. The first indication that melioidosis might be present in this African subregion was provided in 1956 by the isolation of *B. pseudomallei* from a lymph node of a goat in Chad [37]. From 2012 to 2013, prospective screening of blood cultures for *B. pseudomallei* was conducted in Gabon and led to the identification of the first melioidosis case in a diabetic female patient in this country [38], and environmental *B. pseudomallei* could be isolated from different sites. In the course of AMENET, the first environmental pilot studies in the DR Congo indicated the presence of *B. pseudomallei* in soil samples [24] by using direct molecular screening, as recently described [23]. Current activities focus on serological surveys and the extension of environmental screening in various subregions. In parallel, clinical surveillance and laboratory screening for human and animal melioidosis is being implemented.

2.6. Southern Africa

This sub-region seems to contain relatively limited areas of environmental suitability for *B. pseudomallei* [1]. A report from 1956 described the isolation of *B. pseudomallei* from abscesses of mammary glands and kidneys in a goat from South Africa [39].

3. Phenotype, Genomic Diversity, and Phylogenetic Relatedness of *B. pseudomallei* from Africa

At this point in time, the phenotypic characterization of African isolates is essentially restricted to features needed for diagnostic and therapeutic purposes. Wiersinga and colleagues reported that clinical and several environmental features of Gabon isolates showed the typical *B. pseudomallei* diagnostic characteristics, which have also been described in other endemic parts of the world with respect to the API 20NE biochemical profile, colony morphology, antibiotic susceptibility, and *B. pseudomallei*-specific latex agglutination [38]. The known *B. pseudomallei* susceptibility to meropenem, amoxicillin/clavulanic acid, cotrimoxazole and ceftazidime, and characteristic biochemical patterns in respective identification systems, were also reported in isolates from other cases [20,38,40].

As for the phenotypic properties, information on genomic characteristics of *B. pseudomallei* strains from Africa is also based on a limited number of isolates. At this point in time, most available data have been generated using multi-locus sequence typing (MLST), which is a cost-effective and straightforward method for investigating the epidemiology of *B. pseudomallei* [41,42]. The *B. pseudomallei* MLST scheme developed in 2003 is based on seven housekeeping genes and strains are classified according to their allelic profile [43]. Despite the emergence of next generation sequencing (NGS) and its advantages concerning recombination and homoplasy [44,45], MLST still provides valuable insight into the genetic variability of an organism and the geographic distribution/prevalence of different strains, due to its simplicity and sheer amount of deposited STs. As of March 2018, only 26 (0.47%) out of 5494 deposited isolates originate from Africa–compared to 2992 (54.46%) Australian and 906 (16.46%) Thai strains (https://pubmlst.org/bpseudomallei/) [46]. Noteworthily, the African *B. pseudomallei* strains were isolated in as few as eight different countries and do not share a single sequence type (ST) among each other. Furthermore, only four of the 26 STs were also reported in Southeast Asian countries, with none in Australia. While these observations might partially result from the low number of isolates, they already hint at the great genotypic diversity of the African isolates and indicate a segregated, geographically distinct, African subpopulation.

Since the publication of the first closed *B. pseudomallei* genome of the Thai strain K96243 in 2004 [47], the phylogeny of the bacterium has been intensively studied by the emerging NGS methods. At the same time, whole genome sequencing (WGS) offers the advantage of high coverage and, therefore, provides better phylogenetic resolution, which makes it a more robust tool compared to other genetic typing methods that rely on only a few loci [48]. In the first phylogenetic study based on single nucleotide polymorphisms (SNP) of 43 *B. pseudomallei* strains from Asia and Australia, the authors presented strong evidence for an ancestral Australian origin and proposed a single transmission event to Southeast Asia during the glacial periods [45]. Two recent genomic studies, which not only rely on larger datasets but also on more geographically diverse ones, support these findings and further extend them in a global context [49,50]. Phylogenetic analyses show that the South American strains form a sub-cluster within an otherwise African-dominated *B. pseudomallei* clade, which in turn branches from the Asian one [50,51]. Therefore, Sarovich and colleagues hypothesized that *B. pseudomallei* was transmitted from Asia to Africa ~2000 years ago when people from Southeast Asia migrated to Madagascar. Nevertheless, the introduction of *B. pseudomallei* to Africa by birds via the Asia-East Africa flyway is another possibility, which is noted by the authors [49]. Moreover, Chewapreecha et al. estimated the most recent common ancestor for the American strains to be from 1759 or 1806 using the BEAST (Bayesian Evolutionary Analysis by Sampling Trees) method. A time span that coincides with the height of the slave trade (1650–1850) therefore offers a plausible explanation for the onward transmission to the Americas by diseased people or contaminated cargo [50].

It has been argued that the observed difference between predicted and reported meliodosis cases in Africa might not only be due to underreporting and the lack of diagnostic facilities, but it might also be attributed to variations in *B. pseudomallei* virulence [52]. WGS is a well-established technique to address this question on a genetic basis and can further be used to identify geographically-segregated gene variants [50]. For example, a few virulence-associated genes (e.g. *bimA*$_{Bm}$, *fhaB3*) have been described in the literature to correlate with specific clinical presentations and the severity of melioidosis [53]. Therefore, this might account for geographical differences. Additionally, there are reports of African isolates that lack the fimbrial and adhesion virulence protein [52], the type II O-antigenic polysaccharide, or the filamentous hemagglutinin [49]. Even though host and environmental factors are also crucial determinants, it will be most interesting to see how diverse the African *B. pseudomallei* population is and whether bacterial diversity contributes to geographical differences in disease prevalence and outcome. There is no doubt that an extended analysis of more African isolates will not only help to get more detailed insights of *B. pseudomallei* epidemiology and virulence within Africa, but also substantially contributes to our comprehensive understanding of the global evolution and dissemination.

4. Current and Future Challenges

In light of the history of melioidosis in other parts of the world, which shows the degree to which highly-endemic regions may go undetected, and the high case fatality rate of undiagnosed melioidosis, there is an urgent need to define risk areas throughout Africa and the Middle East. The first step should be to conduct serological surveys of humans and animals to estimate the degree of exposure to *B. pseudomallei* in various regions. Based on these results, one can then geographically target raising clinical awareness among infectious disease specialists together with microbiological capacity building, which are both needed to detect cases of melioidosis. For the latter, one can learn from other resource-limited settings in which simple laboratory algorithms for the identification of *B. pseudomallei* from clinical specimens have been successfully applied [54]. Known groups at risk such as diabetics will be targeted first.

Serological surveys should be complemented by environmental studies. It will be necessary to systematically determine the environmental distribution and load of *B. pseudomallei* in the different African regions and habitats. When screening soil samples from Thailand and Vietnam, a recent study demonstrated a higher detection rate using a quantitative multi-target PCR approach compared to culture. Moreover, samples with high PCR signals were more likely to be culture-positive compared to samples with low signals [23]. In the environmental studies conducted in Burkina Faso and Madagascar in the context of AMENET, we can confirm that specific molecular signals are obtained at a significantly higher rate when compared to positive cultures.

In endemic regions, prospective studies are then required to determine the incidence and prevalence of melioidosis in humans and animals. Although the limited available information suggests similar clinical presentations and risk factors in African melioidosis cases as compared to other endemic regions, this has to be verified. In this context, it will be important to assess the virulence traits of African *B. pseudomallei* strains compared to Australian and Asian isolates through WGS and experimental infection models.

The identification of environmental factors determining the presence of *B. pseudomallei* and, thereby, the risk of acquiring infection will be important for any prevention and preparedness strategies. Such factors might be identified by e.g., regressing land use patterns, soil types, and vegetation on results from molecular soil screening and seroprevalence data. Studies on *B. pseudomallei* population structure and phylogenetic relatedness offer the chance to analyze past and contemporary environmental dissemination of this pathogen.

The true magnitude of the melioidosis burden in Africa is still to be determined. However, we can expect it to rise in the coming years on this continent like on the others, due to socio-anthropological changes and the increase of the groups at risk for this disease.

Author Contributions: I.S., K.A., E.K., M.S. (Mamadou Sawadogo), H.S., M.T., E.A., B.Y., L.Y.A.-A., M.S. (Moussa Sanogo), B.B., R.R., C.P.S., M.S.P., E.K.I., J.M., M.O., E.O.-D., and Y.A.-S. participated in activities related to AMENET and conceptualized the AMENET measures described in the manuscript. I.S. coordinated the review. I.S. and G.E.W. wrote the first draft and reviewed the literature. S.L., K.A., J.M., E.B., M.T., L.Y.A.-A., E.O.-D., M.S.P., and Y.A.-S. contributed to drafting and editing. All authors reviewed the final version of the manuscript.

Acknowledgments: We would like to thank the German Federal Ministry of Education and Research for funding AMENET (reference 01DG14011A) in the context of ERAfrica, enabling collaborative projects with the African partner institutions as listed in the affiliations of authors, the Ministère des Ressources Animales et Halieutiques du Burkina Faso and Centre de Recherche Internationale pour la santé (CRIS) for supporting activities in Burkina Faso and Afrique One-ASPIRE for supporting activities in Côte d'Ivoire (DELTAS Africa Initiative [Afrique One-ASPIRE /DEL-15-008]).

Conflicts of Interest: The authors declare no conflict of interest.

References

1. Limmathurotsakul, D.; Golding, N.; Dance, D.A.; Messina, J.P.; Pigott, D.M.; Moyes, C.L.; Rolim, D.B.; Bertherat, E.; Day, N.P.; Peacock, S.J.; et al. Predicted global distribution of *Burkholderia pseudomallei* and burden of melioidosis. *Nat. Microbiol.* **2016**, *1*, 15008. [CrossRef] [PubMed]
2. Katangwe, T.; Purcell, J.; Bar-Zeev, N.; Denis, B.; Montgomery, J.; Alaerts, M.; Heyderman, R.S.; Dance, D.A.; Kennedy, N.; Feasey, N.; et al. Human melioidosis, Malawi, 2011. *Emerg. Infect. Dis.* **2013**, *19*, 981–984. [CrossRef] [PubMed]
3. Birnie, E.; Wiersinga, W.J.; Limmathurotsakul, D.; Grobusch, M.P. Melioidosis in Africa: Should we be looking more closely? *Future Microbiol.* **2015**, *10*, 273–281. [CrossRef] [PubMed]
4. MacLennan, I.S. Melioidosis in the horse. *J. R. Army Vet. Corps* **1953**, *24*, 130–134.
5. Ertug, C. Melioidosis. *Chest* **1961**, *40*, 693–697. [CrossRef]
6. Uraz, G.; Citak, S. The isolation of *Pseudomonas* and other Gram(—) psychrotrophic bacteria in raw milks. *J. Basic Microbiol.* **1998**, *38*, 129–134. [CrossRef]
7. Barbour, E.K.; Nabbut, N.H.; Hamadeh, S.K.; Al-Nakhli, H.M. Bacterial identity and characteristics in healthy and unhealthy respiratory tracts of sheep and calves. *Vet. Res. Commun.* **1997**, *21*, 421–430. [CrossRef] [PubMed]
8. Wernery, R.; Kinne, J.; Haydn-Evans, J.; Ul-Haq, A. Melioidosis in a seven year old camel, a new disease in the United Arab Emirates (UAE). *J. Camel Pract. Res.* **1997**, *4*, 141–143.
9. Pourtaghva, M.; Machoun, A.; Dodin, A. Demonstration of *Pseudomonas pseudomallei* (Whitmore's bacillus) in the mud of Iranian ricefields (author's transl). *Bulletin de la Societe de Pathologie Exotique et de ses Filiales* **1975**, *68*, 367–370. [PubMed]
10. Baharsefat, M.; Amjadi, A.R. Equine melioidosis in Iran. *Arch. Razi Inst.* **1970**, *22*, 209–213.
11. Pourtaghva, M.; Dodin, A.; Portovi, M.; Teherani, M.; Galimand, M. 1st case of human pulmonary melioidosis in Iran. *Bulletin de la Societe de Pathologie Exotique et de ses Filiales* **1977**, *70*, 107–109. [PubMed]
12. Darazam, I.A.; Kiani, A.; Ghasemi, S.; Sadeghi, H.; Alavi, F.; Moosavi, M.J.; Akbari, A.; Shahidi, M.; Jalali, M.; Pourfarziani, V.; et al. Melioidosis: It is not far from here. *Tanaffos* **2011**, *10*, 64–68. [PubMed]
13. Ferry, R.; Poutrel, B.; Bruneau, F. Isolation of Whitmore's bacillus from lesions found in pigs from the Niamey slaughterhouse in Niger. *Bulletin de la Societe de Pathologie Exotique et de ses Filiales* **1973**, *66*, 42–45. [PubMed]
14. Dodin, A.; Ferry, R. Epidemiological studies of the bacillus of Whitmore in Africa. *Bulletin de la Societe de Pathologie Exotique et de ses Filiales* **1974**, *67*, 121–126. [PubMed]
15. Trueba, F.; Blade, J.S.; De Kerangal, X.; Ouedraogo, N.; Borne, M.; Brinquin, L. A man with a saccular aneurysm of the left common iliac artery. *Clin. Infect. Dis.* **2006**, *43*, 945–947. [CrossRef] [PubMed]
16. Galimand, M.; Dodin, A. Focus on melioidosis throughout the world. *Bulletin de la Societe de Pathologie Exotique et de ses Filiales* **1982**, *75*, 375–383. [PubMed]
17. Wall, R.A.; Mabey, D.C.; Corrah, P.T.; Peters, L. A case of melioidosis in West Africa. *J. Infect. Dis.* **1985**, *152*, 424–425. [CrossRef] [PubMed]

18. Cuadros, J.; Gil, H.; Miguel, J.D.; Marabe, G.; Gomez-Herruz, T.A.; Lobo, B.; Marcos, R.; Anda, P. Case report: Melioidosis imported from West Africa to Europe. *Am. J. Trop. Med. Hyg.* **2011**, *85*, 282–284. [CrossRef] [PubMed]

19. Morelli, F.; Smeets, L.; Hobijn, M.; Boom, H. Melioidosis and renal failure in a Dutch man after a trip to Gambia. *Neth. J. Med.* **2015**, *73*, 296–298. [PubMed]

20. Salam, A.P.; Khan, N.; Malnick, H.; Kenna, D.T.; Dance, D.A.; Klein, J.L. Melioidosis acquired by traveler to Nigeria. *Emerg. Infect. Dis.* **2011**, *17*, 1296–1298. [CrossRef] [PubMed]

21. Atsé-Achi, L.Y.; Laboratoire Central Vétérinaire de Bingerville, LANADA, Bingerville, Cote d'Ivoire. Personal communication, 2017.

22. Fertitta, L.; Monsel, G.; Delaroche, M.; Fourniols, E.; Brossier, F.; Caumes, E. Cutaneous melioidosis: Two cases of chronic primary forms. *J. Eur. Acad. Dermatol. Venereol.* **2018**. [CrossRef] [PubMed]

23. Gohler, A.; Trung, T.T.; Hopf, V.; Kohler, C.; Hartleib, J.; Wuthiekanun, V.; Peacock, S.J.; Limmathurotsakul, D.; Tuanyok, A.; Steinmetz, I. Multitarget quantitative PCR improves detection and predicts cultivability of the pathogen *Burkholderia pseudomallei*. *Appl. Environ. Microbiol.* **2017**, *83*. [CrossRef] [PubMed]

24. Steinmetz, I. (Institute of Hygiene, Microbiology and Environmental Medicine, Medical University of Graz, Graz, Austria). Personal communication, 2018.

25. Bremmelgaard, A.; Bygbjerg, I.; Hoiby, N. Microbiological and immunological studies in a case of human melioidosis diagnosed in Denmark. *Scand. J. Infect. Dis.* **1982**, *14*, 271–275. [CrossRef] [PubMed]

26. Batchelor, B.I.; Paul, J.; Trakulsomboon, S.; Mgongo, M.; Dance, D.A. Melioidosis survey in Kenya. *Trans. R. Soc. Trop. Med. Hyg.* **1994**, *88*, 181. [CrossRef]

27. Dance, D. (Lao-Oxford-Mahosot Hospital-Wellcome Trust Research Unit (LOMWRU), Vientiane, Laos). Personal communication, 2018.

28. Frazer, D.N. Melioidosis. *J. R. Army Med. Corps* **1982**, *128*, 123–130. [CrossRef] [PubMed]

29. Almog, Y.; Yagel, Y.; Geffen, Y.; Yagupsky, P. A *Burkholderia pseudomallei* infection imported from Eritrea to Israel. *Am. J. Trop. Med. Hyg.* **2016**, *95*, 997–998. [CrossRef] [PubMed]

30. Girard, G. Can pigs be a healthy carrier of Whitmore's bacillus? *Bulletin de la Societe de Pathologie Exotique et de ses Filiales* **1936**, *29*, 712–716.

31. Rakotondrasoa, A.; Issack, M.; Garin, B.; Biot, F.; Valade, E.; Wattiau, P.; Allou, N.; Belmonte, O.; Bibi, J.; Price, E.; et al. Melioidosis in the western Indian Ocean and the importance of improving diagnosis, surveillance, and molecular typing. *Trop. Med. Infect. Dis.* **2018**, *3*, 30. [CrossRef]

32. Martinet, O.S.; Pac Soo, A.M.; Knezynski, M.; Schlossmacher, P.; Jaffar-Bandjee, C.; Gaüzière, B.A. Melioidosis: Regarding a case acquired in Madagascar and two nosocomial cases [in French]. *Bulletin de la Societe de Pathologie Exotique et de ses Filiales* **2004**, *97*, 366–370.

33. Issack, M.I.; Bundhun, C.D.; Gokhool, H. Melioidosis in Mauritius. *Emerg. Infect. Dis.* **2005**, *11*, 139–140. [CrossRef] [PubMed]

34. Borgherini, G.; Camuset, G.; Foucher, A.; Maiza, J.C.; Thibault, F.M.; Picot, S.; Poubeau, P. The first autochthonous case of human melioidosis in Reunion Island. *Med. Mal. Infect.* **2015**, *45*, 47–49. [CrossRef] [PubMed]

35. Bibi, J.; Biscornet, L.; Bermingham, A.; von Gottberg, A. First identification of *Burkholderia pseudomallei* in Seychelles. In Proceedings of the 1st International Forum Public Health Surveillance and Response in Island Territories, Saint Denis, La Réunion, France, 11–13 June 2013; p. 124.

36. Göhler André, T.T.T.; Kohler, C.; Herinirina, J.N.; Rakotondrainiarivelo, J.P.; Razafindabre, T.; Poppert, S.; Hopf, V.; Rakotozandrindrainy, R.; Steinmetz, I. Molecular and cultural detection of *B. pseudomallei* from soil in Madagascar. In Proceedings of the Abstract Book of the 7th World Melioidosis Congress, Bangkok, Thailand, 18–20 September 2013.

37. Provost, A.; Vigier, M. Isolation in Tchad (Central Africa) of 2 strains of *Malleomyces pseudomallei*. *Annales de l'Institut Pasteur* **1960**, *98*, 461–463. [PubMed]

38. Wiersinga, W.J.; Birnie, E.; Weehuizen, T.A.; Alabi, A.S.; Huson, M.A.; Huis in 't Veld, R.A.; Mabala, H.K.; Adzoda, G.K.; Raczynski-Henk, Y.; Esen, M.; et al. Clinical, environmental, and serologic surveillance studies of melioidosis in Gabon, 2012–2013. *Emerg. Infect. Dis.* **2015**, *21*, 40–47. [CrossRef] [PubMed]

39. Van der Lugt, J.J.; Henton, M.M. Melioidosis in a goat. *J. S. Afr. Vet. Assoc.* **1995**, *66*, 71–73. [PubMed]

40. Morosini, M.I.; Quereda, C.; Gil, H.; Anda, P.; Nunez-Murga, M.; Canton, R.; Lopez-Velez, R. Melioidosis in traveler from Africa to Spain. *Emerg. Infect. Dis.* **2013**, *19*, 1656–1659. [CrossRef] [PubMed]

41. McCombie, R.L.; Finkelstein, R.A.; Woods, D.E. Multilocus sequence typing of historical *Burkholderia pseudomallei* isolates collected in Southeast Asia from 1964 to 1967 provides insight into the epidemiology of melioidosis. *J. Clin. Microbiol.* **2006**, *44*, 2951–2962. [CrossRef] [PubMed]

42. Chantratita, N.; Wuthiekanun, V.; Limmathurotsakul, D.; Vesaratchavest, M.; Thanwisai, A.; Amornchai, P.; Tumapa, S.; Feil, E.J.; Day, N.P.; Peacock, S.J. Genetic diversity and microevolution of *Burkholderia pseudomallei* in the environment. *PLoS Negl. Trop. Dis.* **2008**, *2*, e182. [CrossRef] [PubMed]

43. Godoy, D.; Randle, G.; Simpson, A.J.; Aanensen, D.M.; Pitt, T.L.; Kinoshita, R.; Spratt, B.G. Multilocus sequence typing and evolutionary relationships among the causative agents of melioidosis and glanders, *Burkholderia pseudomallei* and *Burkholderia mallei*. *J. Clin. Microbiol.* **2003**, *41*, 2068–2079. [CrossRef] [PubMed]

44. De Smet, B.; Sarovich, D.S.; Price, E.P.; Mayo, M.; Theobald, V.; Kham, C.; Heng, S.; Thong, P.; Holden, M.T.; Parkhill, J.; et al. Whole-genome sequencing confirms that *Burkholderia pseudomallei* multilocus sequence types common to both Cambodia and Australia are due to homoplasy. *J. Clin. Microbiol.* **2015**, *53*, 323–326. [CrossRef] [PubMed]

45. Pearson, T.; Giffard, P.; Beckstrom-Sternberg, S.; Auerbach, R.; Hornstra, H.; Tuanyok, A.; Price, E.P.; Glass, M.B.; Leadem, B.; Beckstrom-Sternberg, J.S.; et al. Phylogeographic reconstruction of a bacterial species with high levels of lateral gene transfer. *BMC Biol.* **2009**, *7*, 78. [CrossRef] [PubMed]

46. Jolley, K.A.; Maiden, M.C. BIGSdb: Scalable analysis of bacterial genome variation at the population level. *BMC Bioinform.* **2010**, *11*, 595. [CrossRef] [PubMed]

47. Holden, M.T.; Titball, R.W.; Peacock, S.J.; Cerdeno-Tarraga, A.M.; Atkins, T.; Crossman, L.C.; Pitt, T.; Churcher, C.; Mungall, K.; Bentley, S.D.; et al. Genomic plasticity of the causative agent of melioidosis, *Burkholderia pseudomallei*. *Proc. Natl. Acad. Sci. USA* **2004**, *101*, 14240–14245. [CrossRef] [PubMed]

48. Aziz, A.; Sarovich, D.S.; Harris, T.M.; Kaestli, M.; McRobb, E.; Mayo, M.; Currie, B.J.; Price, E.P. Suspected cases of intracontinental *Burkholderia pseudomallei* sequence type homoplasy resolved using whole-genome sequencing. *Microb. Genom.* **2017**, *3*. [CrossRef] [PubMed]

49. Sarovich, D.S.; Garin, B.; De Smet, B.; Kaestli, M.; Mayo, M.; Vandamme, P.; Jacobs, J.; Lompo, P.; Tahita, M.C.; Tinto, H.; et al. Phylogenomic analysis reveals an Asian origin for African *Burkholderia pseudomallei* and further supports melioidosis endemicity in Africa. *mSphere* **2016**, *1*. [CrossRef] [PubMed]

50. Chewapreecha, C.; Holden, M.T.; Vehkala, M.; Valimaki, N.; Yang, Z.; Harris, S.R.; Mather, A.E.; Tuanyok, A.; De Smet, B.; Le Hello, S.; et al. Global and regional dissemination and evolution of *Burkholderia pseudomallei*. *Nat. Microbiol.* **2017**, *2*, 16263. [CrossRef] [PubMed]

51. Price, E.P.; Currie, B.J.; Sarovich, D.S. Genomic insights into the melioidosis pathogen, *Burkholderia pseudomallei*. *Curr. Trop. Med. Rep.* **2017**, *4*, 95–102. [CrossRef]

52. Weehuizen, T.A.F.; Birnie, E.; Ferwerda, B.; Roelofs, J.; de Vos, A.F.; Grobusch, M.P.; Wiersinga, W.J. Differences in inflammation patterns induced by African and Asian *Burkholderia pseudomallei* isolates in mice. *Am. J. Trop. Med. Hyg.* **2017**, *96*, 1365–1369. [CrossRef] [PubMed]

53. Sarovich, D.S.; Price, E.P.; Webb, J.R.; Ward, L.M.; Voutsinos, M.Y.; Tuanyok, A.; Mayo, M.; Kaestli, M.; Currie, B.J. Variable virulence factors in *Burkholderia pseudomallei* (melioidosis) associated with human disease. *PLoS ONE* **2014**, *9*, e91682. [CrossRef] [PubMed]

54. Trinh, T.T.; Hoang, T.S.; Tran, D.A.; Trinh, V.T.; Gohler, A.; Nguyen, T.T.; Hoang, S.N.; Krumkamp, R.; Nguyen, L.T.N.; May, J.; et al. A simple laboratory algorithm for diagnosis of melioidosis in resource-constrained areas: A study from north-central Vietnam. *Clin. Microbiol. Infect.* **2018**, *24*, 84.e1–84.e4. [CrossRef] [PubMed]

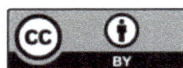

Tropical Medicine and Infectious Disease

MDPI

Review

Melioidosis: An Australian Perspective

Simon Smith [1,2,*], Josh Hanson [1,3,4] and Bart J. Currie [3,5]

1 Department of Medicine, Cairns Hospital, Cairns, QLD 4870, Australia; Joshua.Hanson@health.qld.gov.au
2 James Cook University Clinical School, Cairns Hospital, Cairns, QLD 4870, Australia
3 Global and Tropical Health Division, Menzies School of Health Research, Charles Darwin University, Darwin, NT 0811, Australia; Bart.Currie@menzies.edu.au
4 The Kirby Institute, University of New South Wales, Sydney, NSW 2052, Australia
5 Department of Infectious Diseases, Royal Darwin Hospital, Darwin, NT 0811, Australia
* Correspondence: simon.smith2@health.qld.gov.au; Tel.: +61-0(7)-42260000

Received: 31 January 2018; Accepted: 22 February 2018; Published: 1 March 2018

Abstract: *Burkholderia pseudomallei* is endemic in northern Australia, with cases of melioidosis most commonly occurring during the wet season in individuals with diabetes, hazardous alcohol use, and chronic kidney disease. Pneumonia is the most common presentation and the majority of patients are bacteraemic—however, infection may involve almost any organ, with the skin and soft tissues, genitourinary system, visceral organs, and bone and joints affected most commonly. Central nervous system involvement is rarer, but has a high attributable mortality. Increased awareness of the disease amongst healthcare providers, ready access to appropriate antibiotic therapy and high-quality intensive care services has resulted in a sharp decline in the case fatality rate over the last 20 years. Further improvement in clinical outcomes will require a greater understanding of the disease's pathophysiology, its optimal management, and more effective strategies for its prevention.

Keywords: melioidosis; Australia; tropical medicine

1. History

Melioidosis was initially described in Australia in 1949, following an outbreak in sheep in central west Queensland [1]. The first human case of melioidosis in Australia was described in Townsville, North Queensland from 1950 [2] and cases were subsequently reported in the Northern Territory (NT) from 1960 [3].

Melioidosis is endemic across northern, tropical Australia north of latitude 20° S [4–7], with focal areas of endemicity described in much more southern, temperate regions (latitude 31° S) [8–10]. Outbreaks, related to contaminated water, have been described in pigs in south-east Queensland (latitude 25.5° S) [11] and human and bovine cases have also been identified in the same region [12–14]. Even in dry, arid desert regions of Central Australia, cases of melioidosis have occurred following intense rainfall, highlighting the organism's ability to survive in harsh environments [15].

The incidence of melioidosis differs across northern Australia. In the Top End of the NT, yearly incidence rates range between 5.4 and 50.2/100,000 population [6,16]. Indigenous Australians are disproportionately affected and bear the greatest burden of the disease. During the monsoonal rains of 2009–2010, a wet season with above average rainfall, incidence increased to 102.4/100,000 population in the Top End Indigenous population [16]. In the Torres Strait Islands, the mean incidence is 33.1/100,000 population [17].

Despite the high incidence of disease in northern Australia, background seropositivity rates are relatively low compared to those seen in Southeast Asia, even if a lower indirect haemagglutination assay titre cut-off of 1:40 is used. Rates range from 5 to 12.8%, with the highest identified in Indigenous Australians and people living in rural locations [18,19].

It was previously believed that *Burkholderia pseudomallei* colonised Australia from Southeast Asia, but phylogeographic reconstruction suggests an Australian origin for *B. pseudomallei*, with dispersal into Southeast Asia occurring after one or more introduction events during the last glacial period [20].

B. pseudomallei in northern Australia is genetically diverse; there is significant differentiation between the genotypes present in isolates from Queensland and the Northern Territory [21]. The organism rarely moves across major biogeographic boundaries; however, in Darwin, an Asian *B. pseudomallei* strain, sequence type (ST)-562, has become a common ST affecting patients with melioidosis in this area [22].

2. Melioidosis Cases and the Presence of *B. pseudomallei*

B. pseudomallei has been identified from a number of Australian animals, including goats [23], sheep [1], camels [24], and alpacas [25], all of which are considered to be highly susceptible to melioidosis [26]. Melioidosis commonly presents as mastitis in goats, but zoonotic transmission remains exceedingly rare [26]. Outbreaks have occurred in pigs [11] and cases have been identified in a wide variety of domestic and native Australia animals and birds [27–34]. *B. pseudomallei* has been detected in faecal samples from wallabies and chickens, suggesting that faecal shedding may contribute to the geographical expansion of the disease [35].

Melioidosis in humans is considered an opportunistic infection in Australia, with the vast majority of people having at least one identifiable risk factor. The most common risk factors identified are diabetes mellitus, hazardous alcohol use, chronic lung disease, and chronic kidney disease [6]. In healthy people, death from melioidosis is considered extremely rare if appropriate antibiotics and intensive care support are available [6,17].

In Australia, melioidosis is usually acquired percutaneously or by inhalation. Infection by ingestion is considered unusual, although outbreaks caused by contaminated drinking water supplies have occurred [36,37]. In northern Australia, cases of melioidosis follow a seasonal pattern and are strongly associated with monsoonal rains [17,38,39]. An increase in the dew point, cloud cover, temperature, rainfall, and groundwater have all been associated with an increased risk of the disease [40]. An increase in the number of people with melioidosis pneumonia has been attributed to cyclones and tropical storms in the NT [41] and cyclones coincide with increased melioidosis cases in Western Australia [42]; however, no correlation is seen between melioidosis cases and severe weather events in Far North Queensland (FNQ) [43]. Melioidosis cases associated with severe weather events have been shown to be caused by different *B. pseudomallei* MLST genotypes, suggesting that airborne dissemination may not come from a common source [44].

Pneumonia is the most common presentation of melioidosis in Australia [45]. Bacteraemic presentations vary between 55% and 74% with particularly high rates observed in FNQ [6,17]. While this may partly be explained by differences in case findings, it is yet to be determined if strains in FNQ are intrinsically more virulent.

Genitourinary involvement is common in Australia, with prostate abscesses occurring in up to 21% of males [46]. Imaging is required to confirm the diagnosis; however, the absence of symptoms and normal urinalysis may be sufficient to exclude prostatic involvement [47]. Drainage of prostatic abscesses is usually required to hasten cure and prevent relapse.

Osteomyelitis and septic arthritis occurs in up to 16% of Australian presentations [17]. Operative intervention is often required, with the majority of patients requiring multiple procedures [48].

Paediatric melioidosis is uncommon in Australia and, in Darwin, has traditionally been associated with skin and soft tissue infection [49,50]. In contrast to Southeast Asia, acute suppurative parotitis is extremely rare in Australia [5], which is likely related to ingestion being an uncommon mode of transmission. Case-fatality rates in Darwin children are comparable to that of adults but, in FNQ, the rates of bacteraemia and mortality are much higher—60% and 50%, respectively—with fatal cases occurring despite optimal treatment [51,52]. The explanation for this observation is uncertain, although it may be partly explained by less active case finding in FNQ. Children in Darwin who present with only skin lesions have been shown to sometimes be infected with minority strains that lack the virulence factor filamentous hemagglutinin gene—fhaB3—which may be more common in FNQ strains [53].

Neurological melioidosis (meningoencephalitis and involvement of the brainstem, cerebellum, and spinal cord) occurs in up to 5% of Australian melioidosis cases [54]. *B. pseudomallei* isolates possessing a *B. mallei*—like bimA allele (bim_{Bm}) have been shown to have increased persistence in phagocytic cells, increased virulence, and to be neurotropic and, hence, strongly associated with neurological disease [55,56].

Environmental sampling has identified *B. pseudomallei* from soil and water across northern Australia [57,58]. *B. pseudomallei* has been isolated from groundwater seeps in endemic areas [59] and melioidosis cases have been linked to contaminated drinking well water [60], as well as two documented outbreaks in remote indigenous communities being linked to contaminated water supplies [36,37]. *B. pseudomallei* is seen in undisturbed, heavily grassed areas, but is also associated with the presence of livestock animals [61]. Soil texture and lower pH levels promote growth of the organism [61]. In Australia, soil exposure often occurs in domestic gardens, [6] where, due to the addition of specific fertilisers and imported grasses, more *B. pseudomallei* is seen compared to other environments [61,62]. *B. pseudomallei* has also been isolated from air samples from outside the home of a patient with suspected inhalational melioidosis [63]. Outbreaks have been associated with contaminated wound irrigation fluid, although this is exceptionally rare [64]. Geographical locations of confirmed cases are shown in Figure 1.

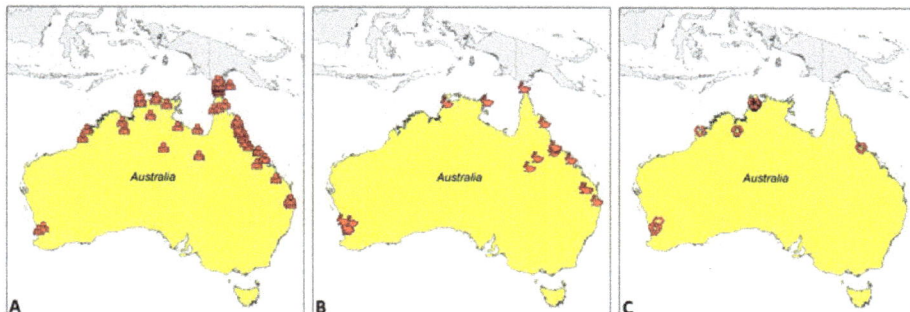

Figure 1. The geographic distribution of confirmed human cases (**A**), animal cases (**B**), and environmental isolates (**C**) of culture-confirmed *B. pseudomallei*.

Mapping shows geographical locations of culture-confirmed *B. pseudomallei* isolates only and does not reflect incidence.

3. Surveillance Systems and Reporting

Human melioidosis is a notifiable disease in the NT, Western Australia and Queensland. Notification usually occurs directly from the microbiology laboratory and public health departments gather information about each case, including occupational or recreational exposure, risk factors, and clinical presentation [7]. In the NT, detailed clinical information has been collected prospectively for over 28 years and a similar database has recently been established in Far North Queensland. Guidelines for the management of animal melioidosis are available, including recommendations for safe disposal of dead affected animals [65].

4. Diagnosis

Clinicians in northern Australia have a high index of suspicion of melioidosis, particularly during the wet season and in people with predisposing risk factors. Culture, the mainstay of diagnosis of melioidosis, is accessible throughout endemic areas of Australia. Vitek 2 (bioMérieux, France)—the automated biochemical system—is routinely used to confirm the isolation of *B. pseudomallei* from cultured specimens [66].

Matrix-assisted laser desorption/ionization time-of-flight (MALDI-TOF) mass spectrometry is available in many Australian laboratories and can be utilised to rapidly identify *B. pseudomallei* from cultured specimens [67]; however, there is a requirement to expand existing databases with pathogens endemic to different localities to help prevent incorrect identification of other *Burkholderia* species.

A lateral flow antigen detection assay has been developed as a rapid diagnostic tool, which is proving to be useful as an adjunct to the diagnosis of melioidosis, however, it is not yet routinely available [68]. Polymerase chain reaction is available in some areas to confirm bacterial isolates from clinical specimens, but is not sensitive or specific enough for routine use directly on clinical samples [69–71].

Serological testing using an indirect haemagglutination assay is available in Australia, but its use is limited in the diagnosis of acute disease in those from endemic locations because of background seropositivity. It is used for identifying people previously exposed to *B. pseudomallei* prior to commencing immunosuppressive treatment or for seroprevalence surveys [72,73].

In northern Queensland, the microbroth dilution method has been used to provide epidemiological cut-off values of clinical isolates of *B. pseudomallei* to meropenem, ceftazidime, trimethoprim-sulfamethoxazole (TMP-SMX) and doxycycline [74]. Meropenem and ceftazidime provide reliable first-line agents against melioidosis, with primary resistance being extremely rare [75,76]. Primary resistance to TMP-SMX in Australian isolates is also extremely rare [77]. Secondary resistance is also uncommon; however, whole-genome sequencing of *B. pseudomallei* isolates from patients receiving intravenous meropenem for melioidosis treatment have exhibited decreased meropenem susceptibility [78]. Additionally, in cystic fibrosis patients, multidrug-resistant *B. pseudomallei* has been identified after prolonged antibiotic therapy [79].

A chest X-ray is performed on all patients with melioidosis. A computed tomography (CT) scan of the abdomen and pelvis is also routinely performed in all adult patients with confirmed or suspected melioidosis to identify abscesses in the prostate, liver, spleen, and kidneys. For pregnant women and children, an abdominal ultrasound is considered a reasonable alternative. In patients with CNS involvement, CT images may be normal and magnetic resonance imaging (MRI) is preferred. MRI often shows extensive hyperintense changes on T2-weighted images; microabscesses, leptomeningeal enhancement, and trigeminal nerve involvement are also common [54,80,81].

5. Treatment

Treatment of melioidosis in Australia consists of an intensive phase with intravenous antibiotics followed by a prolonged eradication phase with oral antibiotics. Meropenem or ceftazidime is used in the intensive phase and both are readily available in Australia, even in remote areas. Additionally, sick patients from rural or remote areas are quickly transferred to referral hospitals or tertiary care centres. Antibiotic regimens are presented in Table 1.

In people with neurological infection, bone or joint infection, genitourinary infection, and skin and soft tissue infections, TMP-SMX is added to the intensive regimen during the intensive phase. Folic acid 5 mg (child: 0.1 mg/kg up to 5 mg) orally, daily, is given to all people receiving TMP-SMX.

Due to concerns regarding adherence to prolonged oral antibiotics, in the NT a longer intensive phase has been developed [10] (Table 2). Using this strategy, the rates of relapse in the NT are very low, even when there is poor adherence to oral eradication therapy [6,53]. A prolonged intensive phase is also used in FNQ, although in this region relapse is more commonly explained by poor initial source control rather than non-adherence to oral eradication therapy [17].

To facilitate adherence to prolonged intravenous antibiotic therapy, ceftazidime administered to outpatients via a peripherally-inserted central catheter using 12-h elastomeric infusers has been widely adopted in Australia and is safe and effective [82].

Table 1. Antibiotic dosing for treatment of melioidosis in Australia.

Phase	Antibiotic	Adult Dose	Child Dose
Intensive	Meropenem	1 g intravenously 8-hourly	25 mg/kg up to 1 g intravenously 8-hourly
		2 g intravenously 8-hourly [1]	50 mg/kg up to 2 g intravenously 8-hourly [1]
Intensive	Ceftazidime	2 g intravenously 6-hourly	50 mg/kg up to 2 g intravenously 6-hourly
Intensive and eradication	Trimethoprim-sulfamethoxazole	≥60 kg: 320 + 1600 mg orally 12-hourly 40–60 kg: 240 + 1200 mg orally 12-hourly	6 + 30 mg/kg up to 240 + 1200 mg orally 12-hourly
Eradication	Amoxicillin-clavulanate	20/5 mg/kg orally 8-hourly	20/5 mg/kg orally 8-hourly
Eradication	Doxycycline	100 mg orally 12-hourly	Not recommended

[1] For cases with neurological involvement.

Table 2. Recommended antibiotic duration for the treatment of melioidosis in Australia.

Site of Infection	Minimum Intensive Phase Duration (Weeks)	Eradication Phase Duration (Months)
Cutaneous infection only	2	3
Bacteraemia without focus	2	3
Pneumonia without lymphadenopathy or ICU admission	2	3
Pneumonia with lymphadenopathy [1] or ICU admission	4	3
Deep seated collection [2]	4 [3]	3
Septic arthritis	4 [3]	3
Osteomyelitis	6	6
Central nervous system infection	8	6
Mycotic aneurysm or other arterial infection	8	6

[1] Defined as any hilar or mediastinal lymph node greater than 10 mm. [2] Involving the liver, spleen, kidneys, or prostate. [3] Start of intensive phase begins after the last drainage or tissue specimen grows *B. pseudomallei*.

Oral eradication therapy is routinely prescribed and TMP-SMX remains the treatment of choice. Oral doxycycline is considered as an alternative for people who cannot tolerate TMP-SMX, while oral amoxicillin-clavulanate may be used as an alternative in pregnant women or young children [83].

Case-fatality rates have decreased dramatically over the last 20 years, and is felt to be due to earlier recognition and diagnosis, ready access to therapy, and improving intensive care unit support [6,17]. Between 1989–1997, up to 92% of critically unwell patients with melioidosis died; however, with the introduction of an intensivist-led model of care and the empirical use of meropenem, case-fatality rates in this patient group dropped to 26% [84]. The reduced case-fatality rate coincided with the introduction of adjunctive treatment with granulocyte colony-stimulating factor (G-CSF); however, the attributable mortality benefit of G-CSF is uncertain [85,86]. In FNQ, G-CSF is not used and mortality rates are comparable to those seen in the NT [17].

6. Awareness and Prevention of Melioidosis

People who are at risk of acquiring melioidosis are advised to wear gardening gloves and footwear when coming into contact with soil [73]. Australian Government authorities provide easily-accessible recommendations on how to prevent melioidosis. This includes advice to remain indoors during wet and windy weather conditions, to wear a mask when using a pressure hose outside and to limit alcohol consumption [87]. A melioidosis awareness campaign in the NT, promulgating the aforementioned recommendations, provided factsheets, posters, and radio announcements to people at risk of acquiring melioidosis, as well as enclosed shoes to particularly vulnerable populations [88].

People receiving long-term haemodialysis are at particular risk of developing melioidosis [89]. In Darwin, prophylaxis using oral TMP-SMX three times per week post-dialysis is a safe and effective way to reduce this risk and is recommended in other areas where melioidosis is prevalent [90]. Melioidosis serology is recommended in all people prior to starting immunosuppressive treatment in the Top End of the NT. If positive, a urine specimen, sputum sample, and throat, rectum and wound swabs should be collected for melioidosis culture to exclude active disease [73]. High-risk immunosuppressed patients are given prophylaxis with daily dosing of oral TMP-SMX for the duration of the wet season.

In animals, strategies to reduce the risk of acquiring disease include limiting their access to high-risk areas and providing sufficient drainage to help avoid surface water accumulation. It is recommended that penned animals are kept on dry solid ground or concrete [91], while unpenned animals should be removed from the area of contamination source and have their water supplies chlorinated [26]. Ultraviolet light sterilisation may also be used to reduce *B. pseudomallei* levels in contaminated well water [60].

7. Major Achievements

The Darwin Prospective Melioidosis Study started on 1 October 1989. Since this time, the programme has documented the many and varied presentations of melioidosis. The program has, in close collaboration with colleagues in Thailand, also undertaken long-term studies, and developed the current treatment guidelines that are used globally, which have helped halve the case fatality rate of melioidosis in northern Australia from 30% to under 15%. Discoveries include the documentation of the spread of melioidosis by introduced grasses and birds. The storage of all isolates with linked patient data will serve as a resource for future research into diagnostics, therapeutics, and vaccines.

Over 1000 *B. pseudomallei* isolates from humans, animals, and the environment across Australia have been submitted to the *B. pseudomallei* MLST database (http://bpseudomallei.mlst.net/). This has permitted the comparison between clinical and environmental isolates, as well as studies of the diversity of *B. pseudomallei* in Australia [92].

8. Current and Future Challenges

Changes in the world's climate is likely to have an effect on the range and transmission of *B. pseudomallei*; a rise in the sea surface and ambient temperature may lead to an increase in melioidosis cases in Australia [40]. The genetic diversity of *B. pseudomallei* populations has been characterised by using multilocus sequence typing (MLST); however, due to its high recombination rate, *B. pseudomallei* isolates may share the same MLST despite being genetically and geographically distinct [93]. Therefore, whole-genome sequencing—which may not always be readily available—is required to identify strain origin in cases where the same ST is identified between geographically-different locations. Geographically-distinct virulence-associated genes have been found to be over-represented in Australian *B. pseudomallei* isolates [94]. The pathogenic nature of most of these virulence factors is not well established and requires further elucidation.

In addition to environmental factors, host factors, including increasing rates of diabetes mellitus and ongoing hazardous alcohol use are expected to increase the population at risk of melioidosis. Further education targeting risk factors and strategies to prevent *B. pseudomallei* exposure are required. In the absence of a suitable vaccine candidate, the use of prophylactic antibiotics to target at-risk populations requires further research.

Extending the intensive phase of intravenous antibiotics in melioidosis has been associated with favourable outcomes and a minimal risk of relapse; therefore, the benefits of, and ongoing need for, prolonged oral antibiotics during the eradication phase for every patient with melioidosis requires further work. The effect of adequate source control on the duration of therapy also requires exploration.

Trop. Med. Infect. Dis. **2018**, *3*, 27

The above challenges will be made possible with continued collaboration both across endemic areas of Australia, as well as with colleagues internationally.

Acknowledgments: The authors would like to thank Prapass Wannapinij for providing the mapping of melioidosis in Australia; Direk Limmathurotsakul and David Dance for coordinating this manuscript; and the numerous laboratory and clinical colleagues supporting the melioidosis work across northern Australia. The work described in this review is supported by the National Health and Medical Research Council (Project Grants 1098337 and 1131932 (the HOT NORTH initiative)).

Author Contributions: All authors contributed equally to this manuscript.

Conflicts of Interest: The authors declare no conflict of interest.

References

1. Cottew, G.S. Melioidosis in sheep in Queensland; a description of the causal organism. *Aust. J. Exp. Biol. Med. Sci.* **1950**, *28*, 677–683. [CrossRef] [PubMed]
2. Rimington, R.A. Melioidosis in north Queensland. *Med. J. Aust.* **1962**, *49*, 50–53. [PubMed]
3. Crotty, J.M.; Bromwich, A.F.; Quinn, J.V.; Brotherton, J. Meliodosis in the Northern Territory: A report of two cases. *Med. J. Aust.* **1963**, *50*, 274–275. [PubMed]
4. Cheng, A.C.; Hanna, J.N.; Norton, R.; Hills, S.L.; Davis, J.; Krause, V.L.; Dowse, G.; Inglis, T.J.; Currie, B.J. Melioidosis in northern Australia, 2001–2002. *Commun. Dis. Intell. Q. Rep.* **2003**, *27*, 272–277. [PubMed]
5. Faa, A.G.; Holt, P.J. Melioidosis in the Torres Strait Islands of Far North Queensland. *Commun. Dis. Intell. Q. Rep.* **2002**, *26*, 279–283. [PubMed]
6. Currie, B.J.; Ward, L.; Cheng, A.C. The epidemiology and clinical spectrum of melioidosis: 540 cases from the 20 year Darwin prospective study. *PLoS Negl. Trop. Dis.* **2010**, *4*, e900. [CrossRef] [PubMed]
7. Hanna, J.N.; Humphreys, J.L.; Brookes, D.L.; Messina, T.; Raulli, A. Melioidosis in north Queensland, 2000–2009. *Commun. Dis. Intell. Q. Rep.* **2010**, *34*, 444–447. [PubMed]
8. Currie, B.; Smith-Vaughan, H.; Golledge, C.; Buller, N.; Sriprakash, K.S.; Kemp, D.J. *Pseudomonas pseudomallei* isolates collected over 25 years from a non-tropical endemic focus show clonality on the basis of ribotyping. *Epidemiol. Infect.* **1994**, *113*, 307–312. [CrossRef] [PubMed]
9. Golledge, C.L.; Chin, W.S.; Tribe, A.E.; Condon, R.J.; Ashdown, L.R. A case of human melioidosis originating in south-west Western Australia. *Med. J. Aust.* **1992**, *157*, 332–334. [PubMed]
10. Chapple, S.N.; Sarovich, D.S.; Holden, M.T.; Peacock, S.J.; Buller, N.; Golledge, C.; Mayo, M.; Currie, B.J.; Price, E.P. Whole-genome sequencing of a quarter-century melioidosis outbreak in temperate Australia uncovers a region of low-prevalence endemicity. *Microb. Genom.* **2016**, *2*, e000067. [CrossRef] [PubMed]
11. Ketterer, P.J.; Webster, W.R.; Shield, J.; Arthur, R.J.; Blackall, P.J.; Thomas, A.D. Melioidosis in intensive piggeries in south eastern Queensland. *Aust. Vet. J.* **1986**, *63*, 146–149. [CrossRef] [PubMed]
12. Scott, I.A.; Bell, A.M.; Staines, D.R. Fatal human melioidosis in south-eastern Queensland. *Med. J. Aust.* **1997**, *166*, 197–199. [PubMed]
13. Munckhof, W.J.; Mayo, M.J.; Scott, I.; Currie, B.J. Fatal human melioidosis acquired in a subtropical Australian city. *Am. J. Trop. Med. Hyg.* **2001**, *65*, 325–328. [CrossRef] [PubMed]
14. Ketterer, P.J.; Donald, B.; Rogers, R.J. Bovine melioidosis in south-eastern Queensland. *Aust. Vet. J.* **1975**, *51*, 395–398. [CrossRef] [PubMed]
15. Yip, T.W.; Hewagama, S.; Mayo, M.; Price, E.P.; Sarovich, D.S.; Bastian, I.; Baird, R.W.; Spratt, B.G.; Currie, B.J. Endemic melioidosis in residents of desert region after atypically intense rainfall in central Australia, 2011. *Emerg. Infect. Dis.* **2015**, *21*, 1038–1040. [CrossRef] [PubMed]
16. Parameswaran, U.; Baird, R.W.; Ward, L.M.; Currie, B.J. Melioidosis at Royal Darwin Hospital in the big 2009-2010 wet season: Comparison with the preceding 20 years. *Med. J. Aust.* **2012**, *196*, 345–348. [CrossRef] [PubMed]
17. Stewart, J.D.; Smith, S.; Binotto, E.; McBride, W.J.; Currie, B.J.; Hanson, J. The epidemiology and clinical features of melioidosis in Far North Queensland: Implications for patient management. *PLoS Negl. Trop. Dis.* **2017**, *11*, e0005411. [CrossRef] [PubMed]
18. Ashdown, L.R.; Guard, R.W. The prevalence of human melioidosis in northern Queensland. *Am. J. Trop. Med. Hyg.* **1984**, *33*, 474–478. [CrossRef] [PubMed]

19. Currie, B.J.; Fisher, D.A.; Howard, D.M.; Burrow, J.N.; Selvanayagam, S.; Snelling, P.L.; Anstey, N.M.; Mayo, M.J. The epidemiology of melioidosis in Australia and Papua New Guinea. *Acta Trop.* **2000**, *74*, 121–127. [CrossRef]

20. Pearson, T.; Giffard, P.; Beckstrom-Sternberg, S.; Auerbach, R.; Hornstra, H.; Tuanyok, A.; Price, E.P.; Glass, M.B.; Leadem, B.; Beckstrom-Sternberg, J.S.; et al. Phylogeographic reconstruction of a bacterial species with high levels of lateral gene transfer. *BMC Biol.* **2009**, *7*, 78. [CrossRef] [PubMed]

21. Cheng, A.C.; Ward, L.; Godoy, D.; Norton, R.; Mayo, M.; Gal, D.; Spratt, B.G.; Currie, B.J. Genetic diversity of *Burkholderia pseudomallei* isolates in Australia. *J. Clin. Microbial.* **2008**, *46*, 249–254. [CrossRef] [PubMed]

22. Price, E.P.; Sarovich, D.S.; Smith, E.J.; MacHunter, B.; Harrington, G.; Theobald, V.; Hall, C.M.; Hornstra, H.M.; McRobb, E.; Podin, Y.; et al. Unprecedented melioidosis cases in northern Australia caused by an Asian *Burkholderia pseudomallei* strain identified by using large-scale comparative genomics. *Appl. Environ. Microbial.* **2016**, *82*, 954–963. [CrossRef] [PubMed]

23. Thomas, A.D.; Spinks, G.A.; D'Arcy, T.L.; Norton, J.H.; Trueman, K.F. Evaluation of four serological tests for the diagnosis of caprine melioidosis. *Aust. Vet. J.* **1988**, *65*, 261–264. [CrossRef] [PubMed]

24. Forbes-Faulkner, J.C.; Townsend, W.L.; Thomas, A.D. *Pseudomonas pseudomallei* infection in camels. *Aust. Vet. J.* **1992**, *69*, 148. [CrossRef] [PubMed]

25. Janmaat, A.; Choy, J.L.; Currie, B.J. Melioidosis in an alpaca (*Lama pacos*). *Aust. Vet. J.* **2004**, *82*, 622–623. [CrossRef] [PubMed]

26. Choy, J.L.; Mayo, M.; Janmaat, A.; Currie, B.J. Animal melioidosis in Australia. *Acta Trop.* **2000**, *74*, 153–158. [CrossRef]

27. Ladds, P.W.; Thomas, A.D.; Pott, B. Melioidosis with acute meningoencephalomyelitis in a horse. *Aust. Vet. J.* **1981**, *57*, 36–38. [CrossRef] [PubMed]

28. Thomas, A.D. Prevalence of melioidosis in animals in northern Queensland. *Aust. Vet. J.* **1981**, *57*, 146–148. [CrossRef] [PubMed]

29. Parkes, H.M.; Shilton, C.M.; Jerrett, I.V.; Benedict, S.; Spratt, B.G.; Godoy, D.; O'Brien, C.R.; Krockenberger, M.B.; Mayo, M.; Currie, B.J.; et al. Primary ocular melioidosis due to a single genotype of *Burkholderia pseudomallei* in two cats from Arnhem Land in the Northern Territory of Australia. *J. Feline Med. Surg.* **2009**, *11*, 856–863. [CrossRef] [PubMed]

30. Ladds, P.W.; Thomas, A.D.; Speare, R.; Brown, A.S. Melioidosis in a koala. *Aust. Vet. J.* **1990**, *67*, 304–305. [CrossRef] [PubMed]

31. Mekisic, A.P.; Wardill, J.R. Crocodile attacks in the Northern Territory of Australia. *Med. J. Aust.* **1992**, *157*, 751–754. [PubMed]

32. Thomas, A.D.; Norton, J.H.; Pott, B.W. Melioidosis in a galah (*Cacatua roseicapilla*). *Aust. Vet. J.* **1980**, *56*, 192–193. [CrossRef] [PubMed]

33. Thomas, A.D.; Wilson, A.J.; Aubrey, J.N. Melioidosis in a sulphur-crested cockatoo (*Cacatua galerita*). *Aust. Vet. J.* **1978**, *54*, 306–307. [CrossRef] [PubMed]

34. Hampton, V.; Kaestli, M.; Mayo, M.; Choy, J.L.; Harrington, G.; Richardson, L.; Benedict, S.; Noske, R.; Garnett, S.T.; Godoy, D.; et al. Melioidosis in birds and *Burkholderia pseudomallei* dispersal, Australia. *Emerg. Infect. Dis.* **2011**, *17*, 1310–1312. [CrossRef] [PubMed]

35. Hoger, A.C.; Mayo, M.; Price, E.P.; Theobald, V.; Harrington, G.; Machunter, B.; Choy, J.L.; Currie, B.J.; Kaestli, M. The melioidosis agent *Burkholderia pseudomallei* and related opportunistic pathogens detected in faecal matter of wildlife and livestock in northern Australia. *Epidemiol. Infect.* **2016**, *144*, 1924–1932. [CrossRef] [PubMed]

36. Currie, B.J.; Mayo, M.; Anstey, N.M.; Donohoe, P.; Haase, A.; Kemp, D.J. A cluster of melioidosis cases from an endemic region is clonal and is linked to the water supply using molecular typing of *Burkholderia pseudomallei* isolates. *Am. J. Trop. Med. Hyg.* **2001**, *65*, 177–179. [CrossRef] [PubMed]

37. Inglis, T.J.; Garrow, S.C.; Henderson, M.; Clair, A.; Sampson, J.; O'Reilly, L.; Cameron, B. *Burkholderia pseudomallei* traced to water treatment plant in Australia. *Emerg. Infect. Dis.* **2000**, *6*, 56–59. [PubMed]

38. Currie, B.J.; Jacups, S.P. Intensity of rainfall and severity of melioidosis, Australia. *Emerg. Infect. Dis.* **2003**, *9*, 1538–1542. [CrossRef] [PubMed]

39. Cheng, A.C.; Jacups, S.P.; Ward, L.; Currie, B.J. Melioidosis and aboriginal seasons in northern Australia. *Trans. R. Soc. Trop. Med. Hyg.* **2008**, *102* (Suppl. 1), S26–S29. [CrossRef]

40. Kaestli, M.; Grist, E.P.M.; Ward, L.; Hill, A.; Mayo, M.; Currie, B.J. The association of melioidosis with climatic factors in Darwin, Australia: A 23-year time-series analysis. *J. Infect.* **2016**, *72*, 687–697. [CrossRef] [PubMed]

41. Cheng, A.C.; Jacups, S.P.; Gal, D.; Mayo, M.; Currie, B.J. Extreme weather events and environmental contamination are associated with case-clusters of melioidosis in the Northern Territory of Australia. *Int. J. Epidemiol.* **2006**, *35*, 323–329. [CrossRef] [PubMed]

42. Inglis, T.J.; O'Reilly, L.; Merritt, A.J.; Levy, A.; Heath, C.H. The aftermath of the Western Australian melioidosis outbreak. *Am. J. Trop. Med. Hyg.* **2011**, *84*, 851–857. [CrossRef] [PubMed]

43. Stewart, J.D.; Smith, S.; Hanson, J. Melioidosis in Far North Queensland is not correlated with severe weather events. *Med. J. Aust.* **2017**, *207*, 394. [CrossRef] [PubMed]

44. Merritt, A.J.; Inglis, T.J.J. The role of climate in the epidemiology of melioidosis. *Curr. Trop. Med. Rep.* **2017**, *4*, 185–191. [CrossRef] [PubMed]

45. Meumann, E.M.; Cheng, A.C.; Ward, L.; Currie, B.J. Clinical features and epidemiology of melioidosis pneumonia: Results from a 21-year study and review of the literature. *Clin. Infect. Dis.* **2012**, *54*, 362–369. [CrossRef] [PubMed]

46. Morse, L.P.; Moller, C.C.; Harvey, E.; Ward, L.; Cheng, A.C.; Carson, P.J.; Currie, B.J. Prostatic abscess due to *Burkholderia pseudomallei*: 81 cases from a 19-year prospective melioidosis study. *J. Urol.* **2009**, *182*, 542–547. [CrossRef] [PubMed]

47. Kozlowska, J.; Smith, S.; Roberts, J.; Pridgeon, S.; Hanson, J. Prostatic abscess due to *Burkholderia pseudomallei*: Facilitating diagnosis to optimize management. *Am. J. Trop. Med. Hyg.* **2017**, *98*, 227–230. [CrossRef] [PubMed]

48. Shetty, R.P.; Mathew, M.; Smith, J.; Morse, L.P.; Mehta, J.A.; Currie, B.J. Management of melioidosis osteomyelitis and septic arthritis. *Bone Jt. J.* **2015**, *97-B*, 277–282. [CrossRef] [PubMed]

49. McLeod, C.; Morris, P.S.; Bauert, P.A.; Kilburn, C.J.; Ward, L.M.; Baird, R.W.; Currie, B.J. Clinical presentation and medical management of melioidosis in children: A 24-year prospective study in the Northern Territory of Australia and review of the literature. *Clin. Infect. Dis.* **2015**, *60*, 21–26. [CrossRef] [PubMed]

50. Sanderson, C.; Currie, B.J. Melioidosis: A pediatric disease. *Pediatr. Infect. Dis. J.* **2014**, *33*, 770–771. [CrossRef] [PubMed]

51. Young, A.; Tacon, C.; Smith, S.; Reeves, B.; Wiseman, G.; Hanson, J. Case report: Fatal pediatric melioidosis despite optimal intensive care. *Am. J. Trop. Med. Hyg.* **2017**, *97*, 1691–1694. [CrossRef] [PubMed]

52. Smith, S.; Stewart, J.D.; Tacon, C.; Archer, N.; Hanson, J. Children with melioidosis in Far North Queensland are commonly bacteraemic and have a high case fatality rate. *Commun. Dis. Intell. Q. Rep.* **2018**, in press.

53. Sarovich, D.S.; Ward, L.; Price, E.P.; Mayo, M.; Pitman, M.C.; Baird, R.W.; Currie, B.J. Recurrent melioidosis in the Darwin prospective melioidosis study: Improving therapies mean that relapse cases are now rare. *J. Clin. Microbial.* **2014**, *52*, 650–653. [CrossRef] [PubMed]

54. Currie, B.J.; Fisher, D.A.; Howard, D.M.; Burrow, J.N. Neurological melioidosis. *Acta Trop.* **2000**, *74*, 145–151. [CrossRef]

55. Sarovich, D.S.; Price, E.P.; Webb, J.R.; Ward, L.M.; Voutsinos, M.Y.; Tuanyok, A.; Mayo, M.; Kaestli, M.; Currie, B.J. Variable virulence factors in *Burkholderia pseudomallei* (melioidosis) associated with human disease. *PLoS ONE* **2014**, *9*, e91682. [CrossRef] [PubMed]

56. Morris, J.L.; Fane, A.; Sarovich, D.S.; Price, E.P.; Rush, C.M.; Govan, B.L.; Parker, E.; Mayo, M.; Currie, B.J.; Ketheesan, N. Increased neurotropic threat from *Burkholderia pseudomallei* strains with a *B. Mallei*-like variation in the bima motility gene, Australia. *Emerg. Infect. Dis.* **2017**, *23*. [CrossRef] [PubMed]

57. Baker, A.; Mayo, M.; Owens, L.; Burgess, G.; Norton, R.; McBride, W.J.; Currie, B.J.; Warner, J. Biogeography of *Burkholderia pseudomallei* in the Torres Strait Islands of northern Australia. *J. Clin. Microbial.* **2013**, *51*, 2520–2525. [CrossRef] [PubMed]

58. Hill, A.A.; Mayo, M.; Kaestli, M.; Price, E.P.; Richardson, L.J.; Godoy, D.; Spratt, B.G.; Currie, B.J. Melioidosis as a consequence of sporting activity. *Am. J. Trop. Med. Hyg.* **2013**, *89*, 365–366. [CrossRef] [PubMed]

59. Baker, A.L.; Ezzahir, J.; Gardiner, C.; Shipton, W.; Warner, J.M. Environmental attributes influencing the distribution of *Burkholderia pseudomallei* in northern Australia. *PLoS ONE* **2015**, *10*, e0138953. [CrossRef] [PubMed]

60. McRobb, E.; Kaestli, M.; Mayo, M.; Price, E.P.; Sarovich, D.S.; Godoy, D.; Spratt, B.G.; Currie, B.J. Melioidosis from contaminated bore water and successful UV sterilization. *Am. J. Trop. Med. Hyg.* **2013**, *89*, 367–368. [CrossRef] [PubMed]

61. Kaestli, M.; Mayo, M.; Harrington, G.; Ward, L.; Watt, F.; Hill, J.V.; Cheng, A.C.; Currie, B.J. Landscape changes influence the occurrence of the melioidosis bacterium *Burkholderiapseudomallei* in soil in northern Australia. *PLoS Negl. Trop. Dis.* **2009**, *3*, e364. [CrossRef] [PubMed]

62. Kaestli, M.; Schmid, M.; Mayo, M.; Rothballer, M.; Harrington, G.; Richardson, L.; Hill, A.; Hill, J.; Tuanyok, A.; Keim, P.; et al. Out of the ground: Aerial and exotic habitats of the melioidosis bacterium *Burkholderia pseudomallei* in grasses in Australia. *Environ. Microbiol.* **2012**, *14*, 2058–2070. [CrossRef] [PubMed]

63. Currie, B.J.; Price, E.P.; Mayo, M.; Kaestli, M.; Theobald, V.; Harrington, I.; Harrington, G.; Sarovich, D.S. Use of whole-genome sequencing to link *Burkholderia pseudomallei* from air sampling to mediastinal melioidosis, Australia. *Emerg. Infect. Dis.* **2015**, *21*, 2052–2054. [CrossRef] [PubMed]

64. Merritt, A.J.; Peck, M.; Gayle, D.; Levy, A.; Ler, Y.H.; Raby, E.; Gibbs, T.M.; Inglis, T.J. Cutaneous melioidosis cluster caused by contaminated wound irrigation fluid. *Emerg. Infect. Dis.* **2016**, *22*, 1420. [CrossRef] [PubMed]

65. Government of Western Australia. Department of Primary Industries and Regional Development. Melioidosis in Animals. Available online: https://www.Agric.Wa.Gov.Au/livestock-biosecurity/melioidosis-animals (accessed on 21 January 2018).

66. Podin, Y.; Kaestli, M.; McMahon, N.; Hennessy, J.; Ngian, H.U.; Wong, J.S.; Mohana, A.; Wong, S.C.; William, T.; Mayo, M.; et al. Reliability of automated biochemical identification of *Burkholderia pseudomallei* is regionally dependent. *J. Clin. Microbial.* **2013**, *51*, 3076–3078. [CrossRef] [PubMed]

67. Inglis, T.J.; Healy, P.E.; Fremlin, L.J.; Golledge, C.L. Use of matrix-assisted laser desorption/ionization time-of-flight mass spectrometry analysis for rapid confirmation of *Burkholderia pseudomallei* in septicemic melioidosis. *Am. J. Trop. Med. Hyg.* **2012**, *86*, 1039–1042. [CrossRef] [PubMed]

68. Robertson, G.; Sorenson, A.; Govan, B.; Ketheesan, N.; Houghton, R.; Chen, H.; AuCoin, D.; Dillon, M.; Norton, R. Rapid diagnostics for melioidosis: A comparative study of a novel lateral flow antigen detection assay. *J. Med. Microbial.* **2015**, *64*, 845–848. [CrossRef] [PubMed]

69. Inglis, T.J.; Merritt, A.; Chidlow, G.; Aravena-Roman, M.; Harnett, G. Comparison of diagnostic laboratory methods for identification of *Burkholderia pseudomallei*. *J. Med. Microbial.* **2005**, *43*, 2201–2206. [CrossRef] [PubMed]

70. Haase, A.; Brennan, M.; Barrett, S.; Wood, Y.; Huffam, S.; O'Brien, D.; Currie, B. Evaluation of PCR for diagnosis of melioidosis. *J. Med. Microbial.* **1998**, *36*, 1039–1041.

71. Kaestli, M.; Richardson, L.J.; Colman, R.E.; Tuanyok, A.; Price, E.P.; Bowers, J.R.; Mayo, M.; Kelley, E.; Seymour, M.L.; Sarovich, D.S.; et al. Comparison of Taqman PCR assays for detection of the melioidosis agent *Burkholderia pseudomallei* in clinical specimens. *J. Med. Microbial.* **2012**, *50*, 2059–2062. [CrossRef] [PubMed]

72. Cheng, A.C.; O'Brien, M.; Freeman, K.; Lum, G.; Currie, B.J. Indirect hemagglutination assay in patients with melioidosis in northern Australia. *Am. J. Trop. Med. Hyg.* **2006**, *74*, 330–334. [PubMed]

73. Davis, J.S.; Currie, B.J.; Fisher, D.A.; Huffam, S.E.; Anstey, N.M.; Price, R.N.; Krause, V.L.; Zweck, N.; Lawton, P.D.; Snelling, P.L.; et al. Prevention of opportunistic infections in immunosuppressed patients in the tropical top end of the Northern Territory. *Commun. Dis. Intell. Q. Rep.* **2003**, *27*, 526–532.

74. Maloney, S.; Engler, C.; Norton, R. Epidemiological cut-off value of clinical isolates of *Burkholderia pseudomallei* from northern Queensland to meropenem, ceftazidime, trimethoprim/sulfamethoxazole and doxycycline by the microbroth dilution method. *J. Glob. Antimicrob. Resist.* **2017**, *10*, 291–294. [CrossRef] [PubMed]

75. Currie, B.J. Melioidosis: Evolving concepts in epidemiology, pathogenesis, and treatment. *Semin. Respir. Crit. Care Med.* **2015**, *36*, 111–125. [CrossRef] [PubMed]

76. Jenney, A.W.; Lum, G.; Fisher, D.A.; Currie, B.J. Antibiotic susceptibility of *Burkholderia pseudomallei* from tropical northern Australia and implications for therapy of melioidosis. *Int. J. Antimicrob. Agents* **2001**, *17*, 109–113. [CrossRef]

77. Crowe, A.; McMahon, N.; Currie, B.J.; Baird, R.W. Current antimicrobial susceptibility of first-episode melioidosis *Burkholderia pseudomallei* isolates from the Northern Territory, Australia. *Int. J. Antimicrob. Agents* **2014**, *44*, 160–162. [CrossRef] [PubMed]

78. Price, E.P.; Smith, M.L.; Paxinos, E.E.; Tallon, L.J.; Sadzewicz, L.; Sengamalay, N.; Baird, R.W.; Currie, B.J.; Sarovich, D.S. Whole-genome sequences of *Burkholderia pseudomallei* isolates exhibiting decreased meropenem susceptibility. *Genome Announc.* **2017**, *5*, e00053-17. [CrossRef] [PubMed]

79. Viberg, L.T.; Sarovich, D.S.; Kidd, T.J.; Geake, J.B.; Bell, S.C.; Currie, B.J.; Price, E.P. Within-host evolution of *Burkholderia pseudomallei* during chronic infection of seven Australasian cystic fibrosis patients. *mBio* **2017**, *8*, e00356-17. [CrossRef] [PubMed]

80. Hsu, C.C.; Singh, D.; Kwan, G.; Deuble, M.; Aquilina, C.; Korah, I.; Norton, R. Neuromelioidosis: Craniospinal MRI findings in *Burkholderia pseudomallei* infection. *J. Neuroimag.* **2016**, *26*, 75–82. [CrossRef] [PubMed]

81. Deuble, M.; Aquilina, C.; Norton, R. Neurologic melioidosis. *Am. J. Trop. Med. Hyg.* **2013**, *89*, 535–539. [CrossRef] [PubMed]

82. Huffam, S.; Jacups, S.P.; Kittler, P.; Currie, B.J. Out of hospital treatment of patients with melioidosis using ceftazidime in 24 h elastomeric infusors, via peripherally inserted central catheters. *Trop. Med. Int. Health* **2004**, *9*, 715–717. [CrossRef] [PubMed]

83. Cheng, A.C.; Chierakul, W.; Chaowagul, W.; Chetchotisakd, P.; Limmathurotsakul, D.; Dance, D.A.; Peacock, S.J.; Currie, B.J. Consensus guidelines for dosing of amoxicillin-clavulanate in melioidosis. *Am. J. Trop. Med. Hyg.* **2008**, *78*, 208–209. [PubMed]

84. Stephens, D.P.; Thomas, J.H.; Ward, L.M.; Currie, B.J. Melioidosis causing critical illness: A review of 24 years of experience from the Royal Darwin Hospital ICU. *Crit. Care Med.* **2016**, *44*, 1500–1505. [CrossRef] [PubMed]

85. Cheng, A.C.; Stephens, D.P.; Anstey, N.M.; Currie, B.J. Adjunctive granulocyte colony-stimulating factor for treatment of septic shock due to melioidosis. *Clin. Infect. Dis.* **2004**, *38*, 32–37. [CrossRef] [PubMed]

86. Cheng, A.C.; Limmathurotsakul, D.; Chierakul, W.; Getchalarat, N.; Wuthiekanun, V.; Stephens, D.P.; Day, N.P.; White, N.J.; Chaowagul, W.; Currie, B.J.; et al. A randomized controlled trial of granulocyte colony-stimulating factor for the treatment of severe sepsis due to melioidosis in Thailand. *Clin. Infect. Dis.* **2007**, *45*, 308–314. [CrossRef] [PubMed]

87. Northern Territory Government. Melioidosis. Available online: https://nt.Gov.Au/wellbeing/health-conditions-treatments/bacterial/melioidosis (accessed on 21 January 2018).

88. Boyd, R.; Mcguinness, S.; Draper, A.; Neilson, M.; Krause, V. *Melioidosis Awareness Campaign*; The Northern Territory Disease Control Bulletin, Centre for Disease Control: Darwin, Australia, 2016; Volume 23, pp. 1–4.

89. Chalmers, R.M.; Majoni, S.W.; Ward, L.; Perry, G.J.; Jabbar, Z.; Currie, B.J. Melioidosis and end-stage renal disease in tropical northern Australia. *Kidney Int.* **2014**, *86*, 867–870. [CrossRef] [PubMed]

90. Majoni, S.W.; Hughes, J.T.; Heron, B.; Currie, B.J. Trimethoprim + sulfamethoxazole reduces rates of melioidosis in high-risk hemodialysis patients. *Kidney Int. Rep.* **2018**, *3*, 160–167. [CrossRef] [PubMed]

91. Fitzpatrick, S.; Kearney, S. Melioidosis. Department of Regional Development, Primary Industry, Fisheries and Resources, Northern Territory Government. Available online: https://dpir.nt.gov.au/__data/assets/pdf_file/0011/232976/840.pdf (accessed on 21 January 2018).

92. McRobb, E.; Kaestli, M.; Price, E.P.; Sarovich, D.S.; Mayo, M.; Warner, J.; Spratt, B.G.; Currie, B.J. Distribution of *Burkholderia pseudomallei* in northern Australia, a land of diversity. *Appl. Environ. Microbial.* **2014**, *80*, 3463–3468. [CrossRef] [PubMed]

93. Aziz, A.; Sarovich, D.S.; Harris, T.M.; Kaestli, M.; McRobb, E.; Mayo, M.; Currie, B.J.; Price, E.P. Suspected cases of intracontinental *Burkholderia pseudomallei* sequence type homoplasy resolved using whole-genome sequencing. *Microb. Genom.* **2017**, *3*. [CrossRef] [PubMed]

94. Chewapreecha, C.; Holden, M.T.; Vehkala, M.; Valimaki, N.; Yang, Z.; Harris, S.R.; Mather, A.E.; Tuanyok, A.; De Smet, B.; Le Hello, S.; et al. Global and regional dissemination and evolution of *Burkholderia pseudomallei*. *Nat. Microbial.* **2017**, *2*, 16263. [CrossRef] [PubMed]

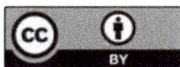

Tropical Medicine and Infectious Disease

MDPI

Review

Melioidosis in Bangladesh: A Clinical and Epidemiological Analysis of Culture-Confirmed Cases

Fazle Rabbi Chowdhury [1,2,3,4,*] [ID], Md. Shariful Alam Jilani [5] [ID], Lovely Barai [6],
Tanjila Rahman [6], Mili Rani Saha [6], Md. Robed Amin [7], Kaniz Fatema [8],
K. M. Shahidul Islam [6], M. A. Faiz [2,9], Susanna J. Dunachie [1,2,3] and David A. B. Dance [1,10,11] [ID]

[1] Centre for Tropical Medicine and Global Health, Nuffield Department of Medicine, University of Oxford, Oxford OX3 7BN, UK; susie.dunachie@ndm.ox.ac.uk (S.J.D.); david.d@tropmedres.ac (D.A.B.D.)
[2] Mahidol Oxford Tropical Medicine Research Unit, Mahidol University, Bangkok 10400, Thailand; drmafaiz@gmail.com
[3] Peter Medawar Building for Pathogen Research, University of Oxford, Oxford OX1 3SY, UK
[4] Department of Medicine, Bangabandhu Sheikh Mujib Medical University, Dhaka 1000, Bangladesh
[5] Department of Microbiology, Ibrahim Medical College, Dhaka 1000, Bangladesh; jilanimsa@gmail.com
[6] Department of Microbiology, BIRDEM General Hospital, Dhaka 1000, Bangladesh; barai_lovely@yahoo.com (L.B.); tanjila_lo@yahoo.com (T.R.); milisaha77@yahoo.com (M.R.S.); kmshahid2000@yahoo.com (K.M.S.I.)
[7] Department of Medicine, Dhaka Medical College, Dhaka 1000, Bangladesh; robedamin@yahoo.com
[8] Department of Critical Care Medicine, BIRDEM General Hospital, Dhaka 1000, Bangladesh; drkanizfatemasb@gmail.com
[9] Dev Care Foundation, Dhaka 1205, Bangladesh
[10] Lao-Oxford-Mahosot Hospital-Wellcome Trust Research Unit (LOMWRU), Vientiane 0100, Laos
[11] Faculty of Tropical Medicine and Infectious Diseases, London School of Hygiene and Tropical Medicine, London WC1E 7HT, UK
*   Correspondence: mastershakil@hotmail.com or fazle.chowdhury@ndm.ox.ac.uk; Tel.: +44-07392-757-139

Received: 10 March 2018; Accepted: 4 April 2018; Published: 9 April 2018

Abstract: Melioidosis is known to occur in Bangladesh, but there are few reports about the condition in the published international literature. We set out to review all known cases of melioidosis in the country to date, using both retrospective and prospective data. A web-based literature search was conducted to identify all published case reports, original articles and conference abstracts. Cases were also included from a prospective study conducted in 2017. Fifty-one cases were identified between 1961 and 2017. Cases have been reported from sixteen out of the 64 districts of Bangladesh. The median age of the patients at presentation was 45 years (IQR 37–52), with a significant male (77%) predominance. Many patients (14/39; 36%) were farmers and 83% had diabetes mellitus. A skin/soft tissue abscess was the most common primary clinical presentation (13/49; 27%), followed by septic arthritis (10/49; 20%), pneumonia, and a deep-seated abscess/organ abscess (7/49; 14%). The major challenges to the diagnosis and treatment of melioidosis in Bangladesh are the lack of resources and the lack of awareness of melioidosis. Capacity development programs are urgently required to define the burden of disease and to tackle the mortality rates.

Keywords: melioidosis; *Burkholderia*; Bangladesh

---

1. Introduction and History of Melioidosis in Bangladesh

Melioidosis is an important cause of infectious disease across Southeast Asia, and it is believed to be a problem in Bangladesh, based on anecdotes and a few case reports [1–3]. The disease is caused by a highly pathogenic, soil-borne, Gram-negative bacterium, *Burkholderia pseudomallei* [4]. Bangladesh is an example of a highly populous, agricultural country where melioidosis may be a significantly underdiagnosed cause of infection and death. A lack of awareness among microbiologists and clinicians and a lack of diagnostic microbiology infrastructure are factors that are likely to lead to the underreporting of melioidosis. The first reported, confirmed case of melioidosis that was acquired from Bangladesh (at that time known as East Pakistan) was a British sailor, who was travelling east of Suez [5]. In October 1960, his ship was carried half a mile inland near Chittagong by a cyclone, and was deposited in a paddy field [5]. The crew stayed there for three months and were repatriated in January 1961. The patient developed symptoms in May in the UK of that year and eventually received a diagnosis of melioidosis based on pus cultures in Liverpool [5]. Several individual case reports/series of melioidosis have been published from Bangladesh since that time. Cases have also been reported among Bangladeshi immigrants presenting in other countries [5–16].

The clinical presentation of melioidosis is widely varied, and a definitive diagnosis requires a skilled microbiology laboratory, making it more difficult to diagnose in low-resource settings such as Bangladesh. Agriculture is the most productive sector of the country's economy, contributing about 30% of the nation's GDP and providing over 90% of Bangladesh's rural employment [17]. A recent modelling study predicted a melioidosis burden of nearly 17,000 cases and 9500 deaths a year in Bangladesh [3,18]. This review identifies 51 cases covering all the published case reports, series, and unpublished cases during the period from 1964 (the case report of the 1961 British sailor) to 2017, with the aim of generating further evidence to increase the awareness of the disease in the national and international healthcare community.

2. Review of Melioidosis Cases and Presence of *B. pseudomallei* in Bangladesh

This was a descriptive study involving both retrospective and prospective data analysis. A web-based literature search was conducted using PubMed, Google Scholar, Medline, ResearchGate, and the Bangladesh Journals Online (BanglaJol) database to identify all published, culture-confirmed case reports of melioidosis in Bangladesh. The key search terms were 'melioidosis', '*Burkholderia*', and 'Bangladesh'. Additional published cases were also identified from the personal EndNote database of one of the authors (D.A.B.D.). We also conducted a prospective study during 2017 in Dhaka to identify cases among patients admitted with an acute febrile illness and included patients confirmed as having culture-positive melioidosis, in this review.

2.1. Published and Unpublished Cases

Overall, we identified 25 case reports/case series, one original article, and three conference abstracts describing cases of culture-confirmed melioidosis in Bangladesh. Of these, one case report, one original article, and two conference abstracts were excluded due to the duplication of data. Additional cases were diagnosed through our research project in 2017. The cases were reported between 1964 and 2017. Of the 24 case reports, twelve described Bangladeshi immigrants diagnosed overseas (UK, Belgium, USA, Cuba, and Kuwait), all of whom had a history of travelling to Bangladesh before their illness [5–16], whereas the rest were diagnosed and reported within Bangladesh [19–31].

2.2. Definitions of Clinical Manifestations:

In this review, major organ involvement and clinical features were classified as follows.

(a) Pulmonary: pneumonia, including complications such as a lung abscess or a pleural effusion.
(b) Musculoskeletal (MSK): septic arthritis, osteomyelitis, and others.
(c) Genitourinary (GU): infection of the urinary and genital tract, including the kidneys.
(d) Neurological: involvement of the brain and spinal cord, including the meninges.
(e) Organ abscess/deep-seated abscess: Abscess involving any solid organ or in any deep-seated site such as the muscles.

(f) Cutaneous: infection and abscess of the skin and subcutaneous tissue.

(g) Bacteraemia without focus: acute sepsis without any specific focus.

2.3. Climate Data

The monthly average mean temperature in degrees Celsius and the monthly average rainfall in millimetres for the years 1961 to 2015 were collected from the climate change knowledge portal of the World Bank [32].

2.4. Statistical Analysis

The results were expressed as median ± interquartile range (IQR) for continuous variables. A choropleth map was drawn using geographic information system (GIS) data to illustrate the distribution of the cases [33]. A choropleth map typically uses either differences in colour value (sometimes in combination with hue) or differences in spacing (e.g., the intensity of a hatched pattern) to represent the differences. The one sample *t*-test was applied to determine the level of significance. Statistical analysis was performed using IBM SPSS Statistics 22 for Windows, and GraphPad Prism 7 was used to display the results. Informed patient consent was obtained from the prospectively studied cases, with ethical permission being granted by the institutional committees of Dhaka Medical College (DMC) and the Bangladesh Institute of Research and Rehabilitation for Diabetes, Endocrine, and Metabolic Disorders (BIRDEM).

2.5. Important Findings

Between 1964 and 2017, 51 cases of culture-positive melioidosis were diagnosed from Bangladesh, with all the published cases listed in Table 1. The median age of the patients at presentation was 45 years (IQR 37–52), with a significant male (79.6%) predominance (Table 2). The oldest patient was 90 years old and the youngest was 8 years old. The median age of the patients in Bangladesh was slightly lower compared to India, Thailand, Taiwan, and Australia [34–37]. However, the male preponderance was higher than the findings from the same countries. A similar male predominance was found in Malaysia [38]. This is probably because in countries such as Bangladesh, males are more involved with outdoor activities. Moreover, the access to healthcare for women is still restricted due to many reasons, including cultural and socioeconomic factors in Bangladesh [39,40].

The majority of the patients for whom data was available (14/39; 36%) were farmers by profession, which is compatible with another hospital-based serosurveillance carried out in Bangladesh in 2010, where farmers had an increased risk of seropositivity (risk ratio = 1.4, 95% CI 1.0–1.8; $p = 0.03$) [41]. The survey recorded 28.9% positivity for *B. pseudomallei* through an indirect haemagglutination assay among 1244 adult febrile patients [41]. However, another study reported 22.6% to 30.8% seropositivity in three districts (Gazipur, Mymensingh, and Sylhet) where melioidosis cases were detected earlier, compared to 9.8% in a district (Kishoreganj) where no melioidosis cases were either detected or reported ($p < 0.01$) [42]. The same study found no significant difference among different occupational groups ($\chi^2 = 3.835$, $p = 0.280$) [42]. Over 88% (23/26) of cases in Bangladesh had a definitive history of soil exposure (Table 2). This is related to the occupational activities of the patients.

Table 1. Reports of all culture-confirmed melioidosis cases from Bangladesh.

Year of Report	Presumed Location of Infection in Bangladesh	Location of Diagnosis	No. of Case/Cases	Reference
1964	Chittagong	UK	1	5
1969	Unknown	UK	1	16
1970	Unknown	UK	1	15
1988	Unknown	Bangladesh	1	30
1991	Sylhet	UK	1	13
1999	Sylhet	UK	3	10
1999	Sylhet	UK	1	14
2000	Unknown	UK	1	12
2001	Sherpur	Bangladesh	1	31
2007	Unknown	Belgium	1	8
2007	Rangpur	Belgium	1	9
2012	Unknown	USA	1	7
2013	Unknown	Bangladesh	1	27
2014	Gazipur, Mymensingh, Tangail, Dhaka, Narayanganj, Khagrachari, Comilla	Bangladesh	15	23
2014	Gazipur	Bangladesh	1	26
2014	Unknown	Kuwait	1	6
2015	Gazipur	Bangladesh	1	19
2015	Gazipur	Bangladesh	1	21
2015	Mymensingh	Bangladesh	1	25
2015	Unknown	Bangladesh	1	24
2015	Gazipur	Bangladesh	1	28
2016	Brahmanbaria	Bangladesh	1	22
2016	Khagrachari	Bangladesh	1	29
2017	Unknown.	Cuba	1	11
2017	Narayanganj, Tangail, Feni, Comilla, Mymensingh, Dhaka, Noakhali, Jamalpur	Bangladesh	11	20

Table 2. Baseline demographic characteristics of the culture-confirmed cases.

Variables	Number (%)	p Value [ⁿ]
Age (years; median, (IQR))	45 (37–52)	
Sex ($n = 51$)		
Men	41 (80)	0.0001
Women	10 (20)	
Occupation ($n = 39$) [Ψ]		
Farmer	14 (36)	
Housewife	8 (21)	
Worker/day labourer	4 (10)	
Unemployed	4 (10)	
Carpenter	2 (5)	
Others	7 (18)	
History of soil/environmental exposure ($n = 26$) [Ψ]		
Yes	23 (88)	0.0001
No	3 (12)	

[Ψ] Variables have missing data. [ⁿ] By one sample *t*-test.

Cases have been reported from sixteen out of 64 districts of Bangladesh, all of which were in the eastern and northern parts of the country (Figure 1). In five patients, the geographic location could not be identified. The highest number of cases (9/46; 18%) were recorded from Gazipur, followed by Tangail (6/46; 12%), Sylhet (5/46; 10%), Mymensingh (4/46; 8%), Feni (4/46; 8%), and others. This study confirms that the Gazipur, Tangail, Sylhet, and Mymensingh districts are hotspots for melioidosis in Bangladesh. Our findings are in consensus with the soil surveillance carried out in these districts in 2011 and confirmed its presence. The isolates were phenotypically identical, arabinose negative and showed a specific 550 bp band in PCR [42]. The reason behind the dearth of cases to the west may be multiple. The agricultural pattern is regionally variable in Bangladesh, especially for rice, which is mainly grown in the north, south, and northeast districts [43]. Moreover, rice is cultivated in two seasons in the north, northeast, and south, but it is cultivated only once a year in the western districts [43]. There is also a clear variation in the pattern of rainfall. High rainfall occurs twice in the northeastern part of the country compared to the west [44]. However, the lack of cases in western Bangladesh could also be due to a lack of diagnosis and/or the underreporting of cases. The communication to the capital from the western and northwestern parts of the country is also more difficult compared to other regions. The infrastructure development index (IDI) is also very poor for those districts [45], so many patients may not travel to Dhaka and other major centres for diagnosis and treatment.

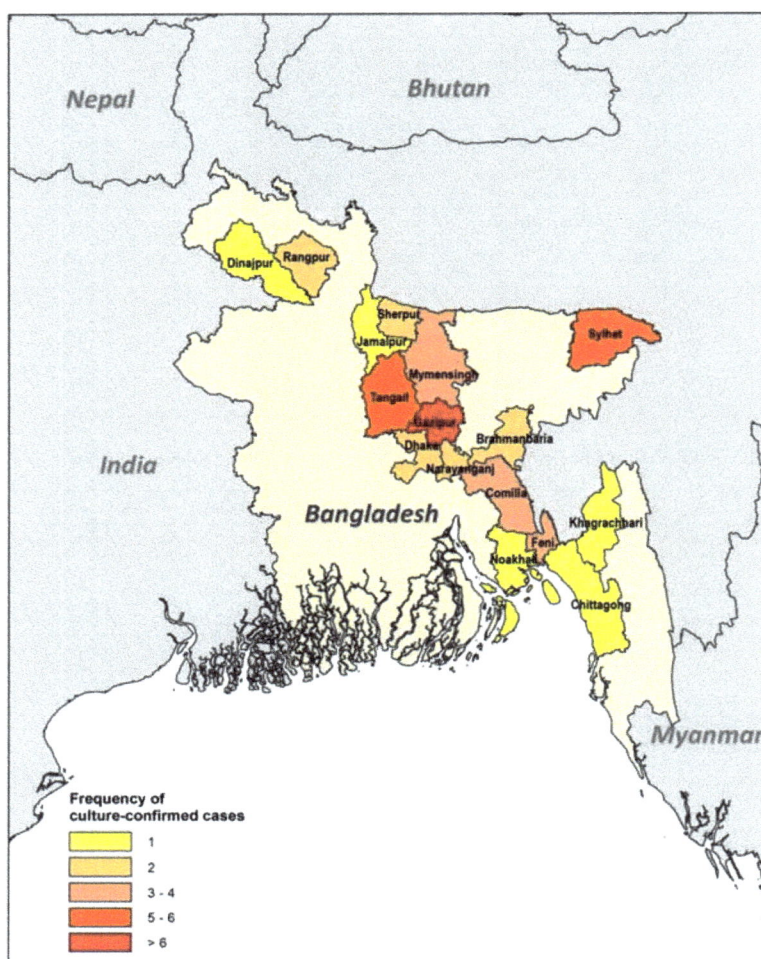

Figure 1. Choropleth map based on GIS data. The map illustrates the frequency by district of culture-confirmed cases of melioidosis (*n* = 46).

In thirty-eight cases, the period between the onset of symptoms and the diagnosis of melioidosis was calculated (Table 3). The median duration was 36 days (IQR 18.75–79.5). Specific risk factors/co-morbidities were identified in forty-eight cases. A high proportion (40/48; 83%) of the cases had diabetes mellitus (Table 3). Among these, 11 were already known to have diabetes at presentation and the rest (29; 76%) were diagnosed after hospital admission. The other comorbidities were smoking (3/48; 6%), chronic kidney disease (CKD; 2/48; 4%), and hypertension (2/48; 4%). We also found alcoholism, ischaemic cardiomyopathy (ICM), and haemoglobin E (HbE) trait in single cases. The presence of *B. pseudomallei* was confirmed in various culture samples. Twenty-three patients (45%) were positive on pus culture. The second most common positive sample was blood (22/51; 43%). Other sources of the bacterium were joint fluid (10/51; 20%), other swabs (6/51; 12%) such as skin, nasotracheal, and tracheal; urine (5/51; 10%) and sputum (3/51; 6%). In total, fourteen patients (27%) died and thirty-seven (73%) survived.

Table 3. Prehospital and laboratory characteristics and clinical outcome of culture-confirmed cases.

Variables [1]	Number (%)
Time between symptom onset and diagnosis (days; median, (IQR))	36 (18.75–79.5)
Risk factors (*n* = 48) [ψ]	
Diabetes mellitus	40 (83)
Chronic kidney disease	2 (4)
Hypertension	2 (4)
Smoking	3 (6)
Others (alcoholism, ICM, Hb ET) [€]	3 (6)
Culture-positive samples (*n* = 51) [ψ]	
Blood	22 (43)
Pus	23 (45)
Joint fluid	10 (20)
Urine	5 (10)
Sputum	3 (6)
Other samples (skin/nasotracheal/tracheal aspirate)	6 (12)
Mortality (*n* = 51) [ψ]	
Survived	37 (73)
Died	14 (27)

[1] Variables have missing data. [ψ] includes multiple positive sites. [€] ICM—ischaemic cardiomyopathy, Hb ET—haemoglobin E trait.

The majority of cases were diagnosed during the rainy season from June to September (Figure 2). The primary clinical presentation and major system involvement of 49 cases are shown in Table 4. In two patients, there was insufficient information in the reports to enable their classification. A skin/soft tissue abscess was the most common primary clinical presentation (13/49; 27%), and none of the patients with localised cutaneous lesions died. The second most common presentation was septic arthritis (10/49; 20%), with one death occurring within this group of patients (a known diabetic woman with CKD who was admitted to hospital with shock and subsequently developed acute-on-chronic renal failure and died). The next most common presentations were pneumonia (7/49; 14%) and a deep-seated abscess/organ abscess (7/49; 14%). Two patients died of pneumonia and one with an organ abscess. Five patients (10%) presented with a urinary tract infection and/or acute kidney injury (AKI), and three of these patients died. All of these cases were admitted with shock and multiple organ involvement. Four (8.1%) patients presented with sepsis without any focus, and three (6%) presented with symptoms and signs suggesting a possible diagnosis of meningitis, although no lumbar punctures were done. All seven of these patients (median age 50 (IQR, 40–59)) were diabetic and developed multiple organ failure during admission and died.

Table 4. Clinical description of culture-confirmed melioidosis cases (*n* = 49).

Clinical Variables	Number (%)	Number of Deaths (%)
Primary Clinical Presentation		
Skin and subcutaneous abscess	13 (27)	0 (0)
Septic arthritis	10 (20)	1 (10)
Pneumonia	7 (14)	2 (29)
Organ abscess/deep-seated abscess	7 (14)	1 (14)
Urinary tract Infection/Acute kidney injury	5 (10)	3 (60)
Sepsis without focus	4 (8)	4 (100)
Meningitis	3 (6)	3 (100)
Major System Involvement $^\Psi$		
Musculoskeletal	21 (43)	1 (5)
Organ abscess/deep-seated abscess	13 (27)	1 (8)
Cutaneous	13 (27)	0 (0)
Pulmonary	10 (20)	2 (20)
Genitourinary	9 (18)	3 (33)
Bacteraemia without focus	4 (8)	4 (100)
Neurological	3 (6)	3 (100)
Total		14 (27)

$^\Psi$ Includes multisystem involvement.

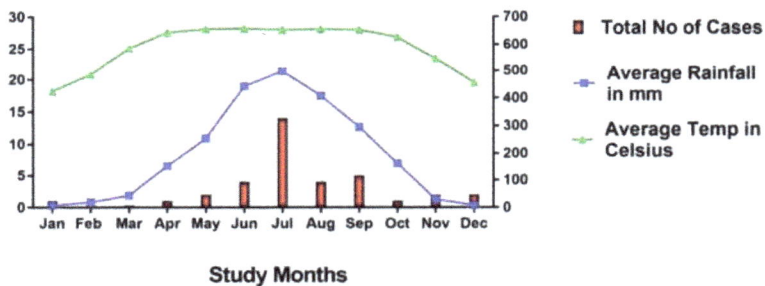

Figure 2. The monthly cases of culture-confirmed melioidosis, the average rainfall in mm, and the average temperature in degrees Celsius. Data represented from 1961 to 2015 [32].

In terms of treatment, 46.3% (19/41) patients were treated with ceftazidime and 41.4% (17/41) received meropenem. Among the cases diagnosed overseas and before 1999, four (9.7%) received cotrimoxazole plus chloramphenicol, and one patient (2.4%) received doxycycline plus amoxicillin/clavulanic acid as intensive phase therapy in this series.

3. Current Recommendations and Availability of Measures against Melioidosis

3.1. Surveillance Systems and Reporting

3.1.1. Human

Melioidosis is not a statutorily notifiable disease in Bangladesh, and there is no formal surveillance system in place for human melioidosis. Reported cases therefore tend to arise from individual researchers who have a specific interest. At present, the health directorate (Ministry of Health and Family Welfare, Bangladesh) has no specific program or operational plan on melioidosis in Bangladesh.

3.1.2. Animal

The infrastructure and facilities for veterinary services and research in Bangladesh are very weak. There is no surveillance system for animal melioidosis currently in place. No veterinary reports have ever been issued from Bangladesh.

3.2. Guidelines

Currently, Bangladesh does not have any national management or treatment guideline for melioidosis. The majority of indigenous cases were diagnosed and treated at BIRDEM General Hospital. The Microbiology Department of BIRDEM hospital follows the Clinical and Laboratory Standard Institute (CLSI) guidelines wherever possible. BIRDEM doctors follow current published treatment guidelines [46].

3.3. Treatment

The antimicrobial susceptibility pattern of clinical isolates showed 100% sensitivity to ceftazidime, imipenem, piperacillin–tazobactam, amoxicillin–clavulanic acid, and tetracycline by both disk diffusion and MIC methods in Bangladesh [47]. Intravenous antibiotics (ceftazidime and meropenem/imipenem) for the acute phase and oral antibiotics for the eradication phase are available in the local market (district and divisional level). Patients usually need to purchase their own drugs for the first two to three days of treatment, and thereafter, they are supplied by the hospital free of cost. It takes some time to order the drug, gain approval from the relevant authority, and obtain a supply from the hospital pharmacy. It is worth mentioning that a free supply of these drugs is only possible in tertiary level hospitals (medical college hospitals), and not in primary (subdistrict) or secondary (district) hospitals. In private clinics, patients need to bear the whole treatment cost. In a developing country such as Bangladesh, it is difficult for many to bear the treatment cost of melioidosis. There is also a dearth of intensive care unit (ICU) beds in tertiary level hospitals in Bangladesh. The moderately high mortality is probably due to late diagnoses, a delayed door-to-needle time for the delivery of appropriate antibiotics, and a lack of ICU care.

4. Awareness of Melioidosis

Awareness of melioidosis among clinicians, microbiologists, and health policymakers is inadequate. Although several case reports have been published in local and international journals, the probability of clinicians considering melioidosis as a diagnosis and requesting the laboratory to look specifically for the bacterium remains low. Public awareness of this organism, particularly among farmers and other high-risk populations, is very low. Recently, the Bangladesh Association for Advancement of Tropical Medicine (BAATM) and the Bangladesh Society of Medicine (BSM) took some special initiatives to raise awareness among clinicians by organising seminars and lectures. David A. B. Dance and Susanna J. Dunachie recently visited Bangladesh on their invitations and conducted seminars in Dhaka. The third South Asian Melioidosis Congress is planned to take place in Bangladesh in 2019, which will further contribute to raising awareness.

5. Major Achievements

So far, the scientists of Ibrahim Medical College and BIRDEM have conducted research on melioidosis in Bangladesh despite the relatively low numbers of cases reported. Doctors at BIRDEM have diagnosed the majority of cases so far in Bangladesh. However, apart from IMC and BIRDEM, microbiologists elsewhere in Bangladesh are unfortunately not currently diagnosing melioidosis. Therefore, we plan to organise capacity development workshops with the support of Mahidol Oxford Research Unit (MORU) and LaoOxford-Mahosot Hospital–Wellcome Trust Research Unit (LOMWRU) for the microbiologists and the clinicians working at tertiary level hospitals in Bangladesh, though funding is currently pending. We also recently completed a prospective study to see if melioidosis is a significant cause of febrile illness in Bangladesh at DMC and BIRDEM in collaboration with the University of Oxford, which will form the basis for a long-term study of melioidosis in Bangladesh.

6. Current and Future Challenges

The major challenges to the diagnosis and the treatment of melioidosis in Bangladesh are a lack of resources and a lack of awareness. Clinicians do not think about this disease in the first instance, and subsequently, microbiologists are not alerted to look specifically for the bacterium. In addition, microbiologists unfamiliar with *B. pseudomallei* are likely to discard the bacterium as a clinically insignificant environmental *Pseudomonas* species. Microbiologists other than those at the BIRDEM laboratory probably do not have the skills, training, and capacity to identify the organism. Therefore, diagnostic capacity development is the key area where immediate attention and funding is required. Awareness-building programs among clinicians are also necessary. Diabetes was found to be the most common risk factor for melioidosis in this series, and this was a similar observation elsewhere. The incidence of diabetes is rapidly increasing in Bangladesh, with 8.4 million people currently living with diabetes [48]. Therefore, we predict that melioidosis could become an enormous clinical challenge in Bangladesh. CKD, hypertension, and smoking were also identified as comorbidities in this series, which are also quite prevalent among Bangladeshi populations. Melioidosis infects both animals and humans. Surveillance among animal populations in the hotspot areas is also required to measure the burden. A One Health approach is needed for the successful mitigation and control of the problem.

Acknowledgments: F.R.C. acknowledge the scholarship (BDCS 2015-44) provided by the Commonwealth Scholarship and Fellowship Plan (CSFP) to undertake PhD at the University of Oxford. S.J.D. is grateful for the support of a Wellcome Trust Intermediate Clinical Fellowship award ref WT100174/Z/12/Z. We especially thank Prapass Wannapinij, senior programmer of MORU, Thailand for preparing the choropleth map for us. We also thank our research assistant Bikash Chandra Das and laboratory assistant Rokibul Hasan for their help during data collection in the prospective cases. We are also grateful to the doctors, technicians, and staff of the Medicine Department, Dhaka Medical College Hospital and Microbiology Department of BIRDEM General Hospital for their support. Finally, we also thank the said hospital administrations for their cooperation.

Author Contributions: F.R.C., S.A.J., S.J.D. and D.A.B.D. conceptualised the study. F.R.C. wrote the first draft of the paper. L.B., T.R., M.R.S., R.A. and K.F. helped to collect and accumulate all the data. F.R.C. and S.J.D. did the statistical analysis. K.M.S.I., M.A.F., S.J.D. and D.A.B.D. revised and edited the primary draft. All authors had a role in reviewing and editing the final version of the report.

Conflicts of Interest: The authors declare no conflict of interest. The funding sponsors had no role in the design of the study; in the collection, analyses, or interpretation of data; in the writing of the manuscript, and in the decision to publish the results.

References

1. Currie, B.J.; Kaestli, M. Epidemiology: A global picture of melioidosis. *Nature* **2016**, *529*, 290–291. [CrossRef] [PubMed]
2. Dance, D.A. Melioidosis as an emerging global problem. *Acta Trop.* **2000**, *74*, 115–119. [CrossRef]
3. Limmathurotsakul, D.; Golding, N.; Dance, D.A.; Messina, J.P.; Pigott, D.M.; Moyes, C.L.; Rolim, D.B.; Bertherat, E.; Day, N.P.; Peacock, S.J.; et al. Predicted global distribution of *Burkholderia pseudomallei* and burden of melioidosis. *Nat. Microbiol.* **2016**, *1*, 15008. [CrossRef] [PubMed]
4. Dance, D.A. Melioidosis. *Curr. Opin. Infect. Dis.* **2002**, *15*, 127–132. [CrossRef] [PubMed]
5. Maegraith, B.G.; Leithead, C.S. Melioidosis: A case-report. *Lancet* **1964**, *1*, 862–863. [CrossRef]
6. Al Shati, M.H.; Joshi, R.M. A 42-year-old farmer from Bangladesh with respiratory failure, septic arthritis, and multiple cavitating consolidations. *Chest* **2014**, *146*, e56–e59. [CrossRef] [PubMed]
7. Christini, A.; King, E. Neck mass in a returning traveler. *JAMA* **2012**, *308*, 2142–2143. [CrossRef] [PubMed]
8. Ezzedine, K.; Heenen, M.; Malvy, D. Imported cutaneous melioidosis in traveler, Belgium. *Emerg. Infect. Dis.* **2007**, *13*, 946–947. [CrossRef] [PubMed]
9. Ezzedine, K.; Malvy, D.; Steels, E.; De Dobbeleer, G.; Struelens, M.; Jacobs, F.; Heenen, M. Imported melioidosis with an isolated cutaneous presentation in a 90-year-old traveller from Bangladesh. *Bull. Soc. Pathol. Exot.* **2007**, *100*, 22–25. [PubMed]

10. Hoque, S.N.; Minassian, M.; Clipstone, S.; Lloyd-Owen, S.J.; Sheridan, E.; Lessing, M.P. Melioidosis presenting as septic arthritis in Bengali men in east London. *Rheumatology* **1999**, *38*, 1029–1031. [CrossRef] [PubMed]

11. Jimenez, R.R.; Garcell, H.G.; Arias, A.V.; Garcia, E.G. Melioidosis in a southeast Asian patient. *Rev. Cuba. Med.* **2017**, *56*, 75–80.

12. Karcher, A.M.; Zaman, A.; Brewis, C.; Fahmy, T. Neck lumps: Expect the unexpected. *Lancet* **2000**, *355*, 1070. [CrossRef]

13. Kibbler, C.C.; Roberts, C.M.; Ridgway, G.L.; Spiro, S.G. Melioidosis in a patient from Bangladesh. *Postgrad. Med. J.* **1991**, *67*, 764–766. [CrossRef] [PubMed]

14. Minassian, M.A.; Gage, A.; Price, E.; Sefton, A.M. Imipenem for the treatment of melioidosis. *Int. J. Antimicrob. Agents* **1999**, *12*, 263–265. [CrossRef]

15. Morrison, I.M. Chronic melioidosis. *Proc. Roy. Soc. Med.* **1970**, *63*, 289–290. [PubMed]

16. Stokes, K.J.; McCarthy, S. *Pseudomonas pseudomallei*: Isolation from a chronic sternal abscess. *J. Med. Lab. Technol.* **1969**, *26*, 199–201. [PubMed]

17. Haradhan, M. Food, agriculture and economic situation of Bangladesh. In Proceedings of the 2nd International Conference on Global Sustainable Development (2nd ICGSD-2013), Kasbit, Pakistan, 5–6 October 2013.

18. Direk, L. Global burden of melioidosis was predicted, what we should do next? In Proceedings of the 8th World Melioidosis Congress, Cebu, Philippines, 7–10 August 2016.

19. Adhikary, P.; Selim, S.; Uddin, N.; Biswas, S.; Basher, A.; Mahmoud, H.; Yusuf, M.A.; Ahsan, H.M.N.; Mowla, S.G.M.; Rahman, M.R. Melioidosis mimicking tuberculosis in an endemic zone: A case report. *Bangladesh J. Infect. Dis.* **2015**, *2*, 23–26. [CrossRef]

20. Afroze, S.R.; Barai, L.; Rahim, M.A.; Haque, H.F.; Afroz, F.; Hoque, M.T.; Ahmed, J.U.; Ahmed, A.K.M.S.; Hossain, M.D.; Rahman, M.R.; et al. Socio-demographic, clinical and laboratory characteristics of melioidosis: Four-year experience of managing consecutive 11 cases in a tertiary care hospital of Bangladesh. *BIRDEM Med. J.* **2017**, *7*, 28–37. [CrossRef]

21. Afroze, S.R.; Rahim, M.A.; Barai, L.; Uddin, K.N. Disseminated melioidosis involving skin and joint: A case report. *Ibrahim Med. Coll. J.* **2015**, *9*, 55–57. [CrossRef]

22. Afroze, S.R.; Rahman, M.R.; Barai, L.; Hossain, M.D.; Uddin, K.N. Successful treatment outcome of primary melioidosis pneumonia—a case report from Bangladesh. *BMC Res. Notes* **2016**, *9*, 100. [CrossRef] [PubMed]

23. Barai, L.; Jilani, M.S.A.; Haq, J.A. Melioidosis—Case reports and review of cases recorded among Bangladeshi population from 1988–2014. *Ibrahim Med. Coll. J.* **2014**, *8*, 25–31. [CrossRef]

24. Fatema, K.; Faruq, M.O.; Ahsan, A.S.M.A.; Ahmed, F.; Saha, D.K.; Afroz, F.; Saha, M. Disseminated meliodosis presenting as septic shock: An endemic disease of Bangladesh. *IJCMAAS* **2015**, *5*, 200–202.

25. Fatema, K.; Ahsan, A.S.M.A.; Barai, L.; Saha, D.K.; Afroze, S.R.; Faruq, M.O.; Ahmed, F.; Saha, M. A case of fatal meliodosis presenting as septic arthritis and septicaemia. *Bangladesh Crit. Care J.* **2015**, *3*, 74–76. [CrossRef]

26. Mahbub, S.; Al-Amin, Z.; Biswas, S.S.; Jamal, M.S.; Halder, S. Melioidosis—A rare infectious disease with atypical presentation. *Bangladesh J. Otorhinolaryngol.* **2014**, *20*, 46–49. [CrossRef]

27. Majumder, M.I.; Haque, M.M.; Ahmed, M.W.; Alam, M.N.; Rahman, M.W.; Akter, F.; Basher, A.; Maude, R.J.; Faiz, M.A. Melioidosis in an adult male. *Mymensingh Med. J.* **2013**, *22*, 413–416. [PubMed]

28. Rahim, M.A.; Afroze, S.R.; Barai, L.; Uddin, K.N. Melioidosis: Truly uncommon or uncommonly diagnosed in Bangladesh? A case report. *Birdem Med. J.* **2015**, *5*, 49–51. [CrossRef]

29. Saha, D.K.; Ahsan, A.S.M.A.; Faruq, M.O.F.; Fatema, K.; Ahmed, F.; Saha, M. Hepatic abscess as presenting feature of melioidosis: A case report. *BIRDEM Med. J.* **2016**, *6*, 43–45. [CrossRef]

30. Struelens, M.J.; Mondol, G.; Bennish, M.; Dance, D.A. Melioidosis in Bangladesh: A case report. *Trans. R. Soc. Trop Med. Hyg.* **1988**, *82*, 777–778. [CrossRef]

31. Uddin, K.N.; Hossain, M.; Mansur, A.; Hoque, M.J.A.; Khan, A.R. Melioidosis–A case report. *J. Bangladesh Coll. Phys. Surg.* **2001**, *19*, 71–74.

32. Average Monthly Temperature and Rainfall for Bangladesh from 1901–2015. Available online: http://sdwebx. worldbank.org/climateportal/index.cfm?page=country_historical_climate&ThisCCode=BGD (accessed on 19 January 2018).

33. University of Waterloo. Global administrative areas (Gadm). In *Global Administrative Areas (GADM)*; Geospatial Center, University of Waterloo: Waterloo, ON, Canada, 2017.

34. Chou, D.; Chung, K.; Chen, C.; Cheung, B.M. Bacteremic melioidosis in southern Taiwan: Clinical characteristics and outcome. *J. Formos. Med. Assoc.* **2007**, *106*, 1013–1022. [CrossRef]

35. Currie, B.J.; Ward, L.; Cheng, A.C. The epidemiology and clinical spectrum of melioidosis: 540 cases from the 20 year Darwin prospective study. *PLoS Negl. Trop. Dis.* **2010**, *4*, e900. [CrossRef] [PubMed]

36. Suputtamongkol, Y.; Chaowagul, W.; Chetchotisakd, P.; Lertpatanasuwun, N.; Intaranongpai, S.; Ruchutrakool, T.; Budhsarawong, D.; Mootsikapun, P.; Wuthiekanun, V.; Teerawatasook, N.; et al. Risk factors for melioidosis and bacteremicmelioidosis. *Clin. Infect. Dis.* **1999**, *29*, 408–413. [CrossRef] [PubMed]

37. Vidyalakshmi, K.; Lipika, S.; Vishal, S.; Damodar, S.; Chakrapani, M. Emerging clinico-epidemiological trends in melioidosis: Analysis of 95 cases from western coastal India. *Int. J. Infect. Dis.* **2012**, *16*, 491–497. [CrossRef] [PubMed]

38. Kingsley, P.V.; Leader, M.; Nagodawithana, N.S.; Tipre, M.; Sathiakumar, N. Melioidosis in Malaysia: A review of case reports. *PLoS Negl. Trop. Dis.* **2016**, *10*, e0005182. [CrossRef] [PubMed]

39. Ahsan, G.; Ahmed, J.; Singhasivanon, P.; Kaewkungwal, J.; Okanurak, K.; Suwannapong, N.; Akarasewi, P.; Majid, M.A.; Begum, V.; Belayetali, K. Gender difference in treatment seeking behaviors of tuberculosis cases in rural communities of Bangladesh. *Southeast Asian J. Trop. Med. Public. Health* **2004**, *35*, 126–135. [PubMed]

40. Hossen, M.A.; Westhues, A. Rural women's access to health care in Bangladesh: Swimming against the tide? *Soc. Work Public Health* **2011**, *26*, 278–293. [CrossRef] [PubMed]

41. Maude, R.R.; Maude, R.J.; Ghose, A.; Amin, M.R.; Islam, M.B.; Ali, M.; Bari, M.S.; Majumder, M.I.; Wuthiekanan, V.; Dondorp, A.M.; et al. Sero-epidemiological surveillance of *Burkholderia pseudomallei* in Bangladesh. *Trans. R. Soc. Trop. Med. Hyg.* **2012**, *106*, 576–578. [CrossRef] [PubMed]

42. Jilani, M.S.A.; Robayet, J.A.; Mohiuddin, M.; Hasan, M.R.; Ahsan, C.R.; Haq, J.A. *Burkholderia pseudomallei*: Its detection in soil and seroprevalence in Bangladesh. *PLoS Negl. Trop. Dis.* **2016**, *10*, e0004301. [CrossRef] [PubMed]

43. Statistics, B.B.O. *Yearbook of Agricultural Statistics-2015*; Government of the People's Republic of Bangladesh: Dhaka, Bangladesh, 2015; pp. 1–575.

44. Chowdhury, M.A.I.; Kabir, M.M.; Sayed, A.F.; Hossain, S. Estimation of rainfall patterns in Bangladesh using different computational methods (arithmetic average, thiessen polygon and isohyet). *J. Biodivers. Environ. Sci.* **2016**, *8*, 43–51.

45. Raihan, S. Infrastructure and growth and poverty in Bangladesh. In *Conference on Infrastructure for Inclusive Growth and Poverty Reduction*; Asian Development Bank: Manilla, Philipines, 2012; pp. 1–38.

46. Wiersinga, W.J.; Currie, B.J.; Peacock, S.J. Melioidosis. *New Engl. J. Med.* **2012**, *367*, 1035–1044. [CrossRef] [PubMed]

47. Dutta, S.; Haq, S.; Hasan, M.R.; Haq, J.A. Antimicrobial susceptibility pattern of clinical isolates of *Burkholderia pseudomallei* in Bangladesh. *BMC Res. Notes* **2017**, *10*, 299. [CrossRef] [PubMed]

48. Akter, S.; Rahman, M.M.; Abe, S.K.; Sultana, P. Prevalence of diabetes and prediabetes and their risk factors among Bangladeshi adults: A nationwide survey. *Bull. World Health Organ.* **2014**, *92*, 204–213. [CrossRef] [PubMed]

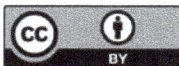

Tropical Medicine and Infectious Disease

MDPI

Review

Melioidosis in Brunei Darussalam

Ketan Pande [1,*] , Khairul Azmi Abd Kadir [1], Rosmonaliza Asli [2] and Vui Heng Chong [2]

1 Department of Orthopaedics, Raja Isteri Pengiran Anak Saleha Hospital, Bandar Seri Begawan BG 1710, Negara Brunei Darussalam; khairulazmiabdkadir@gmail.com
2 Department of Medicine, Raja Isteri Pengiran Anak Saleha Hospital, Bandar Seri Begawan BG 1710, Negara Brunei Darussalam; ROSMONALIZA.ASLI@moh.gov.bn (R.A.); vuiheng.chong@moh.gov.bn (V.H.C.)
* Correspondence: ketanpande@yahoo.com; Tel.: +673-8610747

Received: 30 January 2018; Accepted: 14 February 2018; Published: 19 February 2018

Abstract: Melioidosis continues to be a major health care problem in Brunei Darussalam. The age of patients, gender distribution, risk factors, and clinical presentations are similar to those reported from other countries in the region. The incidence of melioidosis was high during the wet months and in the Temburong district, which has the highest annual rainfall. In spite of adequate facilities for diagnosis and treatment, the mortality remains high (27%). Women and those presenting with septic shock had higher mortality. There is a case for making melioidosis a notifiable disease in Brunei Darussalam. Coordinated efforts between policy-makers and various stakeholders are required to effectively combat the disease.

Keywords: melioidosis; *Burkholderia pseudomallei*; epidemiology; diagnosis; treatment

1. Introduction

Melioidosis is endemic in many countries of Southeast Asia, including Brunei Darussalam and in northern Australia. It is estimated that 40% of all cases occur in the East Asia Pacific region [1].

Brunei Darussalam is a country in Southeast Asia, located in the northeastern part of Borneo island, with geographical coordinates of 4°30′ N 114°40′ E. The country is divided into four districts: Brunei Muara, Tutong, Kuala Belait, and Temburong. The climate in Brunei Darussalam is tropical equatorial and humid subtropical at higher altitudes with heavy rainfall [2]. The annual average rainfall is more than 2300 mm for the whole of Brunei Darussalam and increases inland, with altitude, to more than 4000 mm with maximum rainfall in the Temburong district [3]. The mean monthly rainfall follows seasonal patterns with two maxima and two minima. The first maximum is from October to January, with December being the wettest month, while the second minor maximum is from May to July, with May being relatively wetter [4].

In line with the aims of this special issue on melioidosis, this article addresses various aspects of the disease in Brunei Darussalam. It is divided into the following parts: (i) a review of available literature on melioidosis from Brunei Darussalam; (ii) the current approaches to diagnosis, management, and prevention; (iii) epidemiological study of melioidosis with data obtained from 2015–2016; (iv) melioidosis in animals; and (v) future challenges.

2. Review of Literature from Brunei Darussalam

The first published report on melioidosis (24 cases) in Brunei Darussalam was by Luqman et al. [5]. It was more prevalent in the agricultural districts and in the period (1993, 1994) the rate increased from 2.9 to 5.6/100,000. The majority (79.2%) had risk factors, mostly diabetes mellitus. Septicaemia was the presenting feature in 75% of cases, with 62.6% having multi-organ involvement. The mortality rate was 20.8% and on follow-up, 60% of patients presented with relapse of the disease.

The many and varied radiological manifestations of melioidosis in Brunei Darussalam were reviewed by Lim and Chong [6]. Multiple organ involvement, especially the lungs, liver, and spleen, were common. The 'honeycomb' appearance of abscesses, especially large abscesses and those seen in the liver, was characteristic of melioidosis.

Chong et al. reported the characteristics of pancreatic melioidosis (4/65 cases who had undergone CT imaging, median age 29.5 years (range 25–48 years)). Pancreatic involvement ranged from multi-focal micro-abscesses to focal large abscesses, and associated findings included splenic vein thrombosis, peri-pancreatic inflammation, and peri-pancreatic fat streaking. Pancreatic involvement was typically part of multi-organ involvement [7].

Pande and Hj Abdul Kadir reported their experience with melioidosis affecting the extremities ($n = 14/48$ (29.1%); median age 45 years (range 14–55)). The majority ($n = 13$, 92.8%) were men, with 35.7% ($n = 5$) being expatriates working as labourers. Septic arthritis was the most common presentation ($n = 5$), followed by cellulitis, abscess, and osteomyelitis ($n = 3$ each) [8].

The antibiograms of *Burkholderia pseudomallei* from Brunei Darussalam over a period of ten years (679 isolates from 623 patients) showed that carbapenems, third-generation cephalosporins (ceftazidime), piperacillin, and chloramphenicol had the highest susceptibility rates of between 98% and 100%. Amoxicillin-clavulanic acid had a moderate susceptibility rate (76–100%) and quinolones (ciprofloxacin, 32–68%) and co-trimoxazole (6–54%) had the lowest susceptibility rates. It is, however, recognized that the disk diffusion method overestimates the resistance rate for co-trimoxazole [9]. The gentamicin susceptibility of the isolates was not reported.

A case of right frontal lobe brain abscess due to co-infection with *B. pseudomallei* and *Cryptococcus neoformans* in a patient with underlying systemic lupus erythematosus was reported by Samad et al. [10]. The patient was non-diabetic but was on steroid therapy and the diagnosis was confirmed only after surgical drainage.

Chong et al. reported their experience with urogenital melioidosis ($n = 13$, nine new cases, four relapses; median age 38 (range 29–63 years)). The kidneys were involved in 72.3% followed by the prostate (60%). Testicular and seminal vesicle involvement was noted in one case each. There was no involvement of the gynaecological system [11].

In the clinical case series mentioned above, a male preponderance was noted, with diabetes mellitus being the most common risk factor [7,8,11].

3. Current Approach to Diagnosis, Management, and Prevention

3.1. Microbiological Diagnosis

In Brunei Darussalam, the diagnosis of melioidosis is confirmed by the isolation of *B. pseudomallei* from clinical specimens, such as blood, sputum, abscess aspirates, pericardial fluid, skin lesions, or other clinical specimens. The clinical specimens are collected during the initial admission to the hospital. Positive blood culture bottles are subcultured onto blood agar and MacConkey agar; urine specimens are inoculated onto cystine lactose electrolyte-deficient (CLED) agar; respiratory specimens, onto blood agar, MacConkey agar, and chocolate agar; and pus specimens into cooked meat broth. These are incubated at 37 °C for at least 24 h before being examined. For pus specimens, subsequent subcultures are made from the broth onto blood agar and MacConkey agar and reincubated at 37 °C for at least another 24 h before re-examination. Selective agars, such as those studied by Peacock et al. [12], are not used in Brunei Darussalam, which means that in some cases growth of *B. pseudomallei* may be missed. In a patient with high clinical suspicion of melioidosis, but with negative cultures, reactivity in a *B. pseudomallei* serological test (sent abroad) is taken as a strong evidence of the disease.

The cultures are then examined for colony morphology and Gram-staining. Morphologically, *B. pseudomallei is* identified as large, wrinkled colonies that have a metallic appearance with an earthy odour. On Gram staining, the organism appears as Gram-negative bacilli with bipolar staining, which gives a characteristic 'safety pin' appearance. The cultured colonies are further identified using the

VITEK system, a commercial bacterial identification system. However, it is noted that with the use of the VITEK system there is potential for misidentification of *B. pseudomallei* as *Burkholderia cepacia*, which is regionally dependent [13]. This is of particular significance as the study reporting this was from Malaysian Borneo, on the same island as Brunei Darussalam.

All of the isolated organisms are tested for antibiotic susceptibility using Etest and, at present, the results of susceptibility testing are not validated by an external reference laboratory.

3.2. Management

Patients who are clinically suspected to have melioidosis, particularly those with a background history of uncontrolled diabetes mellitus, are empirically treated with an antibiotic that has activity against *B. pseudomallei*, i.e., either with intravenous (IV) ceftazidime (up to 2 g every 8 h) or, for clinically-severe cases, with IV imipenem (up to 1 g every 8 h) or IV meropenem (up to 1 g every 8 h) while waiting for culture results to become available.

In patients with confirmed *B. pseudomallei* bacteraemia, and in those patients who were empirically treated with either IV imipenem or meropenem and who have been stable for 48 h, the IV antibiotic is de-escalated to IV ceftazidime. Further investigations, like chest radiographs, ultrasound of the abdomen and pelvis, or computed tomography (CT) scan of the thorax, abdomen, and pelvis (CT-TAP), are usually performed to exclude deep-seated infection with organ abscesses that may be drainable.

The antibiotic treatment for melioidosis comprises two phases, i.e., the intensive phase and the eradication phase. In the intensive phase, IV antimicrobial therapy with either IV ceftazidime or IV meropenem or imipenem is recommended for at least 10–14 days for pulmonary disease or if there are no other obvious deep-seated sources. The intensive phase may be extended to at least 4–6 weeks with drainage of deep-seated abscesses. The patient is then continued on to the eradication phase with oral co-trimoxazole (5 mg/kg of the trimethoprim component every 12 h) as the first line antimicrobial therapy for at least 12 weeks in total. If co-trimoxazole is contraindicated or the patient develops adverse reactions to the medication, then the second-line treatment would be with oral co-amoxiclav (625 mg every 8 h) and oral doxycycline (2 mg/kg every 12 h) to complete a total minimum of 12 weeks. However, clinicians need to be aware of the risk of treatment failure with this second-line eradication phase regimen [14,15]. Currently no post-exposure prophylaxis is offered in Brunei Darussalam.

3.3. Preventive Measures

Patients who are admitted with suspected or confirmed pulmonary melioidosis are nursed in droplet isolation for at least 24 h after appropriate antibiotics are commenced.

In the laboratory setting, biosafety level 3 practices are adopted while handling and processing specimens [16].

4. Epidemiological Study of Melioidosis with Data Obtained from 2015–2016

4.1. Material and Methods

All culture-positive cases of melioidosis recorded between January 2015 and December 2016 were retrieved from the electronic database of the Clinical Microbiology Laboratory, Department of Laboratory Services, RIPAS Hospital. All patients were investigated and managed as per the protocol mentioned in the previous section.

Demographic, clinical and diagnostic information (laboratory and imaging) was collected through the Hospital Information Management System (BruHIMS). The study was approved by the Medical and Health Research and Ethics Committee (MHREC).

Data are presented as descriptive statistics. Wherever possible, differences between groups were analysed using the chi-square test. A *p*-value of <0.05 was considered significant.

4.2. Results

4.2.1. Demographics

A total of 115 cases were detected in 2015 (*n* = 46) and 2016 (*n* = 69). There were 84 (73%) male and 31 (27%) female patients with an age range from 2 to 86 years (median 48 years).

There were four (3.5%) patients under the age of 15 years, all with no risk factors, who presented with abscesses in soft tissue (*n* = 3) and neck (*n* = 1). They were admitted in the months of January, April, August, and December.

Excluding a two-year-old expatriate patient, the median age of expatriate patients was 41.5 years (*n* = 25). The age range for Bruneian patients (*n* = 89) was 14 to 86 years with a median age of 52 years.

The ethnic distribution of the cases is given in Table 1.

Table 1. Ethnic distribution of cases of melioidosis.

Country	No.	%
Malay	88	76.5
Chinese: Bruneian	1	0.9
Expatriates	26	22.6
Bangladesh	10	8.7
Indonesia	8	7
India	4	3.5
Philippines	1	0.9
Thailand	1	0.9
Nepal	1	0.9
Malaysia	1	0.9

During 2015–2016, the ethnic distribution of the population of Brunei Darussalam was Malay (65.7%), Chinese (10.3%), and expatriates (23.9%) [17].

The overall incidence rates per 100,000 population in 2015 and 2016 were 11 and 16.3, respectively.

The number of cases and incidence rate per 100,000 population from each of the four districts is presented in Table 2.

Table 2. District-wise incidence of melioidosis/100,000 population for 2015–2016.

District	Pop. 2015	Cases	Inc/100,000	Pop. 2016	Cases	Inc/100,000
Muara	288,400	33	11.44	292,705	51	17.42
Tutong	48,700	9	18.48	49,438	8	16.18
Kuala Belait	69,000	2	2.89	69,992	6	8.57
Temburong	10,400	2	19.23	10,543	4	37.93

Population figures obtained from http://www.depd.gov.bn/sitePages/Population.aspx [17].

The incidence was highest in the Temburong district in both years (Figure 1). Except in the Tutong district, there was an increase in incidence for the remaining districts from 2015 to 2016.

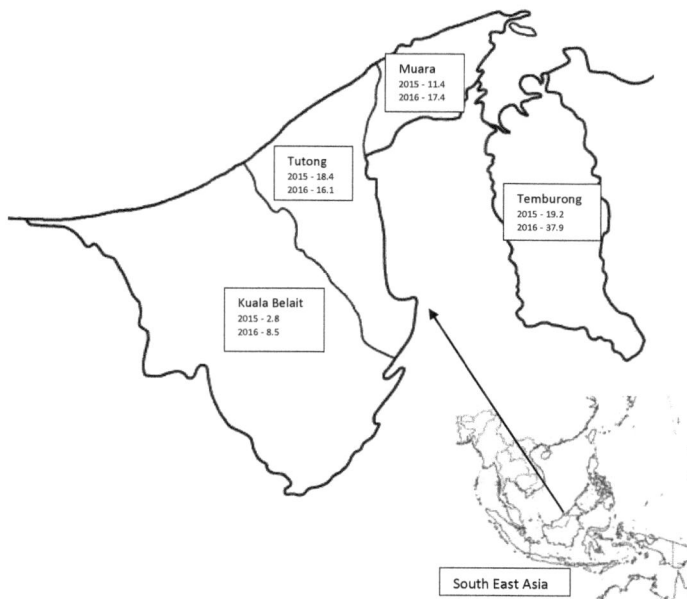

Figure 1. Map showing incidence/100,000 population for 2015 and 2016 by district, Brunei Darussalam.

4.2.2. Month-Wise Number of New Cases

The number of cases (2015 and 2016 combined) according to the month of admission is presented in Figure 2.

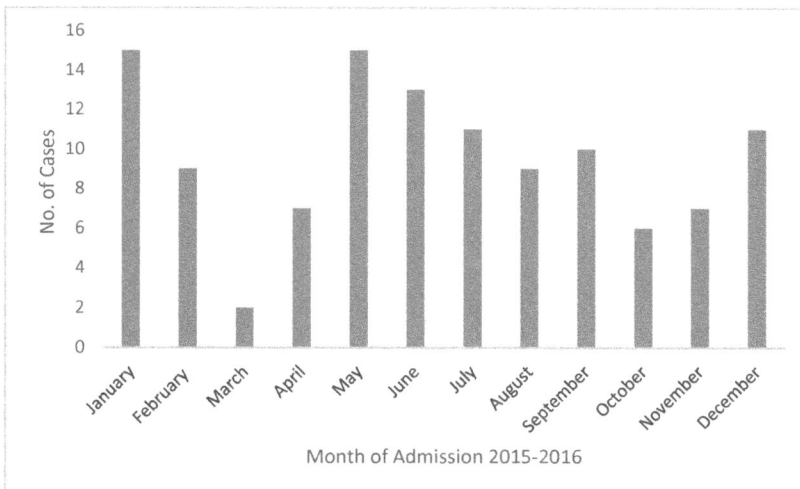

Figure 2. Meliodosis cases by month (2015–2016).

The maximum number of admissions were recorded in the months of January and May with smaller peaks in June, July, and December.

4.2.3. Risk Factors

A number of risk factors were identified and are presented in Table 3.

Table 3. Risk Factors for melioidosis.

Risk Factor	Cases	%
Diabetes mellitus	86	74.8
Chronic renal disease	23	20
Cardiac disease	17	14.8
Lung diseases (COPD/TB)	16	13.9
Excessive alcohol intake	6	5.2
Thalassemia	5	4.3
Malignancy	2	1.7
None	9	7.8

Note: Most of the chronic renal disease patients were those with end-stage renal failure on dialysis and thalassemia patients who were transfusion-dependent and had iron overload.

Diabetes mellitus was the most common risk factor, recorded in 74.8% of cases. More than one risk factor was present in 37.4% of cases, and there was no obvious risk factor seen in 7.8% ($n = 9$).

4.2.4. Clinical Presentations and Diagnosis

Various clinical presentations were recorded (Table 4), pneumonia being the most common (47%). In seven cases (6%) no focus of infection could be found.

Table 4. Clinical presentation of melioidosis.

Presentation	Cases	%
Septic shock	25	21.7
Pneumonia	54	47
Soft tissue abscess	21	18.3
Musculo-skeletal	10	8.7
Neurological	1	0.9
No evidence of primary focus	7	6

Thirteen of 25 cases of septic shock had pneumonia as the primary source of infection, including in the 54 cases of pneumonia.

Internal organ abscesses were most commonly noted in spleen and liver (Table 5).

Table 5. Internal organ abscess in melioidosis.

Organ	Cases	%
Spleen	27	23.5
Liver	20	17.4
Prostate	5	6
Lymph node	4	3.5
Kidney	2	1.7
Parotid	1	0.9
Brain	1	0.9

In most cases (67%), the diagnosis was confirmed by blood culture (Table 6).

Table 6. Source of culture for diagnosis of melioidosis.

Modality	No. of Isolates	%
Blood culture	77	67
Fluid culture	11	9.6
Pus culture	37	32.2

CT-TAP was performed in 50.5% (n = 58) of cases. The reasons for a patient not undergoing CT-TAP were septic shock and serious illness, presentation as cellulitis or soft tissue abscess, and issues with payment for expatriate workers.

4.2.5. Outcome of Treatment

In the years 2015 and 2016, there was an overall mortality of 27% (Table 7). Mortality in patients presenting with septic shock was 64%. The mortality in women was 41.9% (13/31) compared to 21.4% (18/84) in men (p < 0.005).

Table 7. Outcome of treatment of cases.

Outcome	Cases	%
Recovery	79	68.7
Death	31	27
Relapse	5	4.3

Of the five cases with relapse, one patient died during readmission with septic shock (not included in the 31 fatalities).

In 2015, 11 patients (23.9%) were admitted with septic shock and the mortality was 26.1% (n = 12) compared to 14 patients (20%) and 27.5% (n = 19), respectively, in 2016. Five of the nine patients without any risk factors succumbed to the disease.

4.3. Discussion

This is the first detailed epidemiological study of melioidosis from Brunei Darussalam. The data have revealed a slight increase in incidence from 11 to 16 per 100,000 population between 2015 and 2016. It also showed a high number of expatriate workers being affected. Diabetes mellitus and chronic renal disease were the most common risk factors, whilst pneumonia and soft tissue abscess were the most common clinical presentations. The data suggested a possible link with seasonal variation in rainfall with more cases diagnosed in the wet months. Interestingly the highest incidence rate was from the Temburong district, which has the highest annual rainfall. The mortality was 27%, being higher in women and patients presenting with septic shock.

For the purpose of discussion, we have compared our results with other large epidemiological studies from Asia-Pacific published after 2010 [18–25]. Our findings of male preponderance, the median age of patients, diabetes mellitus and chronic renal disease as the most common risk factors, and pneumonia and soft tissue abscesses as the most common presentations, are similar to the studies reviewed.

Though occupational history was not consistently recorded in the hospital notes, similar to a previous study [8], 25 expatriate patients with varied nationalities (median age 41.5 years) were noted. Generally the majority of these were labourers working in the agriculture or construction industries, with a high chance of exposure to contaminated soil and water.

The overall incidences of 11 and 16.3 per 100,000 population in 2015 and 2016, respectively, are considerably higher than those reported from Thailand and Singapore [22,25]. It is important to note that, in Singapore, a recent decrease in incidence was reported [25], while the incidence has remained constant or increased in Australia and Thailand [18,22]. Our rates are comparable to the rate of 16.45/100,000 reported from the state of Kedah, Malaysia by Hassan et al. [21]. In contrast, another study based on the melioidosis registry from the Pahang state of Malaysia reported a much lower rate of 4.3/100,000 (adult 6.0/100,000 and paediatric 1.6/100,000) [26]. This reflects geographical differences, as seen in our study, with different rates between districts, even for a small country.

The current rates reported showed marked increase compared to the incidence rates (2.9 to 5.6/100,000 for 1993 and 1994, respectively) reported by Luqman et al. [5]. The upsurge may well be contributed to by better awareness and improvement in diagnostic facilities. Melioidosis was possibly under-diagnosed and under-reported in the past [27]. Another plausible reason for the upward trend is the rise in the overall population along with an increase in the number of people with risk factors, such as diabetes and chronic kidney disease.

There were four patients (3.5%) under the age of 15 years, comparable to the rate reported by Hassan et al., (5.5%), and higher than the rate reported by How et al., (1.6/100,000) [21,26]. Consistent with reports in the literature, our paediatric patients had no risk factors, presented with soft tissue abscesses, two of them during the wet months of December and January, and recovered completely with treatment [28]. Unlike Kingsley et al., we did not observe any cases of neonatal melioidosis [29].

In the present study, a higher number of cases was observed in the wet months of May to July and December to February, with 64.3% being admitted during these months. The incidence was also higher in the Temburong district, which records the highest rainfall amongst the four districts. A high level of moisture in the soil during months of high rainfall has been reported to correlate with an increased incidence of melioidosis [30,31]. This association has been reported from Australia [18,20], Singapore [25], Malaysia [21], and India [23]. In contrast, Limmathurotsakul et al. reported a negative association between the total annual rainfall and the number of cases in each year of their study from Thailand [22]. However, in this study monthly rainfall data and the number of cases per month were not available. Consistent with an incubation period of a few weeks, the incidence may also be higher in the corresponding period after high rainfall [32].

Diabetes mellitus was recorded as a risk factor in 74.8% of cases, similar to the proportion in India [23] and Malaysia [24]. Other studies have reported it in 39–57% of their cases [18,20–22,25]. In two studies from Australia [18,20], excessive alcohol use was the second most common risk factor. In the present study it was noted in 5.2% of cases but could be underreported due to a reluctance to volunteer such a history. However, the sale of alcohol is banned in Brunei Darussalam and, therefore, our finding is likely to be a true reflection of the real situation.

The number of patients with melioidosis without any risk factors was lower (7.8%, *n* = 9) in the present study compared to other studies (13–22%) [18,20,23,24] but similar to that reported by Kingsley et al. [29]. It has been suggested that individuals with no risk factors have less severe symptoms and mortality is rare [29]. However, in the present study 5/9 patients succumbed to the disease, three of whom presented with septic shock, and two with large soft tissue abscesses suggesting fulminant infection.

Consistent with the studies reviewed, pneumonia was the most common clinical presentation followed by soft tissue abscesses [18,20–25]. Septic shock was the mode of presentation in 21.7% (*n* = 25) cases. In a review of case reports published from Malaysia, a high frequency of primary neurological presentation was noted (7.5%) [29]. The rates reported by other authors [18,21,23,24] and one case in the present study is much lower. This may be due to selection bias in the case reports reviewed.

Internal organ abscesses were most common in the spleen and liver, as noted in the literature [18,21,23,24]; however, the proportion was much higher in the present study. We had only one case of subdural empyema and no cases with mycotic aneurysms or pericardial involvement. The proportion of prostatic abscesses in the present study was 4.3%; there is a wide variation reported in the literature, from 0.3% in Thailand [33], to a high of 20% in Australia [18]. Our finding of the frequency of parotid involvement (*n* = 1, 0.9%) is comparable to other studies [23,24,29], but much lower than that reported in Thai children (20–30%) [34]. We did not find any case with pancreatic involvement in the present study. The four cases previously reported were seen over a period of six years, compared to two years of the present study [7]. Moreover, only about 50% of patients in the present study underwent CT-TAP for various reasons, which could have resulted in under-reporting of internal organ abscesses.

The overall mortality in the present study was 27%, with a higher mortality in women (41.9%) compared to men (21.4%; $p < 0.05$). This association has also been reported by Kingsley et al. [29]. Mortality was also significantly higher in patients who presented with septic shock.

There is a wide variation in the reported mortality in the literature, from 9.5% in India [23], 42.6% in Thailand [22], and between 32–63% in Malaysia [19,21,24]. Decreasing mortality rates have been reported from Australia [18] and Singapore [25]. The reasons put forward for this are access to standardized health care and the institution of prompt treatment according to recommendations [35]. In Singapore, in particular, it is thought to be due to efforts to optimise diabetes care and enhanced environmental and water management [25]. Our current rate is slightly higher than that reported in the earlier study by Luqman et al., (20.3%) [5], possibly due to late presentations and multiple comorbidities.

Five cases (4.3%) had recurrence of the disease, which is a similar rate to that reported by Currie et al. [18]. One of the 31 cases that did not survive also presented with a recurrence. They had underlying risk factors of diabetes mellitus (4/6), malignancy (2/6), and chronic renal disease (1/6). Non-compliance with previous treatment was recorded in two cases. The institution of prompt treatment along international guidelines explains the lower current rate compared to relapses seen in 60% of cases in the past [5].

The strength of the present study is that, owing to the method of data collection, it can be taken as a true reflection of the disease state in the country. A limitation of the study was its retrospective nature. Data, particularly on occupation and alcohol abuse as risk factors, were not adequately recorded.

5. Melioidosis in Animals

All livestock farms in Brunei Darussalam are advised through the Department of Agriculture and Agrifood about good animal husbandry practices as a method of prevention of diseases.

According to the Animal Health and Disease Control Unit under the Livestock and Veterinary Services Division, 93 and 128 goats were treated for presumed melioidosis in 2015 and 2016, respectively. This was based on farmers' complaints and clinical findings, but no bacteriological evidence was obtained. A positive response to treatment was noted in 80% of cases. The high susceptibility of goats to melioidosis has been reported in the literature [36,37].

It has been suggested that goats and humans are exposed to similar levels of *B. pseudomallei* in the environment and, hence, the incidence is likely to be similar [37]. However, data on melioidosis incidence in animals are not available in Brunei Darussalam to confirm this.

In Brunei Darussalam, the goat farms are mostly small, with herds less than 500 head. The goat houses use raised flooring and practice 'cut and carry' grass for feeding to avoid direct contact of animals with the soil. Cattle livestock are imported from Australia, and Sabah and Sarawak in Malaysia, and kept in holding yards for seasonal sales and are then slaughtered shortly afterwards (short-term rearing), so that goats make up the longest-standing ruminant population. Buffaloes are less susceptible to melioidosis, as noted in a review [38].

In late 2016, a few goat and sheep carcasses were submitted for autopsy with lesions suspicious of melioidosis. The farm had recently carried out excavation work, followed by heavy rain. The animals were 2–6 months of age and, hence, thought to be immunocompromised. The bacteriological tests were negative for *B. pseudomallei*. The sick animals from the farm were treated and water was disinfected as a precautionary measure. Workers in the farm and fodder plantation with respiratory symptoms were advised to attend the nearest health centre.

6. Future Direction

It is clear from the Health Information Booklet 2016, published by the Ministry of Health, Brunei Darussalam, that diabetes, pneumonia, and septicaemia are amongst the top 10 causes of death in the country [39]. The number of cases of melioidosis in 2016 (n = 69) was listed after the number of cases of gastroenteritis and food poisoning in the list of waterborne diseases. However, melioidosis does not feature in the list of notifiable diseases in Brunei Darussalam, unlike in Australia [20] and Singapore [25].

Evidence-based guidelines are now available for prevention of melioidosis in endemic areas [40]. Suntornsut et al. explored the barriers in implementing preventive measures for melioidosis and have suggested a number of interventions. Based on these, the authors have recommended a multifaceted intervention involving community and government agencies [41].

Kingsley et al. have stressed the importance of making melioidosis notifiable and starting registries in endemic countries to improve the efforts to effectively control the disease [29]. Through such registries, it will be possible to obtain reliable clinical and epidemiological information, note trends in the incidence, and determine effective treatment and mortality.

Involvement of the various stakeholders that encounter melioidosis in their practice and the formation of a national registry would help to ensure that data collected is complete and standardized. This will allow comparisons and the analysis of trends. Thus, the formation of a regional or international registry would allow the condition to be better studied. If Brunei Darussalam were to follow Australia and Singapore in making the condition a notifiable disease, this would further enhance awareness and this may have an impact on the clinical course of the disease in the future.

Acknowledgments: We are grateful to Diana Dennis and Raihan Zurhairah Bte Hj Zulkipli, Division of Livestock and Veterinary Services, Department of Agriculture and Agrifood, for their input on melioidosis in animals in Brunei Darussalam. We are also grateful to Woo Boon Chu, Clinical Microbiology Laboratory, Department of Laboratory Services, for help with retrieving a list of cases of melioidosis.

Author Contributions: K.P. conducted the data collection and analysis, and the writing and revision of the manuscript; K.A.A.K. conducted the data collection and revision of the manuscript; R.A. wrote and revised the manuscript; and V.H.C. wrote and revised the manuscript.

Conflicts of Interest: The authors declare no conflict of interest.

References

1. Limmathurotsakul, D.; Golding, N.; Dance, D.A.B.; Messina, J.P.; Pigott, D.M.; Moyes, C.L.; Rolim, D.B.; Bertherat, E.; Day, N.P.J.; Peacock, S.J.; et al. Predicted global distribution of *Burkholderia pseudomallei* and burden of melioidosis. *Nat. Microbiol.* **2016**, *1*. [CrossRef] [PubMed]

2. Geography of Brunei. Available online: https://en.wikipedia.org/wiki/Geography_of_Brunei (accessed on 3 January 2018).

3. Rainfall. Available online: https://www.bsp.com.bn/panagaclub/pnhs_old/geology/HTM/OVERVIEW/CLIMATE/RAIN/rain1_1.HTM (accessed on 3 January 2018).

4. Climate. Available online: http://bruneiweather.com.bn/climate (accessed on 3 January 2018).

5. Luqman, N.; On, S.C.; Satyawany, N.; Da, P. Melioidosis in Brunei—epidemiological and clinical profile. *Brunei Int. Med. J.* **1999**, *1*, 291–297.

6. Lim, K.S.; Chong, V.H. Radiological manifestations of melioidosis. *Clin. Radiol.* **2010**, *65*, 66–72. [CrossRef] [PubMed]

7. Chong, V.H.; Lim, K.S.; Sharif, F. Pancreatic Involvement in melioidosis. *JOP* **2010**, *11*, 365–368. [PubMed]

8. Pande, K.C.; Hj Abdul Kadir, K.A. Melioidosis of the extremities in Brunei Darussalam. *Singap. Med. J.* **2011**, *52*, 346–350.

9. Khairul Azmi, A.K.; Sattayavani, M.; Pande, K. Melioidosis: Antibiogram of cases in Brunei Darussalam. *Brunei Int. Med. J.* **2014**, *10*, 19–24.

10. Samad, I.; Wang, M.C.; Chong, V.H. Intracerebral coinfection with *Burkholderia pseudomallei* and *Cryptococcus neoformans* in a patient with systemic lupus erythematosus. *Southeast Asian J. Trop. Med. Public Health* **2014**, *45*, 352–356. [PubMed]

11. Chong, V.H.; Sharif, F.; Bickle, I. Urogenital melioidosis: A review of clinical presentations, characteristic and outcomes. *Med. J. Malays.* **2014**, *69*, 257–260.

12. Peacock, S.J.; Chieng, G.; Cheng, A.C.; Dance, D.A.B.; Amornchai, P.; Wongsuvan, G.; Teerawattanasook, N.; Chierakul, W.; Day, N.P.J.; Wuthiekanun, V. Comparison of Ashdown's medium, *Burkholderia cepacia* medium, and *Burkholderia pseudomallei* selective agar for clinic isolation of *Burkholderia pseudomallei*. *J. Clin. Microbiol.* **2005**, *43*, 5359–5361. [CrossRef] [PubMed]

13. Podin, Y.; Kaestil, M.; McMahon, N.; Hennessy, J.; Ngian, H.U.; Wong, J.S.; Mohana, A.; Wong, S.C.; William, T.; Mayo, M.; et al. Reliability of automated biochemical identification of *Burkholderia pseudomallei* is regionally dependent. *J. Clin. Microbiol.* **2013**, *51*, 3076–3078. [CrossRef] [PubMed]

14. Chetchotisakd, P.; Chierakul, W.; Chaowagul, W.; Anunnatsiri, S.; Phimda, K.; Mootsikapun, P.; Chaisuksant, S.; Pilaikul, J.; Thinkhamrop, B.; Phiphitaporn, S.; et al. Trimethoprim-sulfamethoxazole versus trimethoprim-sulfamethoxazole plus doxycycline as oral eradicative treatment for melioidosis (MERTH): A multicentre, double-blind, non-inferiority, randomised controlled trial. *Lancet* **2014**, *383*, 807–814. [CrossRef]

15. Dance, D. Treatment and prophylaxis of melioidosis. *Int. J. Antimicrob. Agents* **2014**, *43*, 310–318. [CrossRef] [PubMed]

16. Centers for Diseases Control and Prevention. Biosafety in microbiological and biomedical laboratories. Section IV. Laboratory biosafety level criteria. Available online: https://www.cdc.gov/biosafety/publications/bmbl5/bmbl5_sect_iv.pdf (accessed on 9 February 2018).

17. Population. Available online: http://www.depd.gov.bn/sitePages/Population.aspx (accessed on 3 January 2018).

18. Currie, B.J.; Ward, L.; Cheng, A.C. The epidemiology and clinical spectrum of Melioidosis: 540 cases from the 20 year Darwin prospective study. *PLoS Negl. Trop. Dis.* **2010**, *4*, e900. [CrossRef] [PubMed]

19. Deris, Z.Z.; Hasan, H.; Siti Suraiya, M.N. Clinical characteristics and outcomes of bacteraemic melioidosis in a teaching hospital in a northeastern state of Malaysia. *J. Infect. Dev. Ctries.* **2010**, *4*, 430–435. [PubMed]

20. Hanna, J.N.; Humphreys, J.L.; Brookes, D.L.; Messina, T.; Raulli, A. Melioidosis in North Queensland, 2000–2009. *Commun. Dis. Intell.* **2010**, *34*, 444–447.

21. Hassan, M.R.A.; Pani, S.P.; Peng, N.P.; Voralu, K.; Vijayalakshmi, N.; Mehandrakar, R.; Aziz, N.A.; Michael, E. Incidence, risk factors and clinical epidemiology of melioidosis: A complex socio-ecological emerging infectious disease in the Alor Setar region of Kedah, Malaysia. *BMC Infect. Dis.* **2010**, *10*, 302. [CrossRef] [PubMed]

22. Limmathurotsakul, D.; Wongratanacheewin, S.; Teerawattanasook, N.; Wongsuvan, G.; Chaisuksant, S.; Chetchotisakd, P.; Chaowagul, W.; Day, N.P.J.; Peacock, S.J. Increasing incidence of human melioidosis in northeast Thailand. *Am. J. Trop. Med. Hyg.* **2010**, *82*, 1113–1117. [CrossRef] [PubMed]

23. Vidyalakshmi, K.; Lipika, S.; Vishal, S.; Damodar, S.; Chakrapani, M. Emerging clinico-epidemiological trends in melioidosis: Analysis of 95 cases from western coastal India. *Int. J. Infect. Dis.* **2012**, *16*, e491–e497. [CrossRef] [PubMed]

24. Zueter, A.; Yean, C.Y.; Abumarzouq, M.; Rahman, Z.A.; Deris, Z.Z.; Harun, A. The epidemiology and clinical spectrum of melioidosis in a teaching hospital in North-Eastern state of Malaysia: A fifteen-year review. *BMC Infect. Dis.* **2016**, *16*, 333. [CrossRef] [PubMed]

25. Pang, L.; Harris, P.N.A.; Seiler, R.L.; Ooi, P.L.; Cutter, J.; Goh, K.T.; Cook, A.R.; Fisher, D.; Chai, L.Y.A. Melioidosis, Singapore, 2003–2014. *Emerg. Infect. Dis.* **2018**, *24*, 140–143. [CrossRef] [PubMed]

26. How, S.H.; Ng, T.H.; Jamalludin, A.R.; Tee, H.P.; Kuan, Y.C.; Alex, F.; Sc, M.; Aminudin, C.A.; Sapari, S.; Quazi, M.H. Pahang melioidosis registry. *Med. J. Malays.* **2009**, *64*, 27–30.

27. Foong, Y.C.; Tan, M.; Bradbury, R.S. Melioidosis: A review. *Rural Remote Health* **2014**, *14*, 2763. [PubMed]

28. McLeod, C.; Morris, P.S.; Bauert, P.A.; Kilburn, C.J.; Ward, L.M.; Baird, R.W.; Currie, B.J. Clinical presentation and medical management of melioidosis in children: A 24-year prospective study in the Northern Territory of Australia and review of the literature. *Clin. Infect. Dis.* **2015**, *60*, 21–26. [CrossRef] [PubMed]

29. Kingsley, P.V.; Leader, M.; Nagodawithana, N.S.; Tipre, M.; Sathaikumar, N. Melioidosis in Malaysia: A review of case reports. *PLoS Negl. Trop. Dis.* **2016**, *10*, e0005182. [CrossRef] [PubMed]

30. Liu, X.; Pang, L.; Sim, S.H.; Goh, K.T.; Ravikumar, S.; Win, M.S.; Tan, G.; Cook, A.R.; Fisher, D.; Chai, L.Y. Association of melioidosis incidence with rainfall and humidity, Singapore, 2003–2012. *Emerg. Infect. Dis.* **2015**, *21*, 159–162. [CrossRef] [PubMed]

31. Merritt, A.J.; Inglis, T.J.J. The role of climate in the epidemiology of melioidosis. *Curr. Trop. Med. Rep.* **2017**, *4*, 185–191. [CrossRef] [PubMed]

32. Currie, B.J.; Fischer, D.A.; Anstey, N.M.; Jacups, S.P. Melioidosis: Acute and chronic disease, relapse and re-activation. *Trans. R. Soc. Trop. Med. Hyg.* **2000**, *94*, 301–304. [CrossRef]

33. Suputtamongkol, Y.; Hall, A.J.; Dance, D.A.; Chaowagul, W.; Rajchanuvong, A.; Smith, M.D.; White, N.J. The epidemiology of melioidosis in Ubon Ratchatani, northeast Thailand. *Int. J. Epidemiol.* **1994**, *23*, 1082–1090. [CrossRef] [PubMed]

34. Cheng, A.C.; Currie, B.J. Melioidosis: Epidemiology, pathophysiology and management. *Clin. Microbiol. Rev.* **2005**, *18*, 383–416. [CrossRef] [PubMed]

35. Wiersinga, W.J.; Currie, B.J.; Peacock, S.J. Melioidosis. *N. Engl. J. Med.* **2012**, *367*, 1035–1044. [CrossRef] [PubMed]

36. Choy, J.L.; Mayo, M.; Janmaat, A.; Currie, B.J. Animal melioidosis in Australia. *Acta Trop.* **2000**, *74*, 153–158. [CrossRef]

37. Limmathurotsakul, D.; Thammasart, S.; Warrasuth, N.; Thapanagulsak, P.; Jatapai, A.; Pengreungrojanachai, V.; Anun, S.; Joraka, W.; Thongkam koon, P.; Saiyen, P.; et al. Melioidosis in animals, Thailand, 2006–2010. *Emerg. Infect. Dis.* **2012**, *18*, 325–327. [CrossRef] [PubMed]

38. Sprague, L.D.; Neubauer, H. Melioidosis in animals: A review of epizootiology, diagnosis and clinical presentation. *J. Vet. Med.* **2004**, *51*, 305–320. [CrossRef] [PubMed]

39. Health Information Booklet 2016. Available online: www.moh.gov.bn/.../Health%20Indicator%20Booklet/HIB_2016.pdf (accessed on 3 January 2018).

40. Limmathurotsakul, D.; Kanoksil, M.; Wuthiekanun, V.; Kitphati, R.; de Stavola, B.; Day, N.P.J.; Peacock, S.J. Activities of daily living associated with acquisition of melioidosis in northeast Thailand: A matched case-control study. *PLoS Negl. Trop. Dis.* **2013**, *7*, e2072. [CrossRef] [PubMed]

41. Suntornsut, P.; Wongsuwan, N.; Malasit, M.; Kitphati, R.; Michie, S.; Peacock, S.J.; Limmathruotsakul, D. Barriers and recommended interventions to prevent melioidosis in northeast Thailand: A focus group study using the behaviour change wheel. *PLoS Negl. Trop. Dis.* **2016**, *10*, e0004823. [CrossRef] [PubMed]

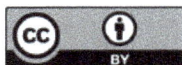

Tropical Medicine and Infectious Disease

MDPI

Meeting Report

A Report from the Cambodia Training Event for Awareness of Melioidosis (C-TEAM), October 2017

Sotharith Bory [1] [iD], Frances Daily [2,*], Gaetan Khim [2], Joanne Letchford [2], Srun Sok [3], Hero Kol [4], Muy Seang Lak [4], Luciano Tuseo [5], Chan Vibol [5], Sopheap Oeng [2] and Paul Turner [6,7] [iD]

[1] Infectious Diseases Unit, Calmette Hospital, Phnom Penh 12201, Cambodia; sotharith_bory@yahoo.com
[2] Diagnostic Microbiology Development Program, Phnom Penh 12302, Cambodia; gaetan.khim@dmdp.org (G.K.); joanne.letchford@dmdp.org (J.L.); oeng.sopheap@dmdp.org (S.O.)
[3] Hospital Services Department, Ministry of Health, Phnom Penh 12152, Cambodia; soksrun@gmail.com
[4] Preventive Medicine Department, Ministry of Health, Phnom Penh 12152, Cambodia; herokol@yahoo.com (H.K.); sreanglak@yahoo.com (M.S.L.)
[5] World Health Organization, Phnom Penh 12302, Cambodia; tuseol@who.int (L.T.); chanv@who.int (C.V.)
[6] Cambodia Oxford Medical Research Unit, Angkor Hospital for Children, Siem Reap 17252, Cambodia; pault@tropmedres.ac
[7] Centre for Tropical Medicine and Global Health, Nuffield Department of Medicine, University of Oxford, Oxford OX3 7FZ, UK
* Correspondence: fdaily@dmdp.org; Tel: +855-12-626-33

Received: 31 January 2018; Accepted: 17 February 2018; Published: 23 February 2018

Abstract: Melioidosis is an endemic infection in Cambodia, a lower middle income SE Asian country. Despite more laboratories isolating and identifying *Burkholderia pseudomallei* in recent years, the infection remains under-recognised and under-diagnosed, particularly in the adult population. Lack of knowledge about the disease and lack of utilization of microbiology laboratories contributes to this, along with laboratory capacity issues. Treatment costs often hamper optimal management. In response to these issues, a national one-health training event was held in October 2017 to raise awareness of the disease amongst clinical, laboratory, and public health professionals. The meeting format, findings, and outcomes are described here.

Keywords: melioidosis; Cambodia; epidemiology

1. Introduction

Melioidosis, infection by the environmental Gram-negative bacterium *Burkholderia pseudomallei*, is an endemic but significantly unrecognized disease in Cambodia, a lower middle income SE Asian country with a population of ~16 million. It was first diagnosed in Phnom Penh in 1928 in a Russian national, although he was almost certainly infected in Thailand [1]. Subsequently, pulmonary melioidosis was described in a resettled refugee who had lived in Thailand for several years before diagnosis [2], and also a porcine outbreak was identified in the 1960s [3]. However, it was not until 2005, that human melioidosis cases began to be regularly identified in-country, initially in children following the establishment of a diagnostic microbiology laboratory at Angkor Hospital for Children, Siem Reap [4]. Since then, significant laboratory capacity building has occurred nationally and several hundred cases in both children and adults have been described [5–9]. Not unexpectedly, mortality is higher in adults (more than 50%) than in children [4,6–8]; however, as with adults, children who are bacteraemic have higher mortality (72%) [8]. Serologic screening using the indirect haemagglutination assay (IHA) revealed that 16% of tested children from Siem Reap province had evidence of exposure to *B. pseudomallei* and the organism was confirmed to be present in rice paddy soil [10].

A recent global mathematical modelling study predicted that in 2015, Cambodia would have had 2083 (95% credible interval 850–5451) melioidosis cases resulting in 1149 (464–3042) deaths [11].

Lack of clinician awareness and limited diagnostic microbiology capacity may explain the discrepancy between the model predictions and the low number of cases confirmed in Cambodia each year.

With aim of improving clinical, laboratory, and public health professional awareness of melioidosis, a national one-health training event was held in Phnom Penh, 17–19 October 2017.

2. The C-TEAM Meeting

There were more than 180 meeting attendees, representing national, provincial and non-governmental hospitals, universities and research institutes, as well as government ministries (Health, Agriculture, Fisheries and Forestry, Environment, Rural Development), international and non-governmental organizations and partners. Hospitals were asked to prepare a summary of melioidosis cases and *B. pseudomallei* isolate numbers prior to the meeting. Where possible, it was requested that data be stratified by date (year), specimen type, and geo-location (home province). Prior to presentation every effort was made to verify the accuracy of the data.

The first day featured plenary talks from international clinical and laboratory melioidosis experts, followed by situation updates from several national, provincial and non-governmental hospitals. Representatives from six major participating hospitals presented data on their clinical and laboratory capacity. In particular, melioidosis case numbers, diagnostic procedures, and treatment regimens were shared. The day concluded with presentations on melioidosis in animals, environmental reservoirs of *B. pseudomallei*, prevention and public engagement activities.

The second and third days featured parallel workshop sessions for clinicians and laboratorians. Cambodian clinicians presented cases to demonstrate the breadth of melioidosis infection, including pneumonia, sepsis, head and neck abscesses, hepatic, splenic, prostatic abscesses, and bone and joint infections. Expert speakers provided commentary on the cases and led discussions around diagnosis and treatment. Particular attention was paid to defining the optimal diagnostic approach and appropriate treatment choices [12,13]. Sessions on the radiologic features and surgical management of melioidosis were included. The recently updated national treatment guidelines were presented and discussed and encouragement was given to participants to collect case data prospectively in the hope of gaining more knowledge about the local epidemiology. Laboratorians gave local situation updates and participated in dry and wet laboratory sessions to gain experience of best practices for safe handling and identification of *B. pseudomallei* from clinical specimens, as well as determination and reporting of appropriate antimicrobial susceptibilities. Identification test demonstrations and hands-on practical sessions included the three-disk test (co-amoxiclav, colistin/polymixin B, and gentamicin) [14], InBios Active Melioidosis Detect lateral flow assay [15], and Mahidol University latex agglutination test [16,17]. There was a demonstration of the advantages of Ashdown's agar and broth, *B. pseudomallei* selective media, for culture of non-sterile site specimens such as throat swabs [18]. Diagnostic Microbiology Development Program (DMDP)-developed standard operating procedures and job aids were shared with meeting participants. Two training videos were prepared for the meeting, providing overviews of specimen processing and identification of *B. pseudomallei* (the Khmer language version can be found at: https://vimeo.com/237880199).

The meeting concluded with an interactive session for clinicians and laboratorians aimed at promoting communication and identification of areas where co-operative efforts between clinical and laboratory teams could be used to improve diagnosis and management patients with melioidosis.

3. Summary of the Current Situation

Since the first national melioidosis conference, held in August 2010, there has been a steady increase in the number of culture confirmed cases from 173 (isolated and identified from five microbiology laboratories since October 2005) to 2592 up to September 2017 (from 17 microbiology laboratories) (Figure 1). Partner organizations, including the DMDP, have worked with the Ministry of Health Bureau of Medical Laboratory Services to improve laboratory diagnostic capacity over this time. Despite the increase, the annual cases remain well below the levels predicted by the mathematical model.

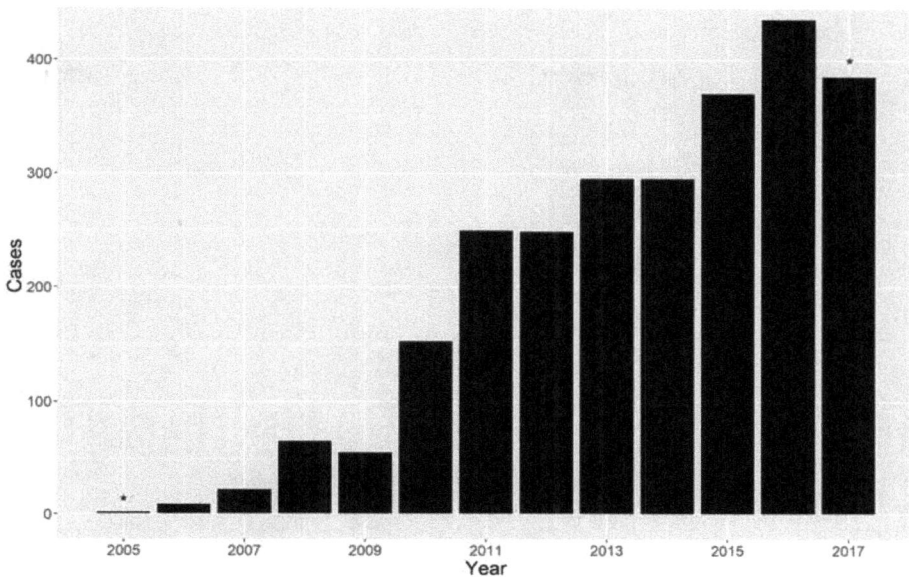

Figure 1. Annual numbers of confirmed melioidosis cases in Cambodia, October 2005–September 2017 (* incomplete years).

To date, the majority of cases have been children (at least 60% (1565/2592), but age data not available for all cases), which is in contrast to other countries where children account for 5–15% of all cases. This is likely due to overrepresentation of cases from three children's hospitals that have well-established microbiology laboratories and clinical diagnostic algorithms. In many hospitals, both public and private, there is as yet no systematic sampling for patients with presumed infections, hence very few microbiology investigations are requested by doctors. In addition, in many hospitals in Cambodia, some patients are required to pay for services including microbiology testing and treatment, which is often cited as a barrier to increasing the number of specimens requested and treating the patient with recommended treatment.

Data on culture-confirmed *B. pseudomallei* cases are not yet routinely collated at a national level. Of data obtainable and presented at the meeting, home province information was only available in one third of patients (34%, 889/2592). Despite this, the data confirm that 23 of 25 provinces have had culture-confirmed cases, suggesting the infection is endemic throughout the country (Figure 2). As soil testing has been limited to one province and no water studies have yet been carried out, it is unknown whether there are areas in the country where the infection is more likely to be acquired.

The month of culture confirmation was available for only one fifth of all cases, but where recorded, the majority of cases (71%, 377/528) occurred during the wet season months of May to October, which is consistent with other endemic areas. Where documented (19% of all cases; 481/2592), adults were more likely to have risk factors than children, with the most common being diabetes mellitus, hazardous alcohol use and corticosteroids. The majority of adults had presented with pneumonia and/or sepsis, whereas children were more likely to have head and neck infections. Both of these findings are consistent with other endemic countries; however, one province had a high number of head and neck presentations in adults (30% of all presentations), which is unusual in this age group.

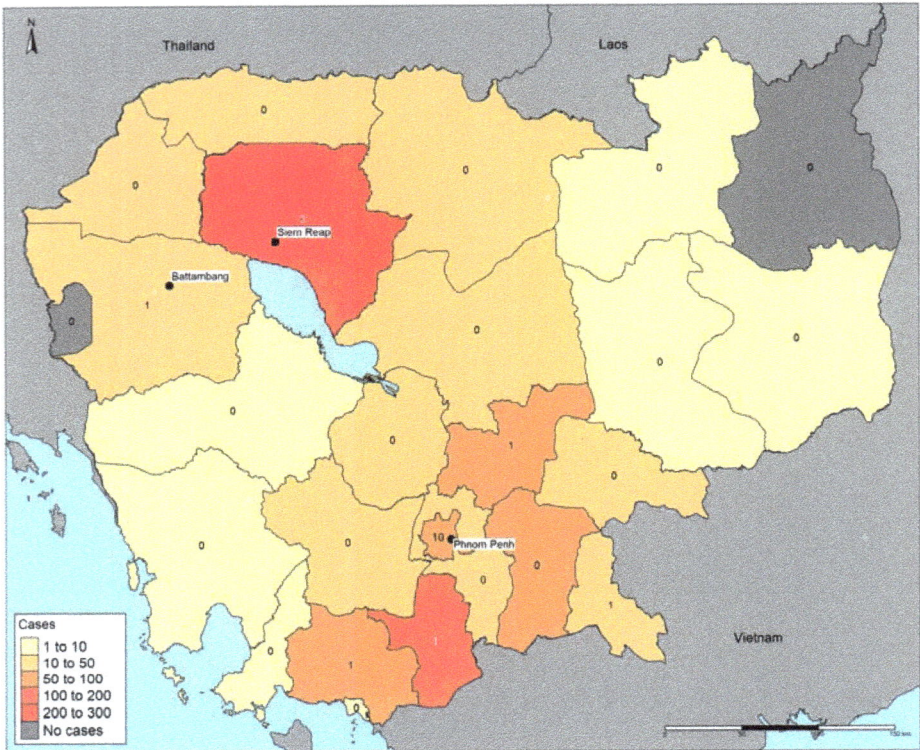

Figure 2. Geographic distribution of melioidosis cases in Cambodia, October 2005–September 2017. Province of residence was available in 889 confirmed cases. Shading represents the total number of culture-confirmed melioidosis cases per province. The numbers represent the count of participating microbiology laboratories per province; however, one was unable to contribute its culture confirmed cases prior to the meeting.

The most common *B. pseudomallei* culture-positive specimen type reported was pus (55%, 1530/2765 specimens) followed by blood culture (34%, 941/765). Only 73 sputum cultures were documented, despite pneumonia being a common clinical presentation. Bronchoalveolar lavage/aspirates were positive in 17 specimens and there were 26 pleural fluid specimens positive for the bacterium. Commonest diagnostic methods in routine use were the three-disc test (82%, 14/17 laboratories) and the bioMerieux API 20NE test strip (59%, 10/17 laboratories). One third (35%, 6/17) of the laboratories reported use of Ashdown selective media, although it is not yet routinely used or readily available in all of these laboratories. Several laboratories reported routinely releasing antibiotic susceptibility data on drugs that are not recommended for melioidosis treatment, such as ceftriaxone, cefuroxime, colistin and fosfomycin. Prior to the meeting, some laboratories were unaware of the limitations of disc diffusion testing for co-trimoxazole [19].

Treatment choice and length of treatment varied between hospitals, with some using ceftriaxone during the initial phase, rather than the recommended ceftazidime. Many hospitals reported they often lack sufficient supplies of ceftazidime and therefore treat patients with inferior drugs (e.g., co-trimoxazole or ceftriaxone) or with shortened courses of ceftazidime. Carbapenems are not readily available in almost all hospitals, so rarely prescribed. Eradication phase options sometimes included co-amoxiclav as first-line treatment, rather than the recommended co-trimoxazole, mostly without consideration of amoxicillin:clavulanate ratio. The length of treatment and follow up during this phase was inconsistent. Outcome data was very incomplete with hospitals often having no information as patients were lost to follow up, or outcome had not been collated.

4. Outcomes and Future Plans

The major outcome of the meeting was the successful drawing together of a broad range of Cambodian health professionals to share knowledge and experience of the epidemiology, clinical and laboratory diagnosis, treatment and prevention of melioidosis. Many of the animal and environmental sector participants heard for the first time about the importance of this disease and were eager to learn more. Local data were collated and presented alongside state-of-the-art lectures from global melioidosis experts. Current challenges in clinical case detection, awareness of risk factors (e.g., diabetes), laboratory diagnosis, treatment and limited collation of epidemiological data were highlighted. Updated national diagnosis and treatment guidelines were showcased. Laboratory staff were made aware of current best practices for safe culture and identification of *B. pseudomallei,* and were provided with key standard operating procedures and job aids. The need for reliable surveillance data was recognised as a priority. It is hoped that the enthusiasm shown by all participants at the meeting will be translated into a sustained effort to improve clinical diagnosis, laboratory confirmation, treatment, outcomes and surveillance of melioidosis in Cambodia moving forwards. Further training workshops, plus development and provision of an information package summarizing the current situation and outstanding challenges to policy makers, clinicians, laboratory technicians and other stakeholders, will consolidate the considerable momentum generated at the C-TEAM meeting.

Acknowledgments: This conference and training event was made possible through the generous support of the Cooperative Biological Engagement Program, Defense Threat Reduction Agency, US Department of Defense, USA. The authors extend their gratitude to all of the institutions who presented and shared data at the meeting. The authors and meeting organisers are extremely grateful for the contributions of Stuart Blacksell (Mahidol-Oxford Tropical Medicine Research Unit, Thailand), Lance Brooks (Cooperative Biological Engagement Program, Defense Threat Reduction Agency, US Department of Defense, USA), Bart Currie (Menzies School of Health Research, Royal Darwin Hospital, Australia), David Dance (Lao-Oxford-Mahosot Hospital-Wellcome Trust Research Unit, Laos), Vicki Krause (Centre for Disease Control, Department of Health, Northern Territory, Australia), Direk Limmathurotsakul (Mahidol-Oxford Tropical Medicine Research Unit, Thailand), Sau Sokunna (Hospital Services Department, Ministry of Health, Cambodia), Martha Stokes (Cooperative Biological Engagement Program, Defense Threat Reduction Agency, US Department of Defense, USA), Pichest Watanapairojrat (Naresuan University, Thailand), Jitraporn Wongwiwatchai (Khon Kaen University, Thailand), and Vanaporn Wuthiekanun (Mahidol-Oxford Tropical Medicine Research Unit, Thailand).

Conflicts of Interest: The authors declare no conflict of interest

References

1. Sourchard, L. Contribution a l'étude de la Mélioidose en Indochine. *Archive des Instituts Pasteurs d'Indochine* **1932**, *16*, 193–219. (In French)
2. Chan, C.K.; Hyland, R.H.; Leers, W.D.; Hutcheon, M.A.; Chang, D. Pleuropulmonary melioidosis in a Cambodian refugee. *Can. Med. Assoc. J.* **1984**, *131*, 1365–1367. [PubMed]
3. Thonn, S.; Lebon, E.; Saphon Triau, R. Note sure une épizootie de mélioïdose porcine au Cambodge. *Rev. Elev. Med. Vet. Pays. Trop.* **1960**, *13*, 175–179. (In French) [CrossRef]
4. Pagnarith, Y.; Kumar, V.; Thaipadungpanit, J.; Wuthiekanun, V.; Amornchai, P.; Sin, L.; Day, N.P.; Peacock, S.J. Emergence of pediatric melioidosis in Siem Reap, Cambodia. *Am. J. Trop. Med. Hyg.* **2010**, *82*, 1106–1112. [CrossRef] [PubMed]
5. Overtoom, R.; Khieu, V.; Hem, S.; Cavailler, P.; Te, V.; Chan, S.; Lau, P.; Guillard, B.; Vong, S. A first report of pulmonary melioidosis in Cambodia. *Trans. Roy. Soc. Trop. Med. Hyg.* **2008**, *102* (Suppl. 1), S21–S25. [CrossRef]
6. Vlieghe, E.; Kruy, L.; De Smet, B.; Kham, C.; Veng, C.H.; Phe, T.; Koole, O.; Thai, S.; Lynen, L.; Jacobs, J. Melioidosis, Phnom Penh, Cambodia. *Emerg. Infect. Dis.* **2011**, *17*, 1289–1292. [CrossRef] [PubMed]

7.   Rammaert, B.; Beaute, J.; Borand, L.; Hem, S.; Buchy, P.; Goyet, S.; Overtoom, R.; Angebault, C.; Te, V.; Try, P.L.; Mayaud, C.; Vong, S.; Guillard, B. Pulmonary melioidosis in Cambodia: a prospective study. *BMC Infect. Dis.* **2011**, *11*. [CrossRef] [PubMed]

8.   Turner, P.; Kloprogge, S.; Miliya, T.; Soeng, S.; Tan, P.; Sar, P.; Yos, P.; Moore, C.E.; Wuthiekanun, V.; Limmathurotsakul, D.; Turner, C.; Day, N.P.J.; Dance, D.A.B. A retrospective analysis of melioidosis in Cambodian children, 2009–2013. *BMC Infect. Dis.* **2016**, *16*. [CrossRef] [PubMed]

9.   Schully, K.L.; Berjohn, C.M.; Prouty, A.M.; Fitkariwala, A.; Som, T.; Sieng, D.; Gregory, M.J.; Vaughn, A.; Kheng, S.; Te, V.; Duplessis, C.A.; Lawler, J.V.; Clark, D.V. Melioidosis in lower provincial Cambodia: A case series from a prospective study of sepsis in Takeo Province. *PLoS Negl. Trop. Dis.* **2017**, *11*, e0005923. [CrossRef] [PubMed]

10. Wuthiekanun, V.; Pheaktra, N.; Putchhat, H.; Sin, L.; Sen, B.; Kumar, V.; Langla, S.; Peacock, S.J.; Day, N.P. *Burkholderia pseudomallei* antibodies in children, Cambodia. *Emerg. Infect. Dis.* **2008**, *14*, 301–303. [CrossRef] [PubMed]

11. Limmathurotsakul, D.; Golding, N.; Dance, D.A.; Messina, J.P.; Pigott, D.M.; Moyes, C.L.; Rolim, D.B.; Bertherat, E.; Day, N.P.; Peacock, S.J.; Hay, S.I. Predicted global distribution of and burden of melioidosis. *Nat. Microbiol.* **2016**, *1*. [CrossRef] [PubMed]

12. White, N.J. Melioidosis. *Lancet* **2003**, *361*, 1715–1722. [CrossRef]

13. Dance, D. Treatment and prophylaxis of melioidosis. *Int. J. Antimicrob. Agents* **2014**, *43*, 310–318. [CrossRef] [PubMed]

14. Trinh, T.T.; Hoang, T.S.; Tran, D.A.; Trinh, V.T.; Gohler, A.; Nguyen, T.T.; Hoang, S.N.; Krumkamp, R.; Nguyen, L.T.N.; May, J.; et al. A simple laboratory algorithm for diagnosis of melioidosis in resource-constrained areas: A study from north-central Vietnam. *Clin. Microbiol. Infect.* **2018**, *24*. [CrossRef] [PubMed]

15. Houghton, R.L.; Reed, D.E.; Hubbard, M.A.; Dillon, M.J.; Chen, H.; Currie, B.J.; Mayo, M.; Sarovich, D.S.; Theobald, V.; Limmathurotsakul, D.; et al. Development of a prototype lateral flow immunoassay (LFI) for the rapid diagnosis of melioidosis. *PLoS Negl. Trop. Dis.* **2014**, *8*. [CrossRef] [PubMed]

16. Anuntagool, N.; Naigowit, P.; Petkanchanapong, V.; Aramsri, P.; Panichakul, T.; Sirisinha, S. Monoclonal antibody-based rapid identification of *Burkholderia pseudomallei* in blood culture fluid from patients with community-acquired septicaemia. *J. Med. Microbiol.* **2000**, *49*, 1075–1078. [CrossRef] [PubMed]

17. Amornchai, P.; Chierakul, W.; Wuthiekanun, V.; Mahakhunkijcharoen, Y.; Phetsouvanh, R.; Currie, B.J.; Newton, P.N.; van Vinh Chau, N.; Wongratanacheewin, S.; Day, N.P.; et al. Accuracy of *Burkholderia pseudomallei* identification using the API 20NE system and a latex agglutination test. *J. Clin. Microbiol.* **2007**, *45*, 3774–3776. [CrossRef] [PubMed]

18. Wuthiekanun, V.; Dance, D.A.; Wattanagoon, Y.; Supputtamongkol, Y.; Chaowagul, W.; White, N.J. The use of selective media for the isolation of *Pseudomonas pseudomallei* in clinical practice. *J. Med. Microbiol.* **1990**, *33*, 121–126. [CrossRef] [PubMed]

19. Dance, D.A.; Davong, V.; Soeng, S.; Phetsouvanh, R.; Newton, P.N.; Turner, P. Trimethoprim/sulfamethoxazole resistance in *Burkholderia pseudomallei*. *Int. J. Antimicrob. Agents* **2014**, *44*, 368–369. [CrossRef] [PubMed]

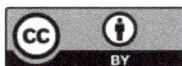

Tropical Medicine and Infectious Disease

MDPI

Review

Melioidosis in Vietnam: Recently Improved Recognition but still an Uncertain Disease Burden after Almost a Century of Reporting

Trung T. Trinh [1,*] [iD], **Linh D. N. Nguyen** [2], **Trung V. Nguyen** [3,4], **Chuong X. Tran** [5], **An V. Le** [6], **Hao V. Nguyen** [7,8], **Karoline Assig** [9], **Sabine Lichtenegger** [9], **Gabriel E. Wagner** [9], **Cuong D. Do** [10] **and Ivo Steinmetz** [9,11] [iD]

1   Institute of Microbiology and Biotechnology, Vietnam National University, Hanoi 100000, Vietnam
2   Department of Academic Affairs, Phan Chau Trinh University, Quang Nam 560000, Vietnam; nguyendongoclinh@gmail.com
3   Department of Medical Microbiology, Hanoi Medical University, Hanoi 100000, Vietnam; nguyen.vu.trung@gmail.com
4   National Hospital for Tropical Diseases, Hanoi 100000, Vietnam
5   Department of Infectious Diseases, Hue University of Medicine and Pharmacy, Hue 530000, Vietnam; xuanchuonghue@gmail.com
6   Department of Medical Microbiology, Hue University of Medicine and Pharmacy, Hue 530000, Vietnam; levanan.hump@gmail.com
7   Department of Infectious Diseases, University of Medicine and Pharmacy, Ho Chi Minh 700000, Vietnam; haodiep61@gmail.com
8   Hospital for Tropical Diseases, Ho Chi Minh 700000, Vietnam
9   Institute of Hygiene, Microbiology and Environmental Medicine, Medical University of Graz, 8010 Graz, Austria; karoline.assig@medunigraz.at (K.A.); sabine.lichtenegger@medunigraz.at (S.L.); gabriel.wagner-lichtenegger@medunigraz.at (G.E.W.); ivo.steinmetz@medunigraz.at (I.S.)
10   Department of Infectious Diseases, Bach Mai Hospital, Hanoi 100000, Vietnam; doduy.cuong@gmail.com
11   Friedrich Loeffler Institute of Medical Microbiology, University Medicine Greifswald, 17475 Greifswald, Germany
*   Correspondence: tttrung@vnu.edu.vn; Tel.: +84-243-7548747

Received: 12 March 2018; Accepted: 30 March 2018; Published: 9 April 2018

Abstract: The first cases of human melioidosis were described in Vietnam in the 1920s, almost a century ago. It was in Vietnam in the thirties that the saprophytic nature of *B. pseudomallei* was first recognized. Although a significant number of French and U.S. soldiers acquired the disease during the Vietnam wars, indigenous cases in the Vietnamese population were only sporadically reported over many decades. After reunification in 1975, only two retrospective studies reported relatively small numbers of indigenous cases from single tertiary care hospitals located in the biggest cities in the South and the North, respectively. Studies from provincial hospitals throughout the country were missing until the Research Network on Melioidosis and *Burkholderia pseudomallei* (RENOMAB) project started in 2014. From then on seminars, workshops, and national scientific conferences on melioidosis have been conducted to raise awareness among physicians and clinical laboratory staff. This led to the recognition of a significant number of cases in at least 36 hospitals in 26 provinces and cities throughout Vietnam. Although a widespread distribution of melioidosis has now been documented, there are still challenges to understand the true epidemiology of the disease. Establishment of national guidelines for diagnosis, management, and reporting of the disease together with more investigations on animal melioidosis, genomic diversity of *B. pseudomallei* and its environmental distribution are required.

Keywords: melioidosis; *Burkholderia pseudomallei*; Vietnam; public awareness; animal; environment

1. Introduction

Although sporadic cases of melioidosis have been reported from Vietnam since the year 1927, the disease has only recently attracted the deserved attention among Vietnamese health care professionals. This neglect is particularly remarkable, given the fact that a fundamental characteristic of *B. pseudomallei*—namely, the environmental reservoir of this pathogen—was demonstrated for the first time in Vietnam [1,2]. Although many melioidosis cases among French and American soldiers were reported during the long-lasting armed conflicts, this had no sustainable effect on the recognition of melioidosis in the indigenous Vietnamese population. In this report, we summarize the history of melioidosis in Vietnam in humans and animals starting almost a century ago and finally describe more recent activities trying to unravel the burden of disease and to increase awareness. We also discuss current knowledge on environmental *B. pseudomallei* in Vietnam, the population structure of Vietnamese *B. pseudomallei* and its phylogenetic relatedness. Finally, we address current and future challenges in prevention and diagnosis of the disease.

2. Review of Melioidosis in Vietnam

2.1. Human Melioidosis

2.1.1. 1920s to 1950s

The first case of human melioidosis in Vietnam was detected in 1925 in an ill-nourished female patient, pregnant in the fifth month, living at Thu Duc, close to Saigon (now Ho Chi Minh City). Six days after onset of symptoms, the patient had a miscarriage and, after 14 days of illness, the patient died [3]. *B. pseudomallei* was isolated from the blood at the Pasteur Institute of Ho Chi Minh City and the identification was confirmed at the Institute for Medical Research, Malaysia [4].

Subsequently cases were reported by Menard in 1928 from Ho Chi Minh City and Tonkin (now Hanoi in the North), as cited by Pons (1930) [5]. Further culture-confirmed cases of melioidosis, including cases related to traffic accidents (see below Section 3) were then reported at Hue city (Central Vietnam) and from the North [1]. In 1947, 28 cases of acute, sub-acute, and chronic melioidosis were described from various hospitals in the South [6]. Of those, only nine cases were Vietnamese patients. The others were 15 Caucasians, 2 black patients, and 1 patient of Chinese and 1 of south Asian descent. Fatal outcomes were reported in 19 out of those 28 cases, although the outcome was not documented for all patients. From 1951 to 1953, five pulmonary cases of melioidosis were diagnosed at hospitals in both southern Vietnam and France. All of the cases were French citizens with a history of residence or station in the region of Vietnam, Laos, and Cambodia [7]. A case of chronic pulmonary melioidosis was also described in a soldier suffering from a chest wound caused by a bullet in Vietnam [8]. Between 1948 and 1954, approximately 100 cases were reported among 400,000 French forces stationed in Vietnam, Laos, and Cambodia, as cited by Sanford (1978) [9]. In 1956, a fatal case of septicemic melioidosis was diagnosed in a 40-year-old south Vietnamese soldier admitted to Cong Hoa Hospital [10].

2.1.2. 1960s to 1980s

It is interesting to note that already in 1967, Mo and Duong stated that the disease was most likely underdiagnosed in hospitals of southern Vietnam and that cases of melioidosis were probably misdiagnosed as tuberculosis or disseminated fungus infections. The authors also mentioned several cases detected annually in different hospitals of the South and described the development of melioidosis in a young soldier after a military operation in a swampy area of the South [11]. With the deployment of the U.S. Armed Forces in Vietnam, melioidosis started to be detected in the U.S. military personnel. As cited by Diamond and Pastore (1967), through February 1967, 35 cases were diagnosed in U.S. troops stationed in Southeast Asia, with 8 fatal cases reported [12]. Those patients were diagnosed because diseased or wounded soldiers were referred to modern hospitals of either Republic of South Vietnam or United States, where microbiological laboratories were available for diagnosis of melioidosis as well as for other infectious diseases. Within the year of 1966, a series of 9 cases of pulmonary melioidosis in U.S. soldiers was described [13]. Another nine cases of melioidosis in U.S. soldiers, including four fatal cases, were diagnosed in Vietnam in Long Binh (now Dong Nai province in the South) [14]. Since more cases of melioidosis were subsequently reported in U.S. soldiers, melioidosis became one of six major tropical infectious diseases for which U.S. physicians needed to maintain a high index of suspicion in febrile soldiers returning from Vietnam [15]. From April 1965 to December 1969, 187 cases with 13 deaths were reported in the U.S. Army personnel stationed in Vietnam. Until the U.S. withdrawal in 1972, approximately two to three culture-confirmed cases were detected among the U.S. soldiers every month [9,16,17]. Serology using indirect hemagglutination (IHA) showed that 8.9% of the sera from the Vietnam veterans had titers of 1:40 or greater [18]. Based on such titers it was estimated by Clayton et al. that approximately 250,000 among three million U.S. Army personnel got infected with *B. pseudomallei* when serving in Vietnam [18,19]. Although these estimates might be interpreted with some cautions considering the limited specificity and sensitivity of the non-standardized IHA test, this study indicated a potential reservoir of latent *B. pseudomallei* infection among personnel returning from Vietnam. Indeed, it became obvious that latent infection and reactivation, sometimes after many years, does occur [20]. This phenomenon led to the melioidosis nickname 'Vietnam Time Bomb' [21]. A possible human-to-human transmission via sexual contact was suggested in the wife of a returning Vietnam veteran with prostatitis due to *B. pseudomallei* infection [22]. Melioidosis was also diagnosed in a newborn whose father had served in Vietnam, although the source of a possible transmission remained unclear [23]. Despite this large number of melioidosis cases related to Vietnam during this period of time, very little information on the disease was reported for the indigenous population (Table 1).

Table 1. Number of indigenous Vietnamese patients with melioidosis and the respective outcome reported over time in medical journals.

Year of Reporting	No. of Patient	No. of Recoveries [a]	No. of Deaths	No. of Unknown Outcome	Reference
1926	1	0	1	0	[3]
1949	9	5	0	4	[6]
1958	1	0	1	0	[10]
1967	1	1	0	0	[11]
1995	7	1	6	0	[24]
1990	1	1	0	0	[25]
1999	9	0	0	9	[26]
2008	55	32	17	6	[27]
2018	70	30	18	22	[28]

[a] Recovery during the study.

2.1.3. 1990s until Present

In 1991, a medical thesis defended at Hanoi Medical University described 16 cases detected in hospitals of Hanoi over a 10-year period from 1980 to 1990, with seven fatal outcomes [29]. A study by Phung et al. (1993) using an IHA test revealed seropositivity in populations living in suburban communities of Hanoi ranging from 6.4% to 31.8%. This study also observed an association of seropositivity with rice farming [30]. In a study on cellular lipid and fatty acid composition of *B. pseudomallei*, seven patients with melioidosis were listed from whom strains were isolated in Vietnam between 1981 and 1991 [24]. In 1999, a retrospective study in the South reported only nine culture-confirmed cases with melioidosis from 3653 blood cultures of febrile patients admitted to the largest hospital for tropical diseases in Ho Chi Minh City from 1992 to 1998 [26]. Antibiotic treatment and patient outcomes were not reported in this study. In 2008, another retrospective study in the largest general hospital in the North reported 55 culture-confirmed cases observed in a period of time from 1997 to 2005. Analysis of clinical data showed that septicemia with pneumonia was the most common clinical presentation and diabetes was the most common risk factor. Seventeen out of

40 septicemic patients died, with nine deaths occurring within 48 h after admission. Based on the residential addresses of the patients, it was concluded that melioidosis is widely distributed and occurs in at least 18 of 25 northern provinces [27]. In the context of the Research Network on Melioidosis and *Burkholderia pseudomallei* (RENOMAB; see below Section 5) that started in 2014, a recent study reported 70 cases detected within seven months at five hospitals in North Central Vietnam. During the study period, the detection rate of *B. pseudomallei* ranged from 3.4% to 10.2% among positive blood cultures in those hospitals. Fifty-eight patients had septicemia. Of the 36 patients with known outcome, 18 patients died, with 6 deaths occurring within 48 h after admission [28]. However, as for other regions, the true burden of melioidosis in North Central Vietnam still needs to be determined (see below Section 7). The few epidemiological data available for Vietnam imply that rice farmers are at particular risk to acquire a *B. pseudomallei* infection [26–28].

2.2. Animal Melioidosis

2.2.1. 1930s to 1960s

At the time when the first human case of melioidosis was detected in Vietnam, the disease was considered to be a zoonosis and animals a reservoir for *B. pseudomallei*. This assumption was based on the observation that *B. pseudomallei* could infect laboratory rodents and its virulence was comparable to *Yesinia pestis*, the causative agent of plague. However, a large microbiological study of more than 20,500 rats collected in southern Vietnam found only one rat to be culture-positive for *B. pseudomallei* as cited by Luong (1956) [31]. None of the 560 wild rats caught in Hanoi were positive for *B. pseudomallei* by culture [1]. Serological studies showed that serum collected from pigs contained antibodies against *B. pseudomallei*, as cited by Luong (1956) [31]. In 1954, melioidosis was detected in rabbits and guinea pigs at the Pasteur Institute of Ho Chi Minh City, as cited by Luong (1961) [32]. In 1955, Luong described culture-confirmed melioidosis cases in pigs at a pig farm near a rubber plantation in Thu Dau Mot (now Ho Chi Minh City), with the isolation of *B. pseudomallei* from creamy pus in lung and spleen abscesses [31]. Using serology and culture methods, several deaths of pigs were confirmed to be caused by melioidosis in the farms at Tan Son Nhat and Gia Dinh (now both are Ho Chi Minh City) [32].

2.2.2. 1970s until Present

In 1971, cases of melioidosis were reported in the U.S. Army dogs in the Republic of South Vietnam. During a six-month period, 31 working dogs died, with four confirmed melioidosis cases. *B. pseudomallei* was cultured from the dogs' lungs and various organs. The dogs came from different units in diverse locations in Vietnam. All of the dogs showed lesions in the lungs, epididymides, and testes [33]. The author stated that melioidosis remained underdiagnosed because bacteriologic cultures were not routinely performed at necropsy of the U.S. Army working dogs and that the disease does not seem to be uncommon in dogs. A serologic surveillance on 64 healthy U.S. military scout and tracker dogs after service in the Republic of South Vietnam showed that 12 (19%) dogs had developed antibodies against *B. pseudomallei*, with IHA titers higher than 1:80 [34]. After reunification in 1975, no further information about melioidosis in pigs or other livestock, as well as dogs, has been reported in Vietnam. Only recently, in the context of RENOMAB, a study carried out by a group at the National Institute of Veterinary Research reported a culture-confirmed melioidosis case of a pig in a farm at Nghe An province in North Central Vietnam [35].

3. *B. pseudomallei* in the Environment

The first experimental indication of the saprophytic nature of *B. pseudomallei* and its environmental reservoir was provided in Vietnam by Vaucel in 1937 [1]. His studies were triggered by the observation that individuals who developed melioidosis after traffic accidents were either immersed for a prolonged time in water of a pond or had a skull wound contaminated with mud. To test the hypothesis that *B. pseudomallei* exists in the environment, Vaucel submerged the scratched abdomen of guinea pigs into water of a pond collected in the North. Five days later, a moribund animal was sacrificed and *B. pseudomallei* was isolated from pus of the liver and spleen and other sites on solid media in pure culture [1]. About 20 years later in 1955, Chambon provided final evidence by directly isolating seven *B. pseudomallei* strains from five environmental samples including pond muds, rice field water, and a sample of pond water collected in the South [2]. In 1961, Luong provided further evidence for environmental *B. pseudomallei,* when two strains were cultured from water samples of a water spinach plantation from southern Vietnam [32].

Apart from this early environmental work, there are only a few more recent studies sampling rice fields for *B. pseudomallei*. In 1991, a study reported the isolation of *B. pseudomallei* from 4 out of 240 soil samples, and 1 out of 190 surface water samples collected in rice fields at four communities surrounding Hanoi was positive for *B. pseudomallei* [30]. Between 1992 and 1998 soil samples were collected from 137 rice fields around Ho Chi Minh City in southern Vietnam and nine fields were found to be positive [26]. The low *B. pseudomallei* detection rate from soil in those sampling studies is likely to be the result of the current culture protocols for environmental *B. pseudomallei* which have a limited sensitivity. It has been shown recently, that a multitarget quantitative PCR approach improves the detection rate and can predict cultivability of *B. pseudomallei* [36]. By using this multitarget qPCR, *B. pseudomallei* was detected in 35 (83.3%) out of 42 soil samples collected at 28 rice fields in southern Vietnam. From those samples, *B. pseudomallei* strains could be isolated from six (14.3%) samples by using conventional culture methods [36].

A recent prediction of the global environmental presence of *B. pseudomallei* at 5×5 km^2 spatial resolution suggested that predominant parts of Vietnam are highly suitable for the environmental occurrence of *B. pseudomallei* [37]. However, mountainous areas near the border with Laos and China, especially in the Northwest region, some regions in the Central Highlands, and a zone involving the lower South Central Coast were found to be less suitable. It will be most important to test these predictions in future environmental studies and also to investigate the environmental factors involved in creating a habitat for *B. pseudomallei* at a high spatial resolution. The country harbors an enormous diversity of habitats ranging from tropical rain forest to dry forest, natural grassland, and agricultural land such as rice paddies to wetland habitats including rivers and lakes and coastal wetlands. Apart from the limited studies on rice fields, there is no information on the potential role of such different habitats as environmental reservoirs for *B. pseudomallei*. Since Vietnam has an enormous north–south expansion, including humid subtropical climate in the north, tropical monsoon climate in the center, and tropical wet and dry climate in the south, the potential influence of climate factors on the environmental presence of *B. pseudomallei* needs to be investigated. For the development of any preventive strategies or environmental countermeasures it will be important to define risk areas for infection and the role of different habitats and climate factors more precisely.

4. Phenotype, Genomic Diversity, and Phylogenetic Relatedness of *B. pseudomallei*

When the first *B. pseudomallei* strain was isolated from clinical specimens in 1925, the occurrence of different morphotypes, in this case rugose and ultra-rugose colonies on agar, were described [4]. As we now know various morphotypes represent a frequent characteristic of this species. Subsequent work demonstrated virulence of clinical and environmental *B. pseudomallei* strains in experimental infections and described antibiotic susceptibility to drugs available at that time [4,8,11,38]. A more recent study with 25 strains from northern Vietnam reported an antibiotic resistance profile that is also found in other endemic areas, with susceptibility to currently-recommended antibiotics for treatment of melioidosis such as ceftazidime, imipenem, meropenem, and co-trimoxazole. Resistance and intermediate resistance to tetracycline were noted for one strain and three strains, respectively [27].

In a study describing physiological and biochemical characteristics of 15 environmental and clinical *B. pseudomallei* strains from northern Vietnam, all strains shared typical *B. pseudomallei* characteristics with respect to motility, salt tolerance, growth temperature, sugar assimilation, cytochrome c oxidase and acid production, and colony morphology on different routine agar media [24]. The composition of cellular lipids and fatty acids were similar among the tested strains [24]. Biochemical and antigenic characteristics typical for *B. pseudomallei* were also described by Phuong et al. (2008) using the API 20 NE system and through agglutination of those strains with a *B. pseudomallei*-specific monoclonal antibody [27].

The *Burkholderia pseudomallei* 'Multi-Locus Sequence Typing' (MLST) database is a rich resource to assess the genomic population structure based on seven housekeeping genes (https://pubmlst.org/bpseudomallei/ [39]. Since the development of the *B. pseudomallei* MLST scheme in 2003 [40], 104 isolates from Vietnam have been deposited in the database (5309 isolates overall) as of 14 February 2018 [27,41]. A total of 61 sequence types (STs) were identified, emphasizing the great genotypic diversity of the sampled population in this region. Of those, 31 STs were uniquely reported in Vietnam so far and most of the remaining STs are shared with neighboring countries like Thailand or Cambodia. The co-occurrence of the latter and the concomitant lack of regional specificity have already been noticed for other STs [41]. As already implied by Phuong et al. (2008), analysis of current *B. pseudomallei* MLST data showed the Vietnamese strains to mainly cluster with other Asian isolates as opposed to the Australian STs.

However, special care must be taken when analyzing *B. pseudomallei* MLST data. Its high recombination rate complicates the inferences of phylogenetic relationships of sequence types (STs) [42,43]. Nevertheless, the unprecedented amount of deposited data and the comparatively cheap prices render it a valuable tool, despite the emergence of next generation sequencing. With the advent of next generation sequencing (NGS), whole genome sequencing (WGS) has proven a powerful tool to study population genetics at a much higher resolution. This was recently shown by De Smet et al. (2015), reporting two strains, which shared one ST due to homoplasy, but could be distinguished by WGS [44].

Phylogentic studies based on single nucleotide polymorphisms (SNP) present strong evidence for an Australian *B. pseudomallei* origin [43,45] and a single transmission event to Southeast Asia [43,46]. In a recent study by Chewapreecha et al. (2017) on the global evolution and prevalence of *B. pseudomallei*, 19 strains from Vietnam (spanning a time period from 1947 to 2011) were subjected to whole genome sequencing and placed in a global context (469 isolates) [46]. A SNP-based phylogenetic analysis of these genomes clearly resolved Australian, Asian, and African/American clusters.

Strains from Vietnam appeared in 7 of 17 Asian subgroups, with most of the other members of the subgroup being from Thailand and Cambodia and belonging to the 'Mekong sub-region'. The other Asian subgroups contained mainly isolates from Malaysia and Singapore ('Malay cluster'). It could be shown that the transitions of *B. pseudomallei* between these two sub-regions was less than within the sub-region. As noted by the authors, this observation might be linked to trading networks and cultural links. Furthermore, the results indicate that the Mekong sub-region might have been a hotspot for the evolution of *B. pseudomallei* in Southeast Asia. Unfortunately, in contrast to other Asian clusters, no time could be estimated for the emergence of the most recent common ancestor of the Vietnam-containing subgroups. Besides, the study also demonstrates the potential of WGS to account for geographical differences in disease outcome, by screening for region-specific (virulence) loci [46]. The insights, based on just 19 Vietnamese isolates, already imply the wealth of information that can presumably be gained from such a high level of resolution. Should more rigorous clinical and environmental sampling schemes be applied and a higher number of strains analyzed, this will likely increase our knowledge of *B. pseudomallei* phylogeny and virulence tremendously. There is no doubt that these are interesting times for studying the genomic diversity of *B. pseudomallei* in Vietnam.

5. Activities to Raise Awareness of Melioidosis in Vietnam and Major Achievements

As in many parts of the world, neither melioidosis nor characteristics of *B. pseudomallei* are mandatory components of curricula at medical universities in Vietnam. This leads to a lack of knowledge among many doctors and other health care professionals about how to diagnose and manage the disease. As outlined above, this limited clinical awareness together with limited laboratory resources result in significant underdiagnosis. This has been very obvious in the central part of Vietnam. Although it is located in the same geographical belt and is close to highly endemic areas of Laos and northeast Thailand, cases of melioidosis were not reported from there until recently.

In 2014, a bilateral project called Research Network on Melioidosis and *Burkholderia pseudomallei* (RENOMAB), sponsored by the German Ministry for Education and Research and the Vietnamese Ministry of Science and Technology, was started. The project involved 40 national and regional hospitals in 27 provinces and cities throughout the country. By organizing a series of workshops on diagnosis of melioidosis for laboratory staff, hundreds of culture-confirmed cases have recently been detected [28]. Two national scientific conferences on melioidosis were organized in order to raise awareness of the disease among infectious disease physicians, microbiological laboratory staff, medical teachers, researchers, and health-care managers.

Active melioidosis case-finding reports were presented at national scientific conferences for infectious and respiratory diseases [47,48]. Scientific papers on melioidosis have started to appear in national journals [49]. The existence of the disease was also broadcasted in a wide range of public media such as hospital web portals, newspapers and television programs. A private Facebook group named Research Network on Melioidosis in Vietnam (Hoi Nghien cuu Melioidosis tai Vietnam) was created and consists of approximately 600 members from the healthcare system interested in melioidosis diagnostics. At the time of writing, 36 hospitals in 26 provinces and cities reported culture-confirmed melioidosis cases (Figure 1). Of these, 28 hospitals detected the first cases of the disease after joining case-finding activities within RENOMAB. This project has shown that melioidosis is widely distributed throughout the country with a potential area of high endemicity in North Central Vietnam [28]. The organization of the 9th World Melioidosis Congress in 2019 in Hanoi will be a golden opportunity to further raise awareness for melioidosis and to promote research on different aspects of epidemiology, diagnosis, and treatment in Vietnam.

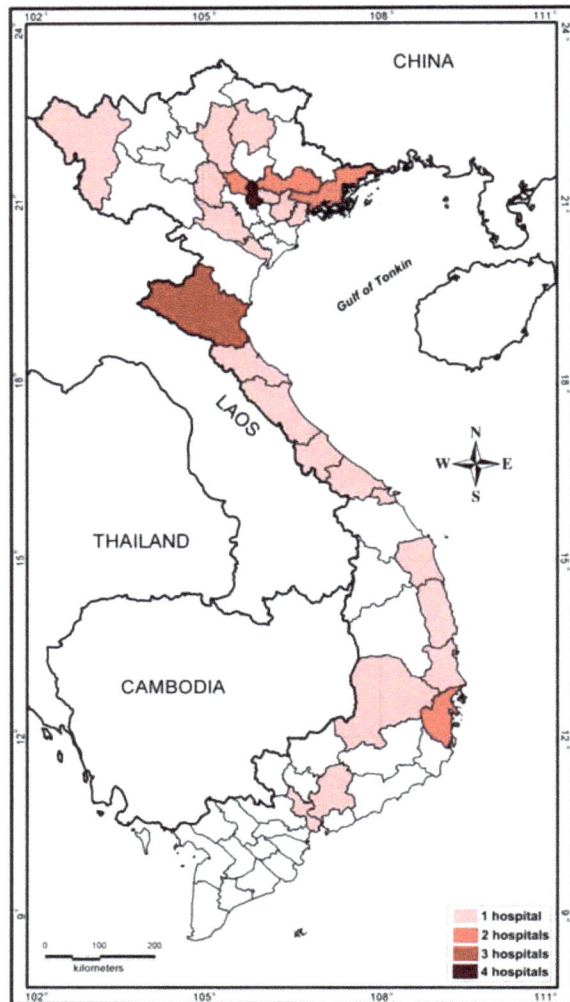

Figure 1. Location of hospitals taking part in the RENOMAB project and reporting culture-confirmed melioidosis cases. All of the *B. pseudomallei* strains were sent to the reference laboratory at the Institute of Microbiology and Biotechnology, Vietnam National University, Hanoi. *B. pseudomallei* identification of bacterial strains was confirmed by using either *recA* sequence analysis or *B. pseudomallei*-specific TTSS1 real-time PCR assay [28]. Border lines of provinces or cities are shown. The color indicates the number of hospitals within the province or city that reported cases of melioidosis. Geographic map was constructed by the MapInfo 7.8 (MapInfo, Troy, NY, USA).

6. Current Recommendations for Diagnosis and Treatment and for Reporting and Prevention

6.1. Diagnosis and Treatment

Currently, there are no official guidelines for diagnosis and treatment of melioidosis issued by the Vietnamese Ministry of Health, and *B. pseudomallei* has not been yet on the list of any national surveillance programs for infectious agents. The current recommendations that have been distributed via seminars, workshops, and national conferences, are based on studies and guidelines from the international literature.

In well-equipped laboratories commercially-available biochemical tests and automated identification systems are routinely used. However, even under such circumstances, a lack of awareness and of additional diagnostic tools can lead to unreliable diagnoses, since misidentification of *B. pseudomallei* has been well documented for such systems [50]. In remote areas where laboratory facilities and resources for consumables are still limited, the identification of bacterial pathogens mostly relies on some basic microbiological tests, and the identification of Gram-negative non-fermenting bacterial species is even more challenging. We therefore recently introduced a simple laboratory algorithm for identification of *B. pseudomallei* from clinical specimens under such resource-constrained conditions. The algorithm makes use of the inherent resistance of *B. pseudomallei* to gentamicin and colistin and the susceptibility to amoxicillin-clavulanic acid [28].

Although the sensitivity and specificity of this algorithm have not been validated yet, compared to more sophisticated identification procedures including selective media such as Ashdown's agar for non-sterile sites, it proved to be an effective and inexpensive procedure leading to the diagnosis of a significant number of melioidosis patients at provincial general hospitals in North Central Vietnam in a short period of time after introduction [28]. We therefore currently recommend the implementation of this simple algorithm in clinical laboratories for a presumptive diagnosis of *B. pseudomallei* from clinical materials. Confirmation of the identification can be obtained in reference laboratories using specific type three secretion system 1 (TTSS1) real-time PCR assays and sequencing of the *recA* gene as reliable target [28].

6.2. Surveillance and Prevention

Melioidosis is not a notifiable disease in Vietnam. There is neither a formal surveillance system for human nor for animal melioidosis in Vietnam. There are also no official recommendations on prevention. The limited epidemiological data available in Vietnam indicate that rice farmers are at a particular risk, similar to other parts of Southeast Asia. At present, it seems plausible to primarily target the rice farming population in terms of better diagnostics and evaluation of possible preventive measures. The majority of them are living in remote areas where the primary healthcare system of the country does not cover microbiological investigations. It is therefore most likely that fatal cases of melioidosis in remote areas are still grossly under recognized.

7. Current and Future Challenges

Although some progress has recently been made in Vietnam to increase awareness of melioidosis and to enhance laboratory skills for identification of *B. pseudomallei* from clinical specimens, there are still significant efforts needed to further improve capacity building in different regions of Vietnam.

Apart from further improving the identification capacity in the laboratories via diagnostic workshops and scientific conferences it will be crucial to generally increase the number of clinical specimens—such as urine, throat swabs, sputum, pus, etc.—to be sent to the laboratory for microbiological investigations. Since bacteremic melioidosis is a common clinical presentation and also associated with a high case fatality rate, increasing the number of blood cultures in patients with prolonged fever has a high priority. There are financial barriers and insurance issues that hinder an appropriate use of blood cultures in the diagnosis not only for melioidosis, but also for other systemic infections, which need to be addressed. Epidemiological studies are needed to determine the true incidence and prevalence of melioidosis in the various regions. The same is true for the veterinary field, where information on melioidosis is still very scarce.

In parallel to capacity building in the clinical laboratory, studies on the environmental distribution of *B. pseudomallei* in Vietnam will be important to define risk areas for the indigenous population more precisely. This information can be used to further target clinical microbiology activities. In addition, serological screening of the indigenous population using newly-developed devices might help to detect exposure to *B. pseudomallei* and to identify possible endemic hot spots.

Acknowledgments: We would like to thank Minh N. Nguyen, at the Faculty of Environmental Science, University of Science, Vietnam National University, Hanoi, for his help in constructing the geographic map. We would like to thank the Vietnamese Ministry of Science and Technology and the German Federal Ministry of Education and Research for co-funding the collaborative RENOMAB project (reference 01DP13007). The National Conferences on Melioidosis were made possible by support from the Vietnam National University, Hanoi; the World Health Organization representative in Vietnam; the Cooperative Biological Engagement Program, Defense Threat Reduction Agency, US Department of Defence, USA; and the US Agency for International Development in Vietnam. The authors and conference organizers are extremely grateful to the valuable contributions of international melioidosis experts, including David Dance (Lao-Oxford-Mahosot Hospital Wellcome Trust Research Unit, Vientiane, Laos), Ploenchan Chetchotisakd (Faculty of Medicine, Khon Kaen University, Thailand), Daniel Altmann (Department of Medicine, Imperial College London, United Kingdom), Direk Limmathurotsakul (Mahidol-Oxford Tropical Medicine Research Unit, Faculty of Tropical Medicine, Mahidol University, Thailand), Wuthiekanun Vanaporn (Mahidol-Oxford Tropical Medicine Research Unit, Faculty of Tropical Medicine, Mahidol University, Thailand), and Bart Currie (Menzies School of Health Research, Charles Darwin University and Royal Darwin Hospital, Australia). We acknowledge all of the hospitals and partners involved in the RENOMAB project.

Author Contributions: T.T.T., I.S., T.V.N., C.D.D., C.X.T., A.V.L. and H.V.N. participated in activities related to RENOMAB and conceived and designed the overall structure of the manuscript. L.D.N.N. and I.S. compiled information from French articles. K.A., S.L. and G.E.W. contributed to drafting Sections 3 and 4 and editing the manuscript. T.T.T., G.E.W. and I.S. wrote the manuscript. All authors approved the final version of the manuscript.

Conflicts of Interest: The authors declare no conflict of interest.

References

1. Vaucel, M. Présence probable du bacille de Whitmore dans l'eau de mare au Tonkin. *Bull. Soc. Pathol. Exot.* **1937**, *30*, 10–15.

2. Chambon, L. Isolement du bacille de Whitmore a partir du milieu extérieur. *Ann. Inst. Pasteur* **1955**, *89*, 229–235.

3. Pons, R.; Advier, M. Melioidosis in Cochin China. *J. Hyg. (Lond.)* **1927**, *26*, 28–30. [CrossRef] [PubMed]

4. Stanton, A.T.; Fletcher, W. Melioidosis: Notes on a culture of *B. whitmori* from Saigon. *J. Hyg. (Lond.)* **1927**, *26*, 31–32. [CrossRef] [PubMed]

5. Pons, R. La Mélioïdose maladie commune à l'homme, aux rongeurs et aux équidés. *Bull. Soc. Pathol. Exot.* **1930**, *23*, 210–215.

6. Alain, M.; Saint-Etienne, J.; Reynes, V. La mélioïdose; considérations étiologiques cliniques et pathogèniques à propos de 28 cas. *Med. Trop.* **1949**, *9*, 119–142.

7. Duroux, A. La mélioïdose pulmonaire. *Poumon Coeur* **1965**, *21*, 355–372. [PubMed]

8. Guillermand, J.; Barrié, J.; Morilleau, R.; Couderc, P. Mélioïdose pulmonaire chronique (Observation anatomoclinique). *Poumon Couer* **1964**, *20*, 269–285.

9. Sanford, J.P. Melioidosis: Forgotten but not gone. *Trans. Am. Clin. Climatol. Assoc.* **1978**, *89*, 201–205. [PubMed]

10. Stein, W.; Duc, N.H.; Low, F.J. Acute melioidosis. *USA Armed Forces Med. J.* **1958**, *9*, 273–276.

11. Mo, H.D.; Cuong, T.H. A typical case of melioidosis in South Vietnam. *Mil. Med.* **1967**, *132*, 98–100.

12. Diamond, H.S.; Pastore, R. Septic arthritis due to *Pseudomonas pseudomallei*. *Arthritis Rheumatol.* **1967**, *10*, 459–466. [CrossRef]

13. Spotnitz, M.; Rudnitzky, J.; Rambaud, J.J. Melioidosis pneumonitis. Analysis of nine cases of a benign form of melioidosis. *JAMA* **1967**, *202*, 950–954. [CrossRef] [PubMed]

14. Weber, D.R.; Douglass, L.E.; Brundage, W.G.; Stallkamp, T.C. Acute varieties of melioidosis occurring in U.S. soldiers in Vietnam. *Am. J. Med.* **1969**, *46*, 234–244. [CrossRef]

15. Deller, J.J. Diseases from Vietnam. *Calif. Med.* **1969**, *111*, 461–466.

16. Sanford, J.P.; Moore, W.L., Jr. Recrudescent melioidosis: A Southeast Asian legacy. *Am. Rev. Respir. Dis.* **1971**, *104*, 452–453. [CrossRef] [PubMed]

17. Everett, E.D.; Nelson, R.A. Pulmonary melioidosis. Observations in thirty-nine cases. *Am. Rev. Respir. Dis.* **1975**, *112*, 331–340. [PubMed]

18. Clayton, A.J.; Lisella, R.S.; Martin, D.G. Melioidosis: A serological survey in military personnel. *Mil. Med.* **1973**, *138*, 24–26. [CrossRef] [PubMed]

19. Morrison, R.E.; Lamb, A.S.; Craig, D.B.; Johnson, W.M. Melioidosis: A reminder. *Am. J. Med.* **1988**, *84*, 965–967. [CrossRef]

20. Koponen, M.A.; Zlock, D.; Palmer, D.L.; Merlin, T.L. Melioidosis. Forgotten, but not gone! *Arch. Intern. Med.* **1991**, *151*, 605–608. [CrossRef] [PubMed]

21. Time Magazine. Diseases: Vietnam's Time Bomb, 10 February 1967. Available online: http://content.time.com/time/magazine/article/0,9171,840848,00.html (accessed on 12 March 2018).

22. McCormick, J.B.; Sexton, D.J.; McMurray, J.G.; Carey, E.; Hayes, P.; Feldman, R.A. Human-to-human transmission of *Pseudomonas pseudomallei*. *Ann. Intern. Med.* **1975**, *83*, 512–513. [CrossRef] [PubMed]

23. Osteraas, G.R.; Hardman, J.M.; Bass, J.W.; Wilson, C. Neonatal melioidosis. *Am. J. Dis. Child.* **1971**, *122*, 446–448. [CrossRef] [PubMed]

24. Phung, L.V.; Tran, T.B.; Hotta, H.; Yabuuchi, E.; Yano, I. Cellular lipid and fatty acid compositions of *Burkholderia pseudomallei* strains isolated from human and environment in Vietnam. *Microbiol. Immunol.* **1995**, *39*, 105–116. [CrossRef] [PubMed]

25. Worthington, M.G.; McEniry, D.W. Chronic melioidosis in a Vietnamese immigrant. *Rev. Infect. Dis.* **1990**, *12*, 966. [CrossRef] [PubMed]

26. Parry, C.M.; Wuthiekanun, V.; Hoa, N.T.; Diep, T.S.; Thao, L.T.; Loc, P.V.; Wills, B.A.; Wain, J.; Hien, T.T.; White, N.J.; et al. Melioidosis in Southern Vietnam: Clinical surveillance and environmental sampling. *Clin. Infect. Dis.* **1999**, *29*, 1323–1326. [CrossRef] [PubMed]

27. Phuong, D.M.; Trung, T.T.; Breitbach, K.; Tuan, N.Q.; Nubel, U.; Flunker, G.; Khang, D.D.; Quang, N.X.; Steinmetz, I. Clinical and microbiological features of melioidosis in northern Vietnam. *Trans. R. Soc. Trop. Med. Hyg.* **2008**, *102*, S30–S36. [CrossRef]

28. Trinh, T.T.; Hoang, T.S.; Tran, D.A.; Trinh, V.T.; Gohler, A.; Nguyen, T.T.; Hoang, S.N.; Krumkamp, R.; Nguyen, L.T.N.; May, J.; et al. A simple laboratory algorithm for diagnosis of melioidosis in resource-constrained areas: A study from north-central Vietnam. *Clin. Microbiol. Infect.* **2018**, *24*, 84.e1–84.e4. [CrossRef] [PubMed]

29. Lam, N.T. Clinical Features and Outcomes of Melioidosis Patients. Bachelor's Thesis, Hanoi Medical University, Hanoi, Vietnam, 1991.

30. Phung, L.V.; Quynh, H.T.; Yabuuchi, E.; Dance, D.A. Pilot study of exposure to *Pseudomonas pseudomallei* in northern Vietnam. *Trans. R. Soc. Trop. Med. Hyg.* **1993**, *87*, 416. [CrossRef]

31. Luong, N.B. A propos d'une épizootie porcine de mélioidose dans une province méridionale du Vietnam. *Bull. Soc. Pathol. Exot.* **1956**, *49*, 25–31.

32. Luong, N.B.; Kim, N.T. La mélioidose porcine au Vietnam. *Off. Int. Epizoot.* **1961**, *56*, 944–976.

33. Stedham, M.A. Melioidosis in dogs in Vietnam. *J. Am. Vet. Med. Assoc.* **1971**, *158*, 1948–1950. [PubMed]

34. Alexander, A.D.; Huxsoll, D.L.; Warner, A.R., Jr.; Shepler, V.; Dorsey, A. Serological diagnosis of human melioidosis with indirect hemagglutination and complement fixation tests. *Appl. Microbiol.* **1970**, *20*, 825–833. [PubMed]

35. Hang, N.T.T.; Hang, T.T.T.; Trung, T.T. Initial investigation of pig with melioidosis caused by *Burkholderia pseudomallei* at Nghe An province. *Vietnam Vet. Assoc. Vet. Sci. Tech.* **2018**, *25*, 48–55.

36. Gohler, A.; Trung, T.T.; Hopf, V.; Kohler, C.; Hartleib, J.; Wuthiekanun, V.; Peacock, S.J.; Limmathurotsakul, D.; Tuanyok, A.; Steinmetz, I. Multitarget quantitative PCR improves detection and predicts cultivability of the pathogen *Burkholderia pseudomallei*. *Appl. Environ. Microbiol.* **2017**, *83*, e03212–e03216. [CrossRef] [PubMed]

37. Limmathurotsakul, D.; Golding, N.; Dance, D.A.; Messina, J.P.; Pigott, D.M.; Moyes, C.L.; Rolim, D.B.; Bertherat, E.; Day, N.P.; Peacock, S.J.; et al. Predicted global distribution of *Burkholderia pseudomallei* and burden of melioidosis. *Nat. Microbiol.* **2016**, *1*, 15008. [CrossRef] [PubMed]

38. Borchardt, K.A.; Stansifer, P.; Albano, P.M. Osteomyelitis due to *Pseudomonas pseudomallei*. *JAMA* **1966**, *196*, 660–662. [CrossRef] [PubMed]

39. Jolley, K.A.; Maiden, M.C. BIGSdb: Scalable analysis of bacterial genome variation at the population level. *BMC Bioinf.* **2010**, *11*, 595. [CrossRef] [PubMed]

40. Godoy, D.; Randle, G.; Simpson, A.J.; Aanensen, D.M.; Pitt, T.L.; Kinoshita, R.; Spratt, B.G. Multilocus sequence typing and evolutionary relationships among the causative agents of melioidosis and glanders, *Burkholderia pseudomallei* and *Burkholderia mallei*. *J. Clin. Microbiol.* **2003**, *41*, 2068–2079. [CrossRef] [PubMed]

41. McCombie, R.L.; Finkelstein, R.A.; Woods, D.E. Multilocus sequence typing of historical *Burkholderia pseudomallei* isolates collected in Southeast Asia from 1964 to 1967 provides insight into the epidemiology of melioidosis. *J. Clin. Microbiol.* **2006**, *44*, 2951–2962. [CrossRef] [PubMed]

42. Vesaratchavest, M.; Tumapa, S.; Day, N.P.; Wuthiekanun, V.; Chierakul, W.; Holden, M.T.; White, N.J.; Currie, B.J.; Spratt, B.G.; Feil, E.J.; et al. Nonrandom distribution of *Burkholderia pseudomallei* clones in relation to geographical location and virulence. *J. Clin. Microbiol.* **2006**, *44*, 2553–2557. [CrossRef] [PubMed]

43. Pearson, T.; Giffard, P.; Beckstrom-Sternberg, S.; Auerbach, R.; Hornstra, H.; Tuanyok, A.; Price, E.P.; Glass, M.B.; Leadem, B.; Beckstrom-Sternberg, J.S.; et al. Phylogeographic reconstruction of a bacterial species with high levels of lateral gene transfer. *BMC Biol.* **2009**, *7*, 78. [CrossRef] [PubMed]

44. De Smet, B.; Sarovich, D.S.; Price, E.P.; Mayo, M.; Theobald, V.; Kham, C.; Heng, S.; Thong, P.; Holden, M.T.; Parkhill, J.; et al. Whole-genome sequencing confirms that *Burkholderia pseudomallei* multilocus sequence types common to both Cambodia and Australia are due to homoplasy. *J. Clin. Microbiol.* **2015**, *53*, 323–326. [CrossRef] [PubMed]

45. Price, E.P.; Sarovich, D.S.; Smith, E.J.; MacHunter, B.; Harrington, G.; Theobald, V.; Hall, C.M.; Hornstra, H.M.; McRobb, E.; Podin, Y.; et al. Unprecedented melioidosis cases in Northern Australia caused by an Asian *Burkholderia pseudomallei* strain identified by using large-scale comparative genomics. *Appl. Environ. Microbiol.* **2016**, *82*, 954–963. [CrossRef] [PubMed]

46. Chewapreecha, C.; Holden, M.T.; Vehkala, M.; Valimaki, N.; Yang, Z.; Harris, S.R.; Mather, A.E.; Tuanyok, A.; De Smet, B.; Le Hello, S.; et al. Global and regional dissemination and evolution of *Burkholderia pseudomallei*. *Nat. Microbiol.* **2017**, *2*, 16263. [CrossRef] [PubMed]

47. Trung, T.T.; Tiep, H.S.; Dao, T.A.; Tram, Q.A.; Vinh, T.T.; Toan, N.T.; Sanh, H.N.; Lien, N.T.N.; Cuong, D.D.; Phuong, D.M.; et al. Melioidosis in north central part of Vietnam: A series of cases detected after raising awareness and introducing a simple laboratory algorithm. In Proceedings of the Annual Congress of Vietnam Respiratory Society, Hanoi, Vietnam, 23–24 September 2016.

48. Huy, N.Q.; Tra, D.T.; Cuong, N.C.; Cuong, D.H. Clinical features, diagnosis and outcomes of patients with melioidosis at Bach Mai hospital from 2012 to 2015. In Proceedings of the National Scientific Conference on Infectious Diseases and HIV/AIDS, Ninhbinh, Vietnam, 7–9 September 2017.

49. Huong, H.T.L.; Vinh, T.D.; Loan, P.T.T.; Nguyet, H.T.A.; Trinh, P.T.T. Case study: Melioidosis (Whitmore's disease). *Cent. Hosp. J. Clin. Med.* **2016**, *38*, 159–167.

50. Hoffmaster, A.R.; AuCoin, D.; Baccam, P.; Baggett, H.C.; Baird, R.; Bhengsri, S.; Blaney, D.D.; Brett, P.J.; Brooks, T.J.; Brown, K.A.; et al. Melioidosis diagnostic workshop, 2013. *Emerg. Infect. Dis.* **2015**, *21*. [CrossRef]

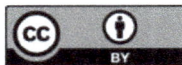

Tropical Medicine and Infectious Disease

MDPI

Review

Melioidosis in Hong Kong

Grace Lui [1,*], Anthony Tam [2], Eugene Y. K. Tso [3], Alan K. L. Wu [4], Jonpaul Zee [5], Kin Wing Choi [6], Wilson Lam [7], Man Chun Chan [8], Wan Man Ting [7] and Ivan F. N. Hung [2,9,10,*]

[1] Department of Medicine and Therapeutics, Faculty of Medicine, Stanley Ho Centre for Emerging Infectious Diseases, The Chinese University of Hong Kong, Hong Kong, China

[2] Department of Medicine, Queen Mary Hospital, Hong Kong, China; antamwf@connect.hku.hk

[3] Department of Medicine and Geriatrics, United Christian Hospital, Hong Kong, China; tsoyke@ha.org.hk

[4] Department of Clinical Pathology, Pamela Youde Nethersole Eastern Hospital, Hong Kong, China; alanklwu@gmail.com

[5] Department of Clinical Pathology, Tuen Mun Hospital, Hong Kong, China; jonpaulzee@gmail.com

[6] Department of Medicine, Alice Ho Miu Ling Nethersole Hospital, Hong Kong, China; choikw1@ha.org.hk

[7] Department of Medicine, Queen Elizabeth Hospital, Hong Kong, China; lwzz04@ha.org.hk (W.L.); twm608@ha.org.hk (W.M.T.)

[8] Department of Medicine and Geriatrics, Princess Margaret Hospital, Hong Kong, China; cmc061@ha.org.hk

[9] Carol Yu Centre for Infection, Department of Medicine, Li Ka Shing Faculty of Medicine, The University of Hong Kong, Hong Kong, China

[10] Department of Clinical Microbiology and Infection Control, The University of Hong Kong-Shenzhen Hospital, Shenzhen 518172, China

* Correspondence: gracelui@cuhk.edu.hk (G.L.); ivanhung@hku.hk (I.F.N.H.); Tel.: +85-23-505-1464 (G.L.); +85-22-255-4049 (I.F.N.H.)

Received: 1 August 2018; Accepted: 21 August 2018; Published: 25 August 2018

Abstract: Melioidosis, although endemic in many parts of Southeast Asia, has not been systematically studied in Hong Kong, which is a predominantly urban area located in the subtropics. This review describes the early outbreaks of melioidosis in captive animals in Hong Kong in the 1970s, as well as the early reports of human clinical cases in the 1980s. A review of all hospitalized human cases of culture-confirmed melioidosis in the last twenty years showed an increasing trend in the incidence of the disease, with significant mortality observed. The lack of awareness of this disease among local physicians, the delay in laboratory diagnosis and the lack of epidemiological surveillance are among the greatest challenges of managing melioidosis in the territory.

Keywords: melioidosis; *Burkholderia pseudomallei*; Hong Kong

1. Introduction

Melioidosis is an emerging infectious disease caused by *Burkholderia pseudomallei* that causes significant morbidity and mortality [1]. Melioidosis was first described in Southeast Asia in the early 1910s [2]. Since then, melioidosis has been well recognized to be highly endemic in northern Australia and many parts of Asia, with the highest prevalence observed in Southeast and South Asia [3,4]. It is being increasingly reported in previously non-endemic regions [4].

Melioidosis is endemic in regions located at tropical latitudes between 20° N and 20° S [1]. However, there is an increasing bulk of evidence of this disease in territories with no previous documentation of melioidosis, as well as an expansion of the geographical areas with a significant burden of the disease outside the tropics, including Southern China [5,6] and Taiwan [7]. Hong Kong is also considered to be situated in an endemic region with high environmental suitability for *B. pseudomallei* [3,4].

Despite its high fatality rate, melioidosis is often a neglected disease. It has been estimated that the disease was regularly under-reported in many countries [4]. *B. pseudomallei* is a natural saprophyte, thus human cases of melioidosis were frequently associated with exposure to soil and contaminated waters in rural areas [8]. Epidemiological studies from urbanized cities like Hong Kong were therefore rarely performed. Melioidosis is currently not a statutorily notifiable disease in Hong Kong, and this disease has never been systematically studied in Hong Kong. Therefore, the local burden of illness is currently largely unknown.

This review aims to provide an overview of melioidosis in Hong Kong. In the first part, the history of melioidosis in humans and animals and evidence of *B. pseudomallei* in the environment, as reported in the literature, is reviewed. In the second part, a review of all clinical cases of culture-confirmed melioidosis managed in public hospitals in Hong Kong in the past 20 years is presented. This is followed by results of a survey performed among local infectious diseases physicians and microbiologists on the local practice of diagnosis and management of melioidosis. Lastly, challenges in the control and clinical management of this disease are discussed.

2. History of Melioidosis in Hong Kong: Presence in Animals, Humans and the Environment

The earliest record of *B. pseudomallei* in Hong Kong came from isolates obtained from bottlenose dolphins and a harbor seal kept in an oceanarium in 1975 and 1976 [9]. This outbreak at the oceanarium caused 24 dolphins to succumb to this illness [10]. Subsequently, *B. pseudomallei* was isolated from other dolphins and numerous other captive sea mammals, including sea lions and pilot whales, as well as birds in a nearby aviary, including zebra doves and scarlet macaws, from 1978 to 2000 [9,11].

A clinical review was performed to evaluate all the melioidosis cases in animals kept at the oceanarium in the period from 1974 to 2003. A total of 49, 31, 16 and 5 cases of melioidosis were recorded in cetaceans, pinnipeds, birds and terrestrial mammals during this period, respectively. All but four succumbed to the disease. Melioidosis caused 55% and 50% of all known causes of deaths in cetaceans and pinnipeds, respectively, during this period [12].

An experimental acellular *B. pseudomallei* vaccine that was tested to be safe and effective in hamsters was given to false killer whales and bottlenose dolphins in the oceanarium from 1986 to 1987. The vaccine produced a high level of specific antibodies in these cetaceans, and was able to reduce mortality in the cetaceans from 45% in 1983 to less than 1% in 1988 [13].

The first human case of melioidosis in Hong Kong was reported in 1983 [14], followed shortly by another five cases reported in 1984 [10]. All these patients were immunocompromised, with either diabetes or had been receiving immunosuppressive therapy for autoimmune diseases. All patients had bacteremia with or without pulmonary involvement. None of them had reported travelling to other endemic areas. Mortality was high, and the majority of them did not receive adequate anti-microbial therapy.

The first serological study was published in 1984, in which 22 elderly patients admitted to a general medical unit of a teaching hospital were screened for hemagglutinating antibodies against lipopolysaccharide antigens of *B. pseudomallei*. 23% of patients in this small cohort had evidence of possible subclinical infection [10,15]. This was followed by another serological survey published in 1987 involving 275 patients with underlying tuberculosis or chronic pulmonary diseases. This study showed that 14% of subjects had serological evidence of exposure to *B. pseudomallei*. Among those with positive antibodies against *B. pseudomallei*, 77% of subjects had not traveled to other endemic areas [15]. This finding, together with the first few human cases described above, produced the earliest evidence that melioidosis was also endemic in Hong Kong, and that human exposure to the bacterium was not at all rare.

Subsequent to those early case reports, eight more human cases of culture-confirmed melioidosis were published from 1987 to 2015 (Table 1). Most of these patients had underlying immunocompromised conditions, including diabetes and hematological malignancies with prolonged neutropenia. One 40-year-old man, with concomitant miliary tuberculosis, was found to have X-linked chronic granulomatous disease. Most patients had bacteremia, pulmonary infection or deep organ abscess. One 82-year-old man developed a mycotic aneurysm in the aortic arch. Such clinical presentation had been reported rarely elsewhere [16]. All of these subsequently reported cases received either intravenous ceftazidime or carbapenem as induction therapy. Three out of these eight patients died due to melioidosis.

There was also a case series published in 2010, describing five patients with autoantibodies against interferon-γ with positive IgG or IgM antibodies against *B. pseudomallei*. All these patients had concomitant non-tuberculous mycobacteriosis, penicilliosis and/or non-typhoidal salmonellosis. None of these patients had a positive culture of *B. pseudomallei* [17].

As in neighboring regions located at similar latitudes, where *B. pseudomallei* had been isolated from the soil [7,18], the bacterium was also isolated from the environment in soil samples in Hong Kong as early as the 1970s [9]. These early reports showed that *B. pseudomallei* was isolated in soil samples taken from sea sludge, farms and a children's playground [10]. In 2000, multiple soil and water samples from an aviary were also found to harbor the bacterium [9]. More recently, among 1400 soil samples collected from the oceanarium in Hong Kong, over a 15-month period, 6.8% of the samples were positive for *B. pseudomallei* by PCR [19].

An epidemiological study, using multilocus sequence typing, on isolates obtained from captive animals and the environment from 1975 to 2000 in Hong Kong, showed that there were two major clusters involving three serotypes. All of these serotypes had been identified in human cases of melioidosis from Hong Kong [9]. The seasonality of melioidosis cases among the captive animals also correlated with the timing of detection of *B. pseudomallei* in soil samples [14]. Such epidemiological data suggested that humans, as in the case of animals, acquired the same strains of *B. pseudomallei* from direct exposure to soil and water [9].

3. Review of Culture-Confirmed Melioidosis Cases in Humans in the Past 20 Years

To determine the burden of illness caused by melioidosis in Hong Kong, a retrospective review of all patients admitted to all public hospitals in Hong Kong with *B. pseudomallei* isolated from one or more clinical specimens during the period from 1998 to 2017, was conducted. In Hong Kong, public hospitals under the Hospital Authority of Hong Kong provide more than 80% of in-patient services to the population in the territory [20]. All patients with one or more clinical specimens with *B. pseudomallei* isolated were identified from the Clinical Data Analysis and Reporting System (CDARS), which is a central computerized database of the Hospital Authority, including patients' demographic characteristics, diagnoses, laboratory data and drug treatment.

A total of 61 culture-confirmed cases of melioidosis was identified during this 20-year period. A progressive increase in the number of cases was observed over this period (Figure 1). 72.1% of the subjects were male, and the median age was 67 (range 8–100, interquartile range 58–83). Only three pediatric cases, with an age between 8 and 17 years, were identified. 60.7% of them had bacteremia, 42.6% had a pulmonary infection, 23.0% had deep organ abscesses (most common being prostate, kidneys, spleen and liver), 11.5% had skin and soft tissue infection and 6.5% had bone and joint infection. A relapse of melioidosis was observed in two patients within 12 months of the initial episode. The overall case fatality rate was 31.1%. Mortality was associated with the presence of bacteremia only (odds ratio 5.14, 95% confidence interval 1.26–21.07, $p = 0.023$).

Table 1. Published reports of culture-confirmed human cases of melioidosis.

Author	Gender/Age	Underlying Diseases	Site of Involvement	Treatment	Outcome
Sridhar 2015 [21]	Male/55	Acute myeloid leukemia with prolonged neutropenia	Bacteremia and pulmonary	Ceftazidime	Died
Sridhar 2015 [21]	Male/57	Follicular lymphoma with prolonged neutropenia	Bacteremia, bursitis and pulmonary	Meropenem, followed by ceftazidime	Died
Li 2015 [22]	Male/82	Coronary artery disease	Mycotic aneurysm and pneumonia	Ceftazidime for 3 weeks, followed by amoxicillin-clavulanate and doxycycline for 3 months	Survived
Lee 2013 [23]	Male/40	X-linked chronic granulomatous disease and concomitant miliary tuberculosis	Not available	Not available	Survived
Woo 2003 [24]	Female/84	Diabetes and bronchiectasis	Bacteremia and pulmonary	Ceftazidime for 2 weeks, followed by amoxicillin-clavulanate for 20 weeks	Survived
Tsang 2001 [25]	Male/51 (Nepalese)	Diabetes	Empyema thoracis	Imipenem for 2 weeks, followed by ciprofloxacin for 7 months, then switched to amoxicillin-clavulanate due to resistance to ciprofloxacin	Survived
Que 1991 [26]	Male/53	Nil	Abscesses in prostate, kidneys, liver, spleen and lungs	Not available	Died
Woo 1987 [27]	Male	Nil	Bacteremia and prostatic abscess	Trimethoprim-sulfamethoxazole	Survived
So 1984 [10]	Female/77	Diabetes	Bacteremia and splenic abscess	Penicillin, gentamicin and metronidazole	Died
So 1984 [10]	Male/62	Diabetes	Bacteremia	Chloramphenicol and tetracycline	Survived
So 1984 [10]	Male/72	Diabetes	Bacteremia and pulmonary	Amikacin	Died
So 1984 [10]	Female/81	Diabetes	Bacteremia and pulmonary	Ampicillin	Died
So 1984 [10]	Male/32	On steroid for pemphigus vulgaris	Bacteremia and pulmonary	Anti-tuberculous drugs	Died
So 1983 [14]	Female/32	Systemic lupus erythematosus, on steroid and azathioprine	Pulmonary	Ceftazidime for 2 months	Survived

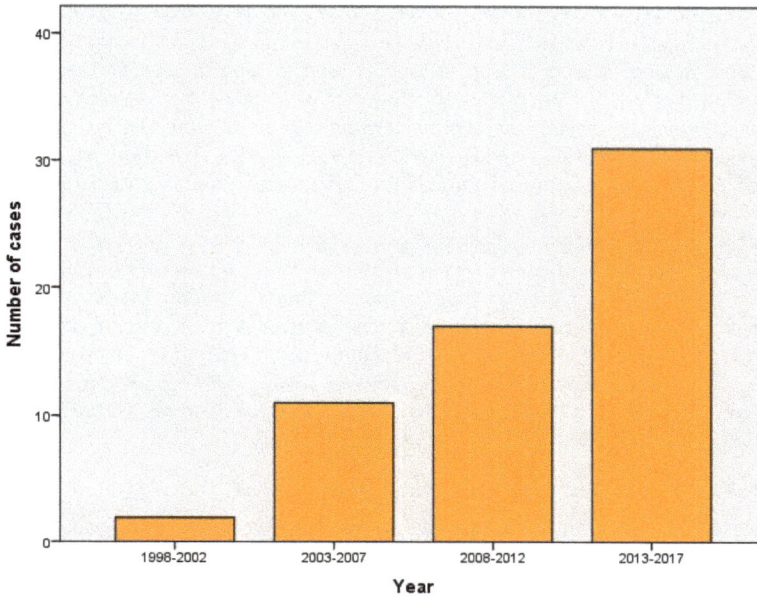

Figure 1. The number of culture-confirmed human cases of melioidosis over a 20-year period.

This series of human cases together with earlier case reports published in the 1980s strongly suggested that melioidosis is endemic in Hong Kong. The saprophytic nature of *B. pseudomallei* has been well recognized since the 1950s [1]. As such, occupational and recreational exposure to soil and contaminated water surfaces, e.g., those working in farms and rice paddies, and those with ingestion or inhalation of food and water contaminated with soil, were consistently described as risk factors for acquiring melioidosis [1,28]. Therefore, not surprisingly, large cohorts of human cases of melioidosis were most commonly reported from rural parts of countries and regions, where primary industry is common [29,30]. Lower incidence of melioidosis was observed in higher-income countries possibly due to lower exposure rates [4]. However, our review and other studies of melioidosis performed in urban cities [31] serve as a good reminder that melioidosis, though less prevalent, should not be neglected in these cities, due to the high mortality and rising incidence. In urbanized areas, working in construction sites, military forces and recreational exposure to soil and contaminated waters have been described as risk factors for acquiring the infection [1,32,33].

We observed a rising trend of culture-confirmed cases over the last 20 years in Hong Kong. An increase in the incidence of human cases of melioidosis has also been reported in Asia in the past decade [4]. For example, Hainan witnessed an increasing trend of annual incidence of melioidosis, with most cases residing in Sanya and Haikou cities [6]. There are several postulations accounting for the rising trend observed in Hong Kong. Improved case detection with better microbiological diagnostic tools is a possibility. Weather changes, through their impacts on environmental contamination, have been shown to cause clustering of human cases of melioidosis [34]. In Hong Kong, the detection rate of *B. pseudomallei* from soil was shown to have significant positive correlation with ambient temperature and relative humidity [19]. Therefore, the significant warming trend and more frequent extreme precipitation events since the 20th century, as reported by the Hong Kong Observatory, could possibly increase human exposure to the bacterium from the environment. The expanding scope of international traveling was proposed to be a source of the importation of cases and the emergence of melioidosis in developed countries as well [4]. Human cases of melioidosis from Hong Kong and other Southeast Asian countries have been shown to share the same serotype [9], supporting the possibility that the disease could be acquired during travel. Lastly, our patients were older than those in other cohorts [29,30], and melioidosis is well recognized to recrudesce after a prolonged period of time [35]. Most of the patients described in the published case reports from Hong Kong had a wide spectrum of underlying immunocompromised conditions (Table 1). Therefore, aging and the increase in immunocompromised diseases and therapies could have contributed to the increase in the incidence of melioidosis by reactivation of the disease after acquisition earlier in life [21,24].

Distinct from the experience in some other Asian countries [36,37], pediatric infections were rare in our cohort. On the other hand, the spectrum of disease involvement observed in our cohort was similar to those described in other studies [35], with bacteremia, pulmonary infection, deep organ abscesses and genitourinary infection being the most common. Bacteremia was present in 61% of cases, and was the major predictor for mortality. The recurrence rate in our cohort was similar to that described previously [35]. Although standard antimicrobial therapy was given to the majority of patients, case fatality rate was still high at 31%. The case fatality rates observed in other developed countries were 14–18% [30,31]. The higher case fatality rate in our cohort could partly be due to the older age of our patients, as compared to most other studies [6,31,38].

4. Current Practice of Management of Melioidosis in Hong Kong

An online survey was performed among local infectious disease physicians and microbiologists from May to July 2018 to evaluate the contemporary local practice in diagnosis and management of melioidosis. The survey was sent to 44 infectious disease physicians and microbiologists, of whom 28 (64%) responded to the survey. They had a median of eight years (interquartile range 3–13) of experience as a specialist. The majority of the respondents (57.1%) had managed 1–2 culture-confirmed cases of melioidosis in the past, while 32.2% had seen three or more cases, and 10.7% had never seen a case.

For laboratory diagnosis, 67.9% of the respondents had access to matrix-assisted laser desorption/ionization time-of-flight mass spectrometry (MALDI-TOF MS) as one of the usual methods of identification of *B. pseudomallei*, while 46.4% and 42.9% regarded biochemical and phenotypic testing and Vitek as the usual methods of identification respectively. 25.0% regarded 16S rRNA sequencing as one of the usual methods of identification. The majority (71.4%) did not find serology to be useful in diagnosing melioidosis, mainly due to the perceived low specificity of the assay. 19.2% of the respondents, however, did believe serology would increase case detection, especially in patients who had negative cultures after antibiotics treatment, and those with compatible epidemiological exposure.

All respondents would prescribe either ceftazidime or meropenem for at least two weeks for the initial treatment of melioidosis. 82.1% of them would choose trimethoprim-sulfamethoxazole, and the remainder amoxicillin-clavulanate, for at least three to six months, as an eradication therapy.

The majority of respondents regarded the lack of awareness among clinicians as the greatest challenge in the management of melioidosis in Hong Kong. The relatively small number of cases in Hong Kong limited the experience and expertise for this disease entity. The low level of clinical suspicion would cause a delay in diagnosis. Respondents were also concerned with the currently available diagnostic tools, and problems of misidentification of *B. pseudomallei* as other *Burkholderia* or *Pseudomonas* species. In terms of treatment, the greatest challenge was ensuring adherence and the management of adverse reactions secondary to prolonged courses of antibiotics.

5. Challenges in the Control and Management of Melioidosis

It is uncertain whether melioidosis is being under-diagnosed in Hong Kong. A recent study estimated that Hong Kong would expect to see 67 new cases of melioidosis annually [4]. This estimation was much higher than the number of cases observed in our review for the last two decades. As reflected in our local survey, under-diagnosis could be due to the low level of clinical suspicion among clinicians. The diagnosis of melioidosis can be difficult in clinical cases, as *B. pseudomallei* might not be readily isolated from clinical specimens [39], or misidentified as other *Burkholderia* species by certain automated systems [40]. Cases diagnosed to be pulmonary tuberculosis or other bacterial cases of pneumonia in Hong Kong have also been suspected to be melioidosis [6,10,15]. Moreover, we have only included culture-confirmed cases in our review; culture-negative cases confirmed only by serological evidence of infection were not included in the analysis. Since we have observed an increasing number of cases over the last 20 years, continual surveillance of this disease in the territory should be implemented.

Improvements in the laboratory diagnosis of melioidosis are urgently needed. Molecular techniques, involving 16S rRNA or *groEL* gene sequencing, would be useful for identification, in particular, to differentiate *B. pseudomallei* from other closely related *Burkholderia* species, including *B. thailandensis* [24,41]. As observed in our survey, MALDI-TOF MS is being increasingly used in Hong Kong microbiology laboratories. This technique has recently been shown to be an accurate method for the identification of *B. pseudomallei* [42]. Preliminary data also showed that profiling metabolites from various lipid classes is a potential biomarker for the diagnosis of melioidosis [39].

The case fatality rate observed in Hong Kong was higher than that observed in other high-income countries. As indicated by the results of our survey, the relatively low number of cases detected in Hong Kong led to a low level of clinical suspicion and possibly a delay in diagnosis. Empirical treatment of melioidosis, for example, is seldom initiated for patients with community-acquired pneumonia in Hong Kong. Awareness of this disease should be raised, and the diagnosis should be particularly considered in patients with compatible clinical manifestations and associated epidemiological risk factors.

The growing number of cases of melioidosis could partially be explained by the aging population and the increase in immunocompromising diseases and therapies. Currently, there is no local guideline in the prevention and management of the disease in patients at high risk of complications and mortality from melioidosis. Recommendations have been issued for the workup of melioidosis in seropositive patients initiating immunosuppressive therapy and symptomatic seropositive immunocompromised patients [36]. Routine serological testing of antibodies against *B. pseudomallei* is currently not performed in immunocompromised patients in Hong Kong. The only published local seroprevalence surveys were done in the 1980s. A study should, therefore, be considered to evaluate the current seroprevalence rate of melioidosis in Hong Kong, and to determine whether routine screening is necessary for immunocompromised patients in Hong Kong.

6. Conclusions

Melioidosis is endemic in the urban city of Hong Kong. Although the observed incidence was lower than in other neighboring countries and regions, there was an increasing number of cases in the last 20 years. Surveillance of the disease should be considered, and more effort should be in place to raise clinicians' awareness of the disease.

Author Contributions: Conceptualization, G.L. and I.F.N.H.; Methodology, G.L., A.T., E.Y.K.T., A.K.L.W., J.Z., W.L., W.M.T., and M.C.C.; Formal Analysis, G.L.; Data Curation, G.L.; Writing-Original Draft Preparation, G.L.; Writing-Review & Editing, E.Y.K.T., A.K.L.W., J.Z., K.W.C., W.L., M.C.C., and I.F.N.H.; Supervision, K.W.C., W.L., and I.F.N.H.

Funding: There is no funding source for this study.

Acknowledgments: We would like to thank all the Infectious Disease physicians and microbiologists who have participated in the survey.

Conflicts of Interest: The authors declare no conflict of interest.

References

1. Cheng, A.C.; Currie, B.J. Melioidosis: Epidemiology, pathophysiology, and management. *Clin. Microbiol. Rev.* **2005**, *18*, 383–416. [CrossRef] [PubMed]
2. Whitmore, A. An account of a glanders-like disease occurring in Rangoon. *Epidemiol. Infect.* **1913**, *13*, 1–34. [CrossRef]
3. Currie, B.J.; Dance, D.A.; Cheng, A.C. The global distribution of *Burkholderia pseudomallei* and melioidosis: An update. *Trans. R. Soc. Trop. Med. Hyg.* **2008**, *102*, S1–S4. [CrossRef]

4. Limmathurotsakul, D.; Golding, N.; Dance, D.A.; Messina, J.P.; Pigott, D.M.; Moyes, C.L.; Rolim, D.B.; Bertherat, E.; Day, N.P.; Peacock, S.J.; et al. Predicted global distribution of *Burkholderia pseudomallei* and burden of melioidosis. *Nat. Microbiol.* **2016**, *1*, 15008. [CrossRef] [PubMed]

5. Dance, D.A. Melioidosis: The tip of the iceberg? *Clin. Microbiol. Rev.* **1991**, *4*, 52–60. [CrossRef] [PubMed]

6. Fang, Y.; Chen, H.; Li, Y.L.; Li, Q.; Ye, Z.J.; Mao, X.H. Melioidosis in Hainan, China: A retrospective study. *Trans. R. Soc. Trop. Med. Hyg.* **2015**, *109*, 636–642. [CrossRef] [PubMed]

7. Su, H.P.; Yang, H.W.; Chen, Y.L.; Ferng, T.L.; Chou, Y.L.; Chung, T.C.; Chen, C.H.; Chiang, C.S.; Kuan, M.M.; Lin, H.H.; et al. Prevalence of melioidosis in the Er-Ren River basin, Taiwan: Implications for transmission. *J. Clin. Microbiol.* **2007**, *45*, 2599–2603. [CrossRef] [PubMed]

8. Suputtamongkol, Y.; Chaowagul, W.; Chetchotisakd, P.; Lertpatanasuwun, N.; Intaranongpai, S.; Ruchutrakool, T.; Budhsarawong, D.; Mootsikapun, P.; Wuthiekanun, V.; Teerawatasook, N.; et al. Risk factors for melioidosis and bacteremic melioidosis. *Clin. Infect. Dis.* **1999**, *29*, 408–413. [CrossRef] [PubMed]

9. Godoy, D.; Randle, G.; Simpson, A.J.; Aanensen, D.M.; Pitt, T.L.; Kinoshita, R.; Spratt, B.G. Multilocus sequence typing and evolutionary relationships among the causative agents of melioidosis and glanders, *Burkholderia pseudomallei* and *Burkholderia mallei*. *J. Clin. Microbiol.* **2003**, *41*, 2068–2079. [CrossRef] [PubMed]

10. So, S.Y.; Chau, P.Y.; Leung, Y.K.; Lam, W.K. First report of septicaemic melioidosis in Hong Kong. *Trans. R. Soc. Trop. Med. Hyg.* **1984**, *78*, 456–459. [CrossRef]

11. Liong, E.; Vedros, N.A.; Hammond, J.K. *Pseudomonas pseudomallei* infection in a dolphin (*Tursiops gilli*): A case report. *Aquat. Mamm.* **1985**, *1*, 20–22.

12. Kinoshita, R.E. Epidemiology of melioidosis in an oceanarium: A clinical, environmental and molecular study. Master's Thesis, University of Hong Kong, Hong Kong, China, 2003.

13. Vedros, N.A.; Chow, D.; Liong, E. Experimental vaccine against *Pseudomonas pseudomallei* infections in captive cetaceans. *Dis. Aquat. Org.* **1988**, *5*, 157–161. [CrossRef]

14. So, S.Y.; Chau, P.Y.; Leung, Y.K.; Lam, W.K.; Yu, D.Y. Successful treatment of melioidosis caused by a multiresistant strain in an immunocompromised host with third generation cephalosporins. *Am. Rev. Respir. Dis.* **1983**, *127*, 650–654. [CrossRef] [PubMed]

15. So, S.Y.; Chau, P.Y.; Aquinas, M.; Gabriel, M.; Lam, W.K. Melioidosis: A serological survey in a tuberculosis sanatorium in Hong Kong. *Trans. R. Soc. Trop. Med. Hyg.* **1987**, *81*, 1017–1019. [CrossRef]

16. Rao, J.; Kaushal, A.S.; Hoong, C.K. Abdominal aortic pseudoaneurysm secondary to melioidosis. *Asian J. Surg.* **2009**, *32*, 64–69. [CrossRef]

17. Tang, B.S.; Chan, J.F.; Chen, M.; Tsang, O.T.; Mok, M.Y.; Lai, R.W.; Lee, R.; Que, T.; Tse, H.; Li, I.W.; et al. Disseminated penicilliosis, recurrent bacteremic nontyphoidal salmonellosis, and burkholderiosis associated with acquired immunodeficiency due to autoantibody against gamma interferon. *Clin. Vaccine Immunol.* **2010**, *17*, 1132–1138. [CrossRef] [PubMed]

18. Ma, G.; Zheng, D.; Cai, Q.; Yuan, Z. Prevalence of *Burkholderia pseudomallei* in Guangxi, China. *Epidemiol. Infect.* **2010**, *138*, 37–39. [CrossRef] [PubMed]

19. Lau, S.K.; Chan, S.Y.; Curreem, S.O.; Hui, S.W.; Lau, C.C.; Lee, P.; Ho, C.C.; Martelli, P.; Woo, P.C. *Burkholderia pseudomallei* in soil samples from an oceanarium in Hong Kong detected using a sensitive PCR Assay. *Emerg. Microbes Infect.* **2014**, *3*, e69. [CrossRef] [PubMed]

20. Kong, X.; Yang, Y.; Gao, J.; Guan, J.; Liu, Y.; Wang, R.; Xing, B.; Li, Y.N.; Ma, W.B. Overview of the health care system in Hong Kong and its referential significance to mainland China. *J. Chin. Med. Assoc.* **2015**, *78*, 569–573. [CrossRef] [PubMed]

21. Sridhar, S.; Teng, J.L.; Lau, S.K.; Woo, P.C. Fatal bacteremic melioidosis in patients with prolonged neutropenia. *Diagn. Microbiol. Infect. Dis.* **2016**, *84*, 258–260. [CrossRef] [PubMed]

22. Li, P.H.; Chau, C.H.; Wong, P.C. Melioidosis Mycotic aneurysm: An uncommon complication of an uncommon disease. *Respir. Med. Case Rep.* **2015**, *14*, 43–46. [CrossRef] [PubMed]

23. Lee, P.P.; Lau, Y.L. Endemic infections in Southeast Asia provide new insights to the phenotypic spectrum of primary immunodeficiency disorders. *Asian Pac. J. Allergy Immunol.* **2013**, *31*, 217–226. [PubMed]

24. Woo, P.C.; Lau, S.K.; Woo, G.K.; Fung, A.M.; Ngan, A.H.; Hui, W.T.; Yuen, K.Y. Seronegative bacteremic melioidosis caused by *Burkholderia pseudomallei* with ambiguous biochemical profile: Clinical importance of accurate identification by 16S rRNA gene and GroEL gene sequencing. *J. Clin. Microbiol.* **2003**, *41*, 3973–3977. [CrossRef] [PubMed]

25. Tsang, T.Y.; Lai, S.T. A case of thoracic empyema due to suppurative melioidosis. *Hong Kong Med. J.* **2001**, *7*, 201–204. [PubMed]

26. Que, T.L.; Chan, Y.F.; Lam, S.Y. Acute disseminated melioidosis presenting as acute retention of urine. *Br. J. Urol.* **1991**, *67*, 556–557. [CrossRef] [PubMed]

27. Woo, M.L.; Chan, P.S.; French, G.L. A case of melioidosis presenting with prostatic abscess in Hong Kong. *J. Urol.* **1987**, *137*, 120–121. [CrossRef]

28. Limmathurotsakul, D.; Kanoksil, M.; Wuthiekanun, V.; Kitphati, R.; deStavola, B.; Day, N.P.; Peacock, S.J. Activities of Daily Living Associated with Acquisition of Melioidosis in Northeast Thailand: A matched case-control study. *PLoS Negl. Trop. Dis.* **2013**, *7*, e2072. [CrossRef] [PubMed]

29. Limmathurotsakul, D.; Wongratanacheewin, S.; Teerawattanasook, N.; Wongsuvan, G.; Chaisuksant, S.; Chetchotisakd, P.; Chaowagul, W.; Day, N.P.; Peacock, S.J. Increasing incidence of human melioidosis in northeast Thailand. *Am. J. Trop. Med. Hyg.* **2010**, *82*, 1113–1117. [CrossRef] [PubMed]

30. Currie, B.J.; Ward, L.; Cheng, A.C. The epidemiology and clinical spectrum of melioidosis: 540 cases from the 20-year Darwin prospective study. *PLoS Negl. Trop. Dis.* **2010**, *4*, e900. [CrossRef] [PubMed]

31. Pang, L.; Harris, P.N.A.; Seiler, R.L.; Ooi, P.L.; Cutter, J.; Goh, K.T.; Cook, A.R.; Fisher, D.; Ann Chai, L.Y. Melioidosis, Singapore, 2003–2014. *Emerg. Infect. Dis.* **2018**, *24*. [CrossRef] [PubMed]

32. Heng, B.H.; Goh, K.T.; Yap, E.H.; Loh, H.; Yeo, M. Epidemiological surveillance of melioidosis in Singapore. *Ann. Acad. Med. Singap.* **1998**, *27*, 478–484. [PubMed]

33. Lim, M.K.; Tan, E.H.; Soh, C.S.; Chang, T.L. *Burkholderia pseudomallei* infection in the Singapore Armed Forces from 1987 to 1994—An epidemiological review. *Ann. Acad. Med. Singap.* **1997**, *26*, 13–17. [PubMed]

34. Cheng, A.C.; Jacups, S.P.; Gal, D.; Mayo, M.; Currie, B.J. Extreme weather events and environmental contamination are associated with case-clusters of melioidosis in the Northern Territory of Australia. *Int. J. Epidemiol.* **2006**, *35*, 323–329. [CrossRef] [PubMed]

35. Ngauy, V.; Lemeshev, Y.; Sadkowski, L.; Crawford, G. Cutaneous melioidosis in a man who was taken as a prisoner of war by the Japanese during World War II. *J. Clin. Microbiol.* **2005**, *43*, 970–972. [CrossRef] [PubMed]

36. Wiersinga, W.J.; Currie, B.J.; Peacock, S.J. Melioidosis. *N. Engl. J. Med.* **2012**, *367*, 1035–1044. [CrossRef] [PubMed]

37. Pagnarith, Y.; Kumar, V.; Thaipadungpanit, J.; Wuthiekanun, V.; Amornchai, P.; Sin, L.; Day, N.P.; Peacock, S.J. Emergence of pediatric melioidosis in Siem Reap, Cambodia. *Am. J. Trop. Med. Hyg.* **2010**, *82*, 1106–1112. [CrossRef] [PubMed]

38. Currie, B.J.; Fisher, D.A.; Howard, D.M.; Burrow, J.N.; Lo, D.; Selva-Nayagam, S.; Anstey, N.M.; Huffam, S.E.; Snelling, P.L.; Marks, P.J.; et al. Endemic melioidosis in tropical northern Australia: A 10-year prospective study and review of the literature. *Clin. Infect. Dis.* **2000**, *31*, 981–986. [CrossRef] [PubMed]

39. Lau, S.K.; Lam, C.W.; Curreem, S.O.; Lee, K.C.; Chow, W.N.; Lau, C.C.; Sridhar, S.; Wong, S.C.; Martelli, P.; Hui, S.W.; et al. Metabolomic profiling of *Burkholderia pseudomallei* Using UHPLC-ESI-Q-TOF-MS reveals specific biomarkers including 4-methyl-5-thiazoleethanol and unique thiamine degradation pathway. *Cell Biosci.* **2015**, *5*, 26. [CrossRef] [PubMed]

40. Lowe, P.; Engler, C.; Norton, R. Comparison of automated and nonautomated systems for identification of *Burkholderia pseudomallei*. *J. Clin. Microbiol.* **2002**, *40*, 4625–4627. [CrossRef] [PubMed]

41. Woo, P.C.; Woo, G.K.; Lau, S.K.; Wong, S.S.; Yuen, K. Single gene target bacterial identification. GroEL gene sequencing for discriminating clinical isolates of *Burkholderia pseudomallei* and *Burkholderia thailandensis*. *Diagn. Microbiol. Infect. Dis.* **2002**, *44*, 143–149. [CrossRef]

42. Suttisunhakul, V.; Pumpuang, A.; Ekchariyawat, P.; Wuthiekanun, V.; Elrod, M.G.; Turner, P.; Currie, B.J.; Phetsouvanh, R.; Dance, D.A.; Limmathurotsakul, D.; et al. Matrix-assisted laser desorption/ionization time-of-flight mass spectrometry for the identification of *Burkholderia pseudomallei* from Asia and Australia and differentiation between *Burkholderia* species. *PLoS ONE* **2017**, *12*, e0175294. [CrossRef] [PubMed]

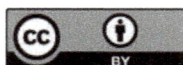

Tropical Medicine and Infectious Disease

MDPI

Review

Melioidosis in the Western Indian Ocean and the Importance of Improving Diagnosis, Surveillance, and Molecular Typing

Andriniaina Rakotondrasoa [1], Mohammad Iqbal Issack [2], Benoît Garin [3], Fabrice Biot [4],
Eric Valade [4], Pierre Wattiau [5], Nicolas Allou [6], Olivier Belmonte [7], Jastin Bibi [8],
Erin P. Price [9] and Jean-Marc Collard [1,*

1   Unité de Bactériologie Expérimentale, Institut Pasteur de Madagascar, Antananarivo 101, Madagascar;
    aina@pasteur.mg
2   Central Health Laboratory, Victoria Hospital, Candos 72211, Mauritius; moissack@yahoo.com
3   Laboratoire Immuno-Hématologie, CHU Pointe-à-Pitre/Abymes 97159, Guadeloupe;
    benoitgarin@gmail.com
4   Unité de Bactériologie/UMR_MD1, Institut de Recherche Biomédicale des Armées, Brétigny sur Orge,
    Ecole du Val-de-Grâce, 91223 Paris, France; fbiot.irba@defense.gouv.fr (F.B.);
    eric.valade@defense.gouv.fr (E.V.)
5   Unit of Foodborne, Highly Pathogenic Bacterial Zoonoses & Antibiotic Resistance, Veterinary and
    Agrochemical Research Center, Brussels 1180, Belgium; Pierre.Wattiau@coda-cerva.be
6   Réanimation polyvalente, Centre Hospitalier Universitaire Félix Guyon, 97499 Saint Denis, France;
    nicolas.allou@hotmail.fr
7   Bactériologie, Centre Hospitalier Universitaire Félix Guyon, 97499 Saint Denis, France;
    olivier.belmonte@chu-reunion.fr
8   Ministry of Health, Public Health Department, Victoria, Seychelles; jastin.bibi@health.gov.sc
9   Faculty of Science, Health, Education and Engineering, University of the Sunshine Coast, Sippy Downs,
    QLD 4556, Australia; eprice@usc.edu.au
*   Correspondence: jmcollard@pasteur.mg; Tel.: +261-20-22-590-19

Received: 18 January 2018; Accepted: 2 March 2018; Published: 7 March 2018

Abstract: Melioidosis, caused by the bacterium *Burkholderia pseudomallei*, is an infectious disease of humans or animals, and the specific environmental conditions that are present in western Indian Ocean islands are particularly suitable for the establishment/survival of *B. pseudomallei*. Indeed, an increasing number of new cases have been reported in this region (Madagascar, Mauritius, Réunion (France), and Seychelles, except Comoros and Mayotte (France)), and are described in this review. Our review clearly points out that further studies are needed in order to investigate the real incidence and burden of melioidosis in the western Indian Ocean and especially Madagascar, since it is likely to be higher than currently reported. Thus, research and surveillance priorities were recommended (i) to improve awareness of melioidosis in the population and among clinicians; (ii) to improve diagnostics, in order to provide rapid and effective treatment; (iii) to implement a surveillance and reporting system in the western Indian Ocean; and (iv) to investigate the presence of *B. pseudomallei* in environmental samples, since we have demonstrated its presence in soil samples originating from the yard of a Madagascan case.

Keywords: Melioidosis; *Burkholderia pseudomallei*; western Indian Ocean; diagnosis; MLST; Madagascar; Mauritius; Réunion; Seychelles

---

1. Introduction and History of Melioidosis in the Western Indian Ocean

Melioidosis (also known as Whitmore's disease or Nightcliff gardener's disease) is an infectious disease that can infect humans or animals. This disease is caused by the bacterium

Burkholderia pseudomallei. A recent study mapped documented human and animal cases and the presence of environmental *B. pseudomallei* in the world, in order to estimate the global burden of melioidosis by a formal modeling framework and assess the environmental suitability for *B. pseudomallei* [1]. Human cases are mainly reported in hyperendemic areas of Southeast Asia and northern Australia, with sporadic reports in parts of the Americas, Africa, Pacific Ocean islands, southern China, Hong Kong and Taiwan, and South Asia. It has been predicted that the specific environmental conditions which are present in western Indian Ocean islands are particularly suitable for the establishment/survival of *B. pseudomallei* [1], and an increasing number of new cases have been reported in this region [2]. A map of the western Indian Ocean with its different islands can be accessed at the website [3]. It was long ago hypothesized that the trade of (healthy or sick) animal carriers could contribute to the spread of the disease to non-endemic areas.

In Thailand, melioidosis is considered a disease predominantly of rice farmers, which is brought about by their frequent exposure to environments containing *B. pseudomallei*. The organism is a saprophyte found in soil and water, and people become infected, particularly after heavy rains, by contact with contaminated soil or water through percutaneous inoculation, by inhalation, or even through ingestion of contaminated water (e.g., aspiration in near-drowning events during flooding or tsunamis, or consumption of unchlorinated water). Person-to-person transmission can occur, albeit very rarely, through contact with blood and body fluids of an infected person. Infected people generally have underlying predisposing conditions, such as diabetes mellitus, renal disease, cirrhosis, thalassemia, cystic fibrosis, chronic obstructive lung disease, or immunosuppressive therapy. Clinical presentations vary widely, and include skin and soft tissue abscesses, pneumonia, and disseminated infection with septic shock, the latter having mortality rates above 80% [4]. The diverse clinical manifestations and the inadequacy of conventional bacterial identification methods render *B. pseudomallei* identification difficult, particularly in regions where this organism is not well-recognized, and could result in a serious underestimation of the disease in low-income countries, where capacity building is needed in the health services, as recently discussed by Limmathurotsakul et al. [1].

In Madagascar, the first isolation of *B. pseudomallei* occurred in Antananarivo in 1932 when Girard, a former Director of the Pasteur Institute of Madagascar, examined a dead guineapig inoculated with a submaxillary node of a slaughtered pig [5].

The presence of this bacterium in Madagascar was also reported later (1977) by Galimand and Dodin working in the 'Whitmore bacillus laboratory' in the Pasteur Institute in Paris. They isolated and identified the bacterium from soil samples originating from the zoo of Antananarivo and from a pig farm in the same city [6]. There are two isolates (770429-id6- and Soil1977-id7-) in the *B. pseudomallei* multilocus sequencing typing (MLST) database (https://pubmlst.org/bpseudomallei/) originating from soil collected from the Antananarivo region in 1977. These isolates correspond to ST-6 (alleles: 1, 1, 7, 2, 4, 5, 1) and ST-27 (alleles: 1, 3, 19, 4, 5, 1, 1), respectively [7]. ST-6 has not been reported in any other isolate to date; however, ST-27 was also found in a 1978 soil sample from Chantilly, France, during a devastating and highly unusual melioidosis outbreak (the so-called 'Affaire du Jardin des Plantes') that lasted several years and that resulted in the death or slaughter of dozens of animals across several zoos and equestrian clubs, probably by the transport of infected animals and/or contaminated manure [8]. A case of animal melioidosis, also related to the French outbreak, occurred in 1979 in a horse that had recently been imported from France into Réunion Island [6]. This epizootic of melioidosis across France and beyond was extraordinary, and greatly extended the known boundaries of this disease, being the first report of this disease in a temperate region [6].

Subsequently, between 2004 and 2017, there were six human cases of melioidosis that were detected and probably acquired in the city of Mahajanga (Madagascar), of which three were diagnosed and treated in Réunion Island in 2004, 2005, and 2016. Considering other islands of the western Indian Ocean, there were two cases in Mauritius in 2004 and 2006, one autochthonous case in 2012, and four imported cases in Réunion Island (three from Madagascar, in 2004, 2005, and 2016 respectively, and one from South Asia in 2017), and finally, two cases in cooks from the same facility in Seychelles in 2013.

These cases are described in more detail in the next section. Since the cases were all investigated separately, some methodologies used for culturing and identifying *B. pseudomallei* were slightly different between the different laboratories concerned. We also describe the isolation of *B. pseudomallei* in the yard of case #9 from Madagascar.

2. Review of the Human Cases

N.B. Cases are numbered chronologically, independently of the country of origin.

2.1. Madagascar

Case #1. The first human case of melioidosis in the region was detected in May 2004 in a 60-year-old Frenchman living in Mahajanga, a city on the northwestern coast of Madagascar, along the Mozambique Channel, who had been transferred to a hospital in Réunion Island. He was admitted to an intensive care unit for management of respiratory distress and septic shock. About 20 or 30 years before the onset of the disease, he had lived for an unknown period of time in Vietnam, where melioidosis is endemic. He was a heavy drinker and smoker with cachexia. Four blood cultures and one bronchoalveolar lavage specimen, taken the first day after admission, were positive for *B. pseudomallei* [9]. The initial treatment was a combination of piperacillin and ciprofloxacin (the initial identification was 'Pseudomonas sp.'), followed by ceftazidime when *B. pseudomallei* was recognized. Interestingly, two secondary cases (cases #2 and #3), acquired 150 and 180 days after the initial case and transmitted by a fiberoptic bronchoscope, were detected. A manufacturing defect rendered the decontamination processes of the bronchoscope insufficiently effective, and culture with subsequent DNA restriction analysis confirmed the secondary transmissions. These nosocomial transmissions concerned an 81-year-old man suffering from a chronic pulmonary disease, and a woman undergoing glucocorticoid therapy for lupus. Both secondary cases were also treated with ceftazidime (120 mg/kg/day) until recovery, followed by trimethoprim/sulfamethoxazole for 20 weeks.

Case #5. The second case in Madagascar was a 58-year-old Frenchman with an unremarkable medical history who had lived for the previous five years in Antananarivo [10]. The patient, a retired manager, had spent most of his life in France, and he had traveled for short periods in Tunisia, Turkey, and Mauritius (six years previously). His first symptoms (high fever with cough) appeared during a two-week holiday trip to Mahajanga in March 2005. He was initially admitted to a hospital in Antananarivo, where he was treated for ten days with amoxicillin/clavulanic acid and levofloxacin after a chest X-ray showed a patchy infiltrate of the right upper and middle lobes. His sputum acid-fast stain was negative. After clinical improvement, the patient was discharged, but five days later he became feverish again, and was referred to a hospital in Réunion Island for further management. Although four blood cultures were negative, *B. pseudomallei* was isolated from his bronchoalveolar lavage. He responded to treatment, which firstly comprised imipenem for two weeks, followed by oral trimethoprim/sulfamethoxazole and doxycycline. He was discharged at day 20 on eradication treatment with trimethoprim/sulfamethoxazole for a further five months.

Cases #8 and #9. The third and fourth cases in Madagascar were rural farmers aged 52 and 45 years, respectively [11]. They were both admitted to the University hospital in Mahajanga with sepsis in July 2012 and in May 2013, respectively. One of them had an opacity in the lower left lung and a pleural effusion, whilst the other developed hepatic failure after one week of admission. They were both suffering from diabetes mellitus, and hepatomegaly and splenomegaly were detected by abdominal ultrasound examination during their hospitalization. The diagnosis of *B. pseudomallei* was possible thanks to a specific research study on melioidosis that was being conducted in this hospital during the period 2012–2013, which supported the purchase of consumables, such as blood culture bottles and culture media (chocolate, blood and Ashdown agars). However, both patients died despite antibiotic treatment.

Case #10. The fifth case in Madagascar was a 44-year-old Frenchman admitted with acute anuria and fever to the emergency service of a Belgian hospital near the French border in March 2013 [12].

He had a severe inflammatory syndrome, spondylodiscitis at L1, lung infiltrates, pyelonephritis, and a prostatic abscess. He was treated with a fluoroquinolone after the isolation of an organism initially identified as *B. cepacia* on a VITEK II instrument (bioMérieux, La Balme-Les-Grottes, France) from his blood cultures. The patient's clinical condition remained stable, with decreasing inflammatory syndrome and fever, and he was discharged for few days until the real causative agent was identified. When *B. pseudomallei* was correctly identified by MALDI-TOF MS using the security-relevant reference library, and subsequently confirmed by a highly-specific PCR assay, the patient was readmitted to the hospital, the antimicrobial treatment was immediately changed (to meropenem 1 g iv t.i.d. and trimethoprim/sulfamethoxazole 2 × 160/800 mg t.i.d.) and his condition improved. Interestingly, the patient, a gardener by profession, reported frequent travels to his secondary residence in Mahajanga, usually for 3 weeks, every 3 or 4 months.

Case #13. The last case from Madagascar was recently described by Allou et al. [2], and concerned a 63-year-old Frenchman, with no significant past medical history, who lived in Madagascar and made frequent trips to Mayotte, an island between Madagascar and Mozambique. After his admission to Mahajanga Hospital, where he was treated with ofloxacin for cough and fever lasting one week, his condition worsened (vomiting, dehydration, deterioration of consciousness) and he was transferred to an ICU at Saint Denis Hospital, Réunion Island, with septic shock and coma on admission. Briefly, a total body-computed tomography (TB-CT) scan showed multiple bilateral lung abscesses, a liver abscess, splenomegaly, and hepatomegaly. Despite immediate antimicrobial treatment (meropenem, colistin, amikacin), the evolution was marked by multiple organ failure and the patient died on day one. Blood cultures and respiratory samples were positive for a *Burkholderia* identified as *B. thailandensis* by a MALDI-TOF mass spectrometer (Bruker Biotyper, Bruker Daltonics, Bremen, Germany) but confirmed later as *B. pseudomallei* by qPCR targeting three genetic markers of the type III secretion system (*orf1*, *orf13*, and *BsSCU2*). It is noteworthy that *B. pseudomallei* was not at that time included in the IVD MALDI Biotyper database but in a separate database (SR: security-relevant) which was not available at the hospital. The strain was susceptible in vitro to ticarcillin/clavulanic acid, trimethoprim/sulfamethoxazole, and ceftazidime, and was resistant to meropenem and levofloxacin. The meropenem resistance (MIC = 12 mL/L) was unusual, and the presence of a possible metallo β-lactamase (MBL) was investigated with the RUO Etest MBL MP/MPI US 8/2 (bioMérieux, La Balme-Les-Grottes, France), but failed. The higher MIC values to different antibiotics suggested that this resistance could be due to a non-specific mechanism, such as efflux or impermeability.

The six cases are summarized in Table 1. After investigations, all cases were likely to have been acquired in Mahajanga, a favorite tourist destination in Madagascar located on the country's northwestern coast on the Mozambique Channel (15°43′ S, 46°18′ E), 550 km from Antananarivo. Typing of strains isolated from five human cases by multilocus sequencing typing (MLST; Godoy et al. [7]) showed new sequence types (STs), all of which were possibly related to each other (varying by 1, 2, or 3 alleles, depending on the combinations).

Table 1. Case descriptions of patients who acquired melioidosis after visiting Mahajanga, Madagascar.

Year	2004	2005	2012	2013	2013	2016
Case	#1	#5	#8	#9	#10	#13
Reference	[9]	[10]	[11]	[11]	[12]	[2]
Sex	Male	Male	Male	Male	Male	Male
Age	60	58	52	45	44	63
Strain ID (sequence type) *	4419 (ST-1260)	4420 (ST-1433)	3240 (ST-1053)	3241 (ST-1054)	4416 (ST-1043)	2017-012 (ST1430)
Allele profile	1, 12, 34, 2, 5, 2, 1	4, 1, 34, 2, 5, 2, 1	4, 12, 3, 2, 5, 2, 1	4, 12, 34, 1, 5, 2, 1	4, 1, 3, 2, 5, 2, 1	4, 2, 3, 1, 5, 2, 1
Occupation	Not known	Retired	Rural rice farmer	Rice, sugar cane, and tobacco farmer	Gardener	Not known
Risk factors	Heavy drinker (1 L/day) and smoker (20 cigarettes/day); cachexia	Smoker (35 cigarette packs/year); unremarkable medical history	Diabetes	Diabetes. A history of furunculosis for several months	No diabetes mellitus	
1st admission	CHD Félix Guyon, Saint Denis, Réunion Island (24.05.2004)	Hospital in Antananarivo (March 2005)	Androva University Hospital in Mahajanga (July 2012)	Androva University Hospital in Mahajanga (May 2013)	CHU-AP, Mons, Belgium (16.03.2013)	CHD Félix Guyon, Saint Denis, Réunion Island
2nd admission		Groupe Hospitalier Sud Réunion, Saint Pierre, Réunion Island			CHU-AP, Mons, Belgium (April 2013) due to identification of the causative agent and symptoms	
Previous history	Lived in Madagascar (Mahajanga); lived for an unknown period of time in Vietnam 20 or 30 years before the onset of the disease	Spent most of his life in France but lived for the past 5 years in Madagascar before hospitalisation in Antananarivo. He had also travelled for short periods in Tunisia, Turkey and Mauritius. The first symptoms appeared during the last days of a stay (couple of weeks) in Mahajanga			Frequent travels to Mahajanga for entertainment (beach sports and fishing) lasting usually for 3 weeks every 3 or 4 months including during the rainy season	Had consulted the Hospital in Mahajanga 4 days before being admitted to CHD Félix Guyon, Saint Denis
Outcome	Discharged	Clinical improvement and discharged	Died 3 days later	Died 2 weeks after admission and two days after ceftazidime treatment	Discharged a few days after his clinical status remained stable, with decreasing inflammatory syndrome and fever.	Died on day 1 after his admission

* According to the *B. pseudomallei* multilocus sequencing typing (MLST) database (https://pubmlst.org/bpseudomallei/).

2.2. Soil Investigation in Mahajanga, Madagascar, in the Yard of Case #10

A soil investigation was carried out in the yard of the fifth case from Madagascar (#10). His house in Mahajanga was located on the seashore (separated by an asphalted road). Mahajanga (sometimes spelled Majunga) has a tropical wet and dry/savanna climate (Köppen-Geiger classification [13], with a pronounced dry season in the low-sun months, no cold season, and a wet season in the high-sun months (from November to April) (http://www.mahajanga.climatemps.com/). Sampling and culture of *B. pseudomallei* isolates from soil was done according to Appendix B. In brief, a total of 11 soil and water samples (Figure A1) were collected, among which was A12, a dark, dry, turf-like soil sold as fertilizer/manure by a local supplier. Sandy soil samples A4, A5, and A7-9 had been augmented with the dark soil A12.

The soil samples were processed as described in Appendix B, and subsequent cultures were spread on Ashdown's agar plates (supplemented with colistin 50 mg/L) which were incubated at 37 °C. The plates were examined on a daily basis. Colonies with morphology typical for *B. pseudomallei* (pink/purple, flat, slightly dry, wrinkled-smooth but with surface roughness in the outer half of the colonies) were subcultured onto chocolate agar plates. Only samples A4, A8, and A12 gave rise to *B. pseudomallei*-like colonies on Ashdown medium. Identification of those isolates was confirmed by MALDI-TOF mass spectrometry (Bruker Biotyper, Bruker Daltonics, Germany) using the security-relevant database (*B. pseudomallei* with scores >2) and by PCR amplification targeting a genetic marker of the type III secretion system1 (TTS-1; 115-base-pair region within *orf2*) [14]. The three isolates were tested by disk diffusion on agar, and were found to be susceptible in vitro to amoxicillin/clavulanic acid, ceftazidime, imipenem, trimethoprim/sulfamethoxazole, levofloxacin, chloramphenicol, minocycline, but resistant to meropenem, according to the recommendations of the Antibiogram Committee of the French Society of Microbiology (CA-SFM guidelines 2015 for *Burkholderia cepacia*).

Total DNA was also extracted from 20 g of soil as described in Appendix B. As with the culture results, only soil samples A4, A8, and A12 were positive by PCR amplification for *B. pseudomallei*. MLST of soil isolates identified two novel STs: ST-1430 (4, 2, 3, 1, 5, 2, 1) and ST-1431 (1, 2, 3, 1, 5, 1, 1) from A12 and A4, respectively (Table 2). The isolate from sample A8 is still under investigation. The isolate from case #10 (the owner of the yard where the *B. pseudomallei* isolates were found) was also novel, being ST-1043 (4, 1, 3, 2, 5, 2, 1), which shares five alleles with soil isolate A12, but only two with soil isolate A4.

A consecutive investigation to trace back the origin of the fertilizer identified its origins as the surrounds of the Amborovy airport (15°40′56.59″ S, 46°22′20.50″ E); however, none of four soil samples taken from this location were positive for *B. pseudomallei*, either by culture or PCR.

Further genotyping (or WGS) of *B. pseudomallei* strains from the western Indian Ocean island region will play an important role in unraveling historical and contemporary epidemiological investigations in this region. Of historical importance are the postulated links between animal cases in Paris and Réunion Island and the presence of *B. pseudomallei* in the Antananarivo zoo in the 1970s [6,8], which are thought to illustrate the potential for *B. pseudomallei* to be disseminated across large geographic distances via infected animals or manure. It was previously reported that *B. pseudomallei* was transported from France to Réunion Island in the 1970s via an infected horse, which became ill with melioidosis after its arrival [6]. Although it has long been assumed that this horse contracted melioidosis in France, molecular characterization of this isolate would help to establish whether the horse in fact acquired *B. pseudomallei* from the environment in the Indian Ocean. In another instance, MLST characterization of *B. pseudomallei* isolates has enabled us to identify ST-27 isolates from both the Paris zoo outbreak and a 1977 soil isolate obtained from a zoo in Antananarivo. This previously unreported ST overlap suggests the possibility of transmission of *B. pseudomallei* between these two regions. However, it is not known whether ST-27 was introduced into France via Madagascar, or vice versa. Another possibility that should be considered is that of laboratory cross-contamination. On a contemporary level, molecular fingerprinting of *B. pseudomallei* from the western Indian Ocean island region will enhance surveillance measures, public health, and veterinary awareness of the disease, and epidemiological investigation to identify *B. pseudomallei* 'hotspots'.

Table 2. Genetic typing of *B. pseudomallei* isolated from patients in the western Indian Ocean, and from the soil from the yard of case 9, Mahajanga, Madagascar.

Case [Ref.]	Year	Place of Diagnosis	City (Country) Visited within 12 Months of Diagnosis	Allele Profile							MLST Type	Remark
#1 [1]	2004	Réunion Island	Mahajanga (Madagascar)	1	12	34	2	5	2	1	1260	
#2 [1]	2004	Réunion Island *	0									Not typed, nosocomial cases
#3 [1]	2004	Réunion Island *	0									Not typed, nosocomial cases
#4 [5]	2004	Mauritius	0	4	12	34	2	5	2	1	1549	ST1549 is a single locus variant of ST1053 (case #8), ST1054 (case #9), ST1260 (case #1), and 1433 (case #5)
#5 [10]	2005	Madagascar (1st admission)/Réunion Island (2nd admission)	Antananarivo and Mahajanga (Madagascar)	4	1	34	2	5	2	1	1433	ST1433 is a single locus variant of ST1549 (case #4)
#6 [This study]	2006	Mauritius	Bangladeshi worker									Not typed
#7 [6]	2012	Réunion Island	None									Not typed
#8 [11]	2012	Madagascar	Mahajanga (Madagascar)	4	12	3	2	5	2	1	1053	ST1053 is a single locus variant of ST1043 (case #10), ST1432 (case #11), ST1549 (case #4)
#9 [11]	2013	Madagascar	Mahajanga (Madagascar)	4	12	34	1	5	2	1	1054	ST1054 is a single locus variant of ST1433 (case #5), ST1549 (case #4)
#10 [12]	2013	Belgium	Mahajanga (Madagascar)	4	1	3	2	5	2	1	1043	ST1043 is a single locus variant of ST1053 (case #8), ST1432 (case #11), ST1433 (case #5)
#11 [7]	2013	Seychelles **	Unknown	4	2	3	2	5	2	1	1432	ST1432 is a single locus variant of ST1043 (case #10), ST1430 (soil E1)
#12 [7]	2013	Seychelles **	Unknown									Not typed
#13 [1]	2016	Réunion Island	Mahajanga (Madagascar)	4	2	3	1	5	2	1	1430	Same ST than E1. ST1430 is a single locus variant of ST1432 (case #11).
#14 [1]	2017	Réunion Island	Southeast Asia									Not typed
Environmental isolates												
E1 [This study]	2014	Soil from the garden of case 9 (A4)	N/A	4	2	3	1	5	2	1	1430	Same ST as case #13. ST1430 is a single locus variant of ST1432 (case #11).
E2 [This study]	2014	Soil from the garden of case 9 (A8)	N/A									Typing in progress
E3 [This study]	2014	Soil from the garden of case 9 (A12)	N/A	1	2	3	1	5	1	1	1431	

* Cases #2 and #3 were two nosocomial cases acquired from an endoscope used for Case 1. ** Cases #11 and #12 were two cooks from the same facility, hospitalized at the same time.

2.3. Mauritius

Case #4. The first recorded case of melioidosis in Mauritius occurred in January 2004 [15] when a 40-year-old woman on immunosuppressive treatment for systemic lupus erythematosus (SLE) was admitted to hospital with fever, nausea, and vomiting. She was initially started on ciprofloxacin, and was changed to cefotaxime and metronidazole after 48 h because of persistent fever. However, she developed cellulitis of her leg, became increasingly drowsy and confused, and passed away a week later. Her blood cultures became positive after 5 days of incubation, and by the time the organism was identified as *B. pseudomallei* by API 20NE and consistent with phenotypic characteristics, the patient had died. She lived in a low-socioeconomic suburb of Port Louis, and had never travelled abroad. According to her mother, her residence became very muddy at times of heavy rainfall and, although January is generally a wet month in Mauritius, January 2004 was wetter than average. The clinical isolate was subsequently referred to US Centers for Disease Control and Prevention for MLST genotyping, where it was found to be a novel ST, ST-1549 (alleles: 4, 12, 34, 2, 5, 2, 1).

Case #6. In 2006, *B. pseudomallei* was isolated from a swab from the leg wound of a Bangladeshi worker, who had been in Mauritius for less than one year and was admitted for a non-healing wound. The laboratory was prompted into speciating the organism by API 20E because of its positive oxidase test, colistin and aminoglycoside resistance, and the appearance of wrinkled colonies after 48 h. The patient was not diabetic and not generally unwell. He was treated with intravenous meropenem and oral trimethoprim/sulfamethoxazole. He was lost for follow-up, possibly because he returned to Bangladesh. It was difficult to obtain a clear history from the patient because of language difficulties, and although he stated that he had sustained the wound when he had fallen off his bed in Mauritius, it is possible that he acquired the infection in Bangladesh, with reactivation of infection from a latent focus occurring several months later. Since then, there have been no further documented cases of melioidosis in Mauritius.

2.4. Réunion Island

Case #7. In addition to the three imported cases from Madagascar described hereinabove (cases #1, #5 and #13), an autochthonous case was hospitalized in Réunion Island in 2012 [16]. A 57-year-old patient presenting with type 2 diabetes mellitus and hypertension was admitted to Saint-Pierre Hospital with fever (39 °C), an elevated C-reactive protein (248 mg/L), and acute urinary retention requiring the placement of a urinary catheter. Empirical ceftriaxone treatment was initiated, based on an early diagnosis of acute bacterial prostatitis (tender and enlarged prostate without any other physical abnormalities). The urine and three blood cultures were positive for *B. pseudomallei* using the Vitek Compact (bioMérieux, La Balme-Les-Grottes, France). The bacterium was reported as being sensitive to ceftazidime, imipenem, doxycycline, and resistant to all aminoglycosides and colistin according to EUCAST criteria [18]. The therapy was switched to iv ceftazidime and doxycycline. When he recovered he was discharged, but used a peripheral catheter to complete a 4-week course of ceftazidime, and oral doxycycline and trimethoprim/sulfamethoxazole were given to complete 5 months of eradication treatment. The identification of *B. pseudomallei* was confirmed by MALDI-TOF mass spectrometer (MS) (Bruker Biotyper, Bruker Daltonics, Bremen, Germany), PCR targeting type III secretion system genes, and 16S rDNA sequencing. This patient had always lived in Réunion Island, except for three trips of one week to Mauritius five years before becoming ill. No risk factors for exposure were identified.

Case #14. The last reported case (2017) was an imported case in a 40-year-old man who lived in Indonesia, and was working as a fitter's mate on a cruise ship, which stopped in southeast China and Singapore before cruising to Réunion Island [2]. He had no significant past medical history but developed a fever 15 days after departure from Singapore, and was treated with amoxicillin/clavulanic acid. Five days later, when his condition worsened, he was transported by helicopter from the ship to Saint Denis hospital, Réunion Island. He was admitted with fever (40.6 °C), extensive skin pustules on the face, hepatomegaly, septic shock, and multiple organ failure, requiring intubation.

TB-CT scan revealed cerebral venous thrombosis, multiple bilateral lung abscesses, a liver abscess, splenomegaly, and hepatomegaly. Despite immediate antimicrobial therapy with high doses of meropenem (continuous treatment 6 g/day) and amikacin, blood cultures remained positive until day 10. A second TB-CT scan and magnetic resonance imaging of the brain were performed, which showed two subdural empyemas (of 9.5 mm). Antibiotic treatment was changed to ceftazidime (12 g/day by continuous infusion) and the patient's condition improved on day 15, and he was discharged from the ICU on day 70. The last imaging (day 63) showed a reduction in the size of the bilateral lung abscesses, an almost complete regression of the splenic and hepatic abscesses, and a significant reduction of the cerebral abscesses. Blood cultures, respiratory samples and skin abscesses were positive for a *Burkholderia* species identified as *B. thailandensis* by MALDI-TOF MS but confirmed as *B. pseudomallei* by qPCR targeting three genetic markers of the type III secretion system (*orf1*, *orf13*, and *BsSCU2*), as previously reported (see case #13 from Madagascar). The strain was susceptible in vitro to amoxicillin/clavulanic acid (2/1) (MIC of 2 mg/L), ceftazidime (MIC of 1 mg/L), meropenem (MIC of 0.75 mg/L), imipenem (MIC of 0.38 mg/L), trimethoprim/sulfamethoxazole (1/19) (MIC of 0.064 mg/L), and doxycycline (MIC of 0.25 mg/L).

2.5. Seychelles

In January 2013, two patients were hospitalized at Seychelles Hospital with a history of fever, cough, shortness of breath, and chest pain. Their condition deteriorated after admission and they were transferred to the ICU [17]. They were both cooks from the same facility and both had a history of illicit substance abuse. The Seychellois, who had no history of travel, passed away, whereas the other cook, who survived, was from Mauritius, but had been in the Seychelles for the previous ten years. The initial diagnosis was MERS-CoV, legionellosis, or possible tuberculosis. Lung and blood samples were sent to the Health Protection Agency in England and to the National Institute for Communicable Diseases in South Africa for investigation. Samples from both patients grew *B. pseudomallei*, confirmed by qPCR and serology (high IgG titers consistent with a recent infection). The bacterial isolates were sensitive to a wide range of antibiotics, and one of the isolates had a novel ST, ST-1432 (4, 2, 3, 2, 5, 2, 1). A third possible case, who worked at the same premises but not in the kitchen, was identified through active case finding. This third patient originally came from Madagascar. He had equivocal antibody results (1:4000) suggestive of possible exposure to *B. pseudomallei*. The possibility of a point source of contamination was investigated, but no common source of infection was identified.

2.6. Genetic and Genomic Relatedness between Strains Isolated in the Western Indian Ocean

In recent years, whole-genome sequencing (WGS) has become a cost-effective method for strain genotyping, including for MLST. Using WGS data for phylogenomic analyses has also been instrumental in unravelling the early origins of *B. pseudomallei* in Australia, and its subsequent dissemination to tropical regions across the globe, including the western Indian Ocean region. Three studies to date have used WGS to investigate *B. pseudomallei* strains from western Indian Ocean islands [19–21]. Sarovich and colleagues [19] were the first to identify an Asian origin for the Madagascan *B. pseudomallei* strains included in the phylogenetic analysis. Their study showed that the introduction of this bacterium into Madagascar was likely associated with the migration of Austronesian peoples (or their animals) from Indonesian Borneo approximately 2000 years ago [19]. *B. pseudomallei* was subsequently transmitted from the western Indian Ocean region to mainland Africa, and then the Americas, during the Atlantic slave trade [19,20]. The mechanism/s of *B. pseudomallei* dissemination to other western Indian Ocean islands is not yet well understood, but it is likely that it has also been anthropogenically driven. It is also unknown how many of the Indian Ocean islands harbor *B. pseudomallei*, with confirmed cases found only in the most populous islands (Madagascar, Mauritius, Réunion Island, and Seychelles).

Table 2 presents the ST and alleles for 8/13 cases identified in the western Indian Ocean, as well as for the two soil isolates from the garden of case#10 from Mahajanga, Madagascar. MLST analyses have shown that there is no ST overlap between islands, and the STs identified on these islands are not found elsewhere, with the exception of ST-1053, which has been located in both Madagascar [19] and in an imported American case thought to have originated in Ghana [21], although the possibility that this patient had travelled to Madagascar cannot be ruled out. It is also important to stress that the ST of case #13 (hospitalized in Saint Denis, La Réunion, but originally from Mahajanga, Madagascar) and E1 (soil from Mahajanga, Madagascar) are identical (ST-1430), indicating the possibility that the Mahajanga environment was the source of infection in case #13.

3. Current Recommendations and Availability of Measures against Melioidosis

So far, only sporadic melioidosis has been reported in this region, but the increasing number of reported cases ([2], this study) should raise awareness among all those working in the healthcare sector and public health policy makers of the possibility of melioidosis, especially during the rainy season. Doctors and laboratory staff should know how to confirm the diagnosis and treat the disease. Indeed, the association between rainfall and melioidosis has been well demonstrated in hyperendemic regions, with 75% and 85% of cases occurring during the wet season in northeastern Thailand and northern Australia [22,23]. The contaminated soil in the garden of case #10 highlights the risk of occupational or recreational exposure to *B. pseudomallei*, and predisposing risk factors, such as diabetes mellitus, chronic lung or renal diseases, hazardous alcohol use, or thalassaemia, should be considered when gardening or cultivating in endemic zones. Additionally, *B. pseudomallei* has been reported to infect a wide range of animals, such as horses, sheep, goats, cattle, pigs or cats, with anecdotal reports of transmission from animals to humans [22]. Contaminated secretions and excreta represent a possible source of exposure or environmental contamination. As the bacterium typically enters the body through pre-existing cutaneous lesions, including minor trauma such as insect bites, and develops in the wound, contact with contaminated waste may represent an underestimated source of infection.

As with many other tropical regions, melioidosis is probably considerably underreported in the western Indian Ocean islands, and fostering its reporting within national surveillance systems would help to improve monitoring of the incidence of this disease in the western Indian Ocean. Soil (including domestic yards and gardens [24]), surface water and animal waste sampling to test for the presence of *B. pseudomallei* could also be proposed, especially in and around the city of Mahajanga, which has been associated with all the cases from Madagascar. In addition, a seroprevalence survey could be undertaken among all farmers and gardeners in this area.

4. Awareness of Melioidosis

To improve prevention and control of melioidosis, we recommend that physicians consider melioidosis in the differential diagnosis of patients with (1) acute febrile illnesses; (2) risk factors for melioidosis [22] (impaired neutrophil function, diabetes mellitus, pre-existing renal or lung diseases, malignancy, thalassemia and/or excessive alcohol consumption); and (3) compatible occupational or recreational exposure history (soil and water exposure: i.e., farmers, gardeners). However, healthy people can also get the disease if they are infected with a high bacterial load, such as contact with muddy soil without good hand and foot protection. Clinical manifestations are broad, and range from subclinical infection to localized abscess formation, pneumonia, and systemic sepsis. Pneumonia is the most commonly recognized presentation of melioidosis associated with high fever, significant muscle aches, and chest pain [25]. Melioidosis could easily be confused with tuberculosis or even plague, particularly in Madagascar, where this disease is prevalent, or with pneumonia caused by other pathogens. Acute melioidosis septicemia is the most severe form of the infection. It presents as a typical sepsis syndrome with hypotension, high cardiac output, and low systemic vascular resistance. In many cases, a primary focus in the soft tissues or lungs can be found. The syndrome, usually in patients with underlying risk factors, is characteristically associated with multiple abscesses involving soft tissues, the lung, the liver, and spleen. Blood culture is an effective way to diagnose many melioidosis cases, as 50% or more of infections have bacteremia [26].

With the exception of a localized hospital-based study of patients with hyperthermia ($\geq$39 °C), with or without shivering and septic shock, in Mahajanga in 2012, which led to the recognition of cases #8 and #9, no systematic case finding of *B. pseudomallei* infection has been conducted in the western Indian Ocean islands. Generally, there is no awareness of melioidosis in the population and among clinicians, because its diagnosis has been rare, despite the very high prevalence of diabetes in Mauritius. Some laboratory technicians and the clinical microbiologists who diagnosed the cases described above are aware that *B. pseudomallei* is a possibility when they isolate an oxidase-positive Gram-negative bacillus that is resistant to colistin and aminoglycosides, and which produces wrinkled colonies and/or has an earthy smell. However, this knowledge is not universal.

5. Current and Future Challenges

Further studies are needed in order to investigate the true burden of melioidosis in the western Indian Ocean, and especially Madagascar, since it is likely to be higher than currently reported. This could be done by enhancing diagnostic microbiology provision and surveillance systems, training and education of healthcare staff, serological studies and environmental investigations.

Acknowledgments: Authors would like to address a special thank you to all the doctors and medical assistants from the CHU de Mahajanga. We also specially thank Jay Gee, CDC, USA for important information about the sequence types. A part of this work (which took place in Madagascar) was financed by Institut Pasteur à Paris: ACIP2011. We also thank Le Dispositif Prioritaire de Recherche et d'Enseignement en partenariat One Health—Océan Indien for allowing some of the authors to meet and discuss this manuscript.

Conflicts of Interest: The authors declare no conflict of interest.

Appendix A

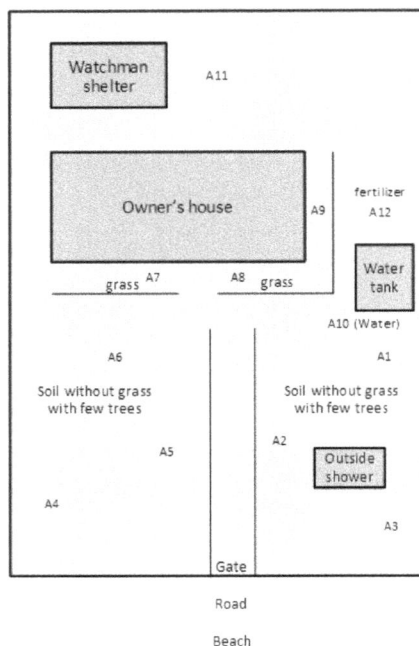

Figure A1. Schematic representation of the estate and yard of the fifth case from Mahajanga, Madagascar (#10). The estate is located along the seashore (separated by an asphalted road).

Appendix B. Materials and Methods

Appendix B.1. Soil Sampling and Culture of B. pseudomallei from Soil and Water

Eleven soil samples and one artesian well water sample were taken from the yard of case #10—(Mahajanga, Madagascar) in 2014 (see Figure A1, Appendix A), one year after the owner fell sick.

Soils: Twenty grams of each soil sample, identified as A1 to A10 and A12, were shaken at 220 rpm at 37 °C for 24 h in 20 mL of distilled water. Ten ml of supernatant were removed and were placed into 30 mL of modified Ashdown's broth (+colistin 50 mg/L). After 48 h, 10 µL of supernatant were spread on modified Ashdown's medium (+gentamicin at 8 mg/L). The plates were examined on a daily basis. Colonies with morphology typical for *B. pseudomallei* were subcultured onto chocolate agar.

B. pseudomallei colonies were identified by basic screening tests (Gram stain, oxidase test), rapid detection of the capsular polysaccharide (CPS) produced by *B. pseudomallei* (Active Melioidosis Detect™ (AMD) rapid test (*InBios*)) [27], MALDI-TOF mass spectrometry, and molecular identification based on the amplification of the *B. pseudomallei* specific target TTS1 (see below).

Water: Sample A10 comprised 1 liter of water from the artesian well. The water was filtered through a membrane (pore size 0.45 µm, diameter 47 mm) on a filtration ramp (Combisart Multi-Branch Systems Manifolds, Sartorius, Göttingen, Germany). The membrane was subsequently placed in Ashdown broth (supplemented with colistin 50 mg/L). After incubation for 48 h, the membrane was transferred onto an Ashdown agar plate (containing gentamicin at 8 mg/L) and incubated for 48 h. No suspicious colonies of *B. pseudomallei* were detected.

Appendix B.2. Molecular Detection of B. pseudomallei from Soil

DNA was extracted from 20 g of soil as previously described [28]: In brief, 20 g of soil was incubated for 48 h with shaking at 37 °C in 20 mL of selective modified Ashdown's broth [29] containing colistin; the sample was then centrifuged twice, and the pellet processed for DNA extraction using a modified protocol of the PowerSoil DNA isolation kit (MoBio Laboratories, Carlsbad, NM, USA). Modifications included the addition of 0.8 mg of aurintricarboxylic acid (ATA) and 20 µL of proteinase K (20 mg/mL). DNA was eluted in 100 µL of 10mM Tris HCl. *B. pseudomallei* DNA was detected by conventional PCR targeting a 115 bp stretch of the *B. pseudomallei* specific *orf2* of type III secretion system (TTS1) as described below. Briefly, 4 µL of DNA were amplified in duplicates in 25 µL volumes.

Appendix B.3. Identification of B. pseudomallei Isolates by PCR

The PCR was conducted in a final reaction volume of 25 µL containing 2 µL of DNA, 0.5 U of FIREPol DNA polymerase, 1× FIREPol Master Mix Ready to Load (2.5 mM MgCl₂), 100 µM of dNTP (Solis Biodine, Tartu, Estonia), and 200 nM of each primer. Primers used to amplify a 548 bp of the *B. pseudomallei* TTS1 gene were BPTT4176F (CGTCTCTATACTGTCGAGCAATCG) and BPTT4290R (CGTGCACACCGGTCAGTATC) [14]. The PCR was performed on a thermocycler (Multigene, Labnet, Woodbridge, NJ, USA) with an initial denaturing step at 95 °C for 1 min, an extension step at 95 °C for 60 s, 54 °C for 60 s, and 72 °C for 2 min for 30 cycles; and a final extension step at 72 °C for 10 min. Samples were separated by agarose gel electrophoresis, stained with ethidium bromide, and visualized with the gelscan (Infinity, VX2-1126MX, Montreal Biotech, Dorval, QC, Canada).

Appendix B.4. MLSTF

The molecular typing tool multilocus sequence typing (MLST), based on sequence polymorphisms in seven genetically stable housekeeping genes, was developed by Brian Spratt at Imperial College London as the initial phylogenetic tool for population analysis of *B. pseudomallei* [7].

PCR conditions were as follows: for each locus, the PCR mixture contained 0.5 U FIREPol DNA polymerase (Solis Biodine, Tartu, Estonia), 200 nM of primers, 1× buffer master mix FIREPol Master Mix Ready to Load (2.5 mM MgCl₂), 100 µM of dNTP, and 2 µL of extracted DNA in reaction volumes

25 µL. These were carried out in a 96-well plate format, with initial denaturation at 95 °C for 4 min, followed by 30 cycles of 95 °C for 30s, 62 °C for 30 s, and 72 °C for 60 s. The samples were maintained at 72 °C for a further 10 min, cooled to 4 °C, and stored at −20 °C. The DNA fragments were sent for sequencing (each strand; forward and reverse) to Beckman Coulter with the primers used in the initial PCR amplification.

For each locus, sequences obtained were analyzed using the MLST database containing the sequences of alleles, allelic profiles, and information about the *Burkholderia* isolates, with analysis tools. This tool is stored on a publicly-available web-based database, allowing comparisons to be made between isolates from different laboratories (https://pubmlst.org/bpseudomallei/). MLST is the gold standard for comparison of isolates from different geographical locations due to high inter-laboratory reproducibility.

References

1. Limmathurotsakul, D.; Golding, N.; Dance, D.A.; Messina, J.P.; Pigott, D.M.; Moyes, C.L.; Rolim, D.B.; Bertherat, E.; Day, N.P.; Peacock, S.J.; et al. Predicted global distribution of *Burkholderia pseudomallei* and burden of melioidosis. *Nat. Microbiol.* **2016**, *1*, 15008. [CrossRef] [PubMed]
2. Allou, N.; Martinet, O.; Allyn, J.; Bouchet, B.; Jaffar-Bandjee, M.-C.; Galas, T.; Traversier, N.; Belmonte, O. Emergence of melioidosis in the Indian Ocean region: Two new cases and a literature review. *PLoS Negl. Trop. Dis.* **2017**, *11*, e0006018. [CrossRef] [PubMed]
3. The Map of Western Indian Ocean. Available online: https://www.lib.utexas.edu/maps/islands_oceans_poles/indian_ocean_w_96.jpg (accessed on 1 March 2018).
4. Leelarasamee, A. Recent development in melioidosis. *Curr Opin Infect Dis.* **2004**, *17*, 131–136. [CrossRef] [PubMed]
5. Girard, G. Can pigs be a healthy carrier of Whitmore's bacillus? *Bull. Soc. Pathol. Exot.* **1936**, *29*, 712–716.
6. Gallimand, M.; Dodin, A. A review of melioidosis worldwide. *Bull. Soc. Pathol. Exot.* **1982**, *75*, 375–383.
7. Godoy, D.G.; Randle, A.J.; Simpson, D.M.; Aanensen, T.L.; Pitt, R.; Kinoshita; Spratt, B.G. Multilocus sequence typing and evolutionary relationships among the causative agents of melioidosis and glanders, *Burkholderia pseudomallei* and *Burkholderia mallei*. *J. Clin. Microbiol.* **2003**, *41*, 2068–2079. [CrossRef] [PubMed]
8. Mollaret, H.H. L'affaire du Jardin des Plantes ou comment la mélioïdose fit son apparition en France. *Med. Mal. Infect.* **1988**, *11*, 643–654. (In French) [CrossRef]
9. Martinet, O.; Soo, A.M.P.; Knezynski, M.; Schlossmacher, P.; Jaffar-Bandjee, C.; Gaüzière, B.A. Melioidosis: About an acquired case in Madagascar and two nosocomial cases. *Bull. Soc. Pathol. Exot.* **2004**, *97*, 366–370.
10. Borgherini, G.; Poubeau, P.; Paganin, F.; Picot, S.; Michault, A.; Thibault, F.; Arvin Berod, C. Melioidosis: An imported case from Madagascar. *Internat. Soc. Trav. Med.* **2006**, *13*, 318–320. [CrossRef] [PubMed]
11. Garin, G.; Djaomazala, I.; Dubois-Cauwelaert, N.; Mahafaly; Raharimanga, V.; Ralison, F.; Herindrainy, P.; Andriamalala, N.C.; Sarovich, D.S.; Mayo, M.; et al. Autochthonous melioidosis in humans, Madagascar, 2012 and 2013. *Emerg. Infect. Dis.* **2014**, *20*, 1739–1741. [CrossRef] [PubMed]
12. Rossi, C.; Vallet, M.; Pierard, M.; Wattiau, P. Melioidosis—Belgium ex Madagascar. Available online: https://www.promedmail.org/post/1687746 (accessed on 8 January 2018).
13. Köppen Climate Classification. Available online: https://www.britannica.com/science/Koppen-climate-classification (accessed on 1 March 2018).
14. Novak, R.T.; Glass, M.B.; Gee, J.E.; Gal, D.; Mayo, M.J.; Currie, B.J.; Wilkins, P.P. Development and evaluation of a real-time PCR assay targeting the type III secretion system of *Burkholderia pseudomallei*. *J. Clin. Microbiol.* **2006**, *44*, 85–90. [CrossRef] [PubMed]
15. Issack, M.I.; Bundhun, C.D.; Gokhool, H. Melioidosis in Mauritius. *Emerg. Infect. Dis.* **2005**, *11*, 139–140. [CrossRef] [PubMed]
16. Borgherini, G.; Camuset, G.; Foucher, A.; Maiza, J.C.; Thibault, F.M.; Picot, S.; Poubeau, P. The first autocthonous case of human melioidosis in Réunion Island. *Med. Mal. Inf.* **2015**, *45*, 47–49. [CrossRef] [PubMed]
17. Bibi, J.; Biscornet, L.; Bermingham, A.; von Gottberg, A. First identification of *Burkholderia pseudomallei* in Seychelles. In Proceedings of the 1st International Forum Public Health Surveillance and Response in Island Territories, Saint Denis, La Réunion, 11–13 June 2013; p. 124.

18. The European Committee on Antimicrobial Susceptibility Testing-EUCAST. Available online: http://www. eucast.org/ (accessed on 1 March 2018).

19. Sarovich, D.S.; Garin, B.; De Smet, B.; Kaestli, M.; Mayo, M.; Vandamme, P.; Jacobs, J.; Lompo, P.; Tahita, M.C.; Tinto, H.; et al. Phylogenomic analysis reveals an Asian origin for African *Burkholderia pseudomallei* and further supports melioidosis endemicity in Africa. *mSphere* **2016**, *1*, e00089-15. [CrossRef] [PubMed]

20. Chewapreecha, C.; Holden, M.T.; Vehkala, M.; Välimäki, N.; Yang, Z.; Harris, S.R.; Mather, A.E.; Tuanyok, A.; De Smet, B.; Le Hello, S.; et al. Global and regional dissemination and evolution of *Burkholderia pseudomallei*. *Nat. Microbiol.* **2017**, *2*, 16263. [CrossRef] [PubMed]

21. Gee, J.E.; Gulvik, C.A.; Elrod, M.G.; Batra, D.; Rowe, L.A.; Sheth, M.; Hoffmaster, A.R. Phylogeography of *Burkholderia pseudomallei* isolates, Western Hemisphere. *Emerg. Infect. Dis.* **2017**, *23*, 1133–1138. [CrossRef] [PubMed]

22. Cheng, A.C.; Currie, B.J. Melioidosis: Epidemiology, pathophysiology, and management. *Clin. Microbiol. Rev.* **2005**, *18*, 383–416. [CrossRef] [PubMed]

23. White, N.J. Melioidosis. *Lancet* **2003**, *361*, 1715–1722. [CrossRef]

24. Kaestli, M.; Harrington, G.; Mayo, M.; Chatfield, M.D.; Harrington, I.; Hill, A.; Munksgaard, N.; Gibb, K.; Currie, B.J. What drives the occurrence of the melioidosis bacterium *Burkholderia pseudomallei* in domestic gardens? *PLoS Negl. Trop. Dis.* **2015**, *9*, e0003635. [CrossRef] [PubMed]

25. Keluangkhot, V.; Pethsouvanh, R.; Strobel, M. Melioidosis. *Med. Mal. Infect.* **2005**, *35*, 469–475. [CrossRef] [PubMed]

26. Vlieghe, E.; Kruy, L.; De Smet, B.; Kham, C.; Veng, C.H.; Phe, T.; Koole, O.; Thai, S.; Lynen, L.; Jacobs, J. Melioidosis, Phnom Penh, Cambodia. *Emerg. Infect. Dis.* **2011**, *17*, 1289–1292. [CrossRef] [PubMed]

27. Houghton, R.L.; Reed, D.E.; Hubbard, M.A.; Dillon, M.J.; Chen, H.; Currie, B.J.; Mayo, M.; Sarovich, D.S.; Theobald, V.; et al. Development of a prototype lateral flow immunoassay (LFI) for the rapid diagnosis of melioidosis. *PLoS Negl. Trop. Dis.* **2014**, *8*, e2727. [CrossRef] [PubMed]

28. Kaestli, M.; Mayo, M.; Harrington, G.; Ward, L.; Hill, J.; Watt, F.; Cheng, A.C.; Currie, B.J. Landscape changes influence the occurrence of the melioidosis bacterium *Burkholderia pseudomallei* in soil in northern Australia. *PLoS Negl. Trop. Dis.* **2009**, *3*, e364. [CrossRef] [PubMed]

29. Kaestli, M.; Mayo, M.; Harrington, G.; Hill, J.; Watt, F.; Gal, D.; Currie, B.J. Sensitive and specific DNA extraction and real-time PCR for detection of *Burkholderia pseudomallei* in the soil in tropical northern Australia. *Appl. Environ. Microbiol.* **2007**, *73*, 6891–6897. [CrossRef] [PubMed]

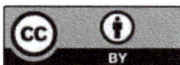

Tropical Medicine and Infectious Disease

MDPI

Article

Emergence of Melioidosis in Indonesia and Today's Challenges

Patricia M. Tauran [1,2,*], Sri Wahyunie [3], Farahanna Saad [4], Andaru Dahesihdewi [5], Mahrany Graciella [6], Munawir Muhammad [7], Delly Chipta Lestari [8], Aryati Aryati [9], Ida Parwati [10], Tonny Loho [11], Dewi Indah Noviana Pratiwi [12], Vivi Keumala Mutiawati [13], Ricke Loesnihari [14], Dewi Anggraini [15], Siwipeni Irmawanti Rahayu [16], Wahyu Nawang Wulan [2], Ungke Antonjaya [2], David A. B. Dance [17,18,19], Bart J. Currie [20], Direk Limmathuthurosakul [18,21], Mansyur Arif [1,2], Abu Tholib Aman [2,22,†], Ni Nyoman Sri Budayanti [23,†] and Diah Iskandriati [24,†] for Indonesia Melioidosis Network

[1] Department of Clinical Pathology, Faculty of Medicine, Universitas Hasanuddin/Dr. Wahidin Sudirohusodo Hospital, Makassar 90245, Indonesia; mansyurarif64@gmail.com
[2] Indonesia Research Partnership on Infectious Diseases (INA-RESPOND), Jakarta 10560, Indonesia; wwahyunawang@gmail.com (W.N.W.); ungkeajy@gmail.com (U.A.); abutholibaman@ugm.ac.id (A.T.A.)
[3] Laboratory of Clinical Pathology, Abdul Wahab Sjahranie Hospital, Samarinda 75123, Indonesia; ayusriwahyunie@gmail.com
[4] Laboratory of Clinical Pathology, Tarakan Hospital, Jakarta10150, Indonesia; farasaad@yahoo.com
[5] Department of Clinical Pathology, Faculty of Medicine, Universitas GadjahMada/Sardjito Hospital, Yogyakarta 55281, Indonesia; adahesihdewi@yahoo.com
[6] Laboratory of Clinical Pathology, Prof. Dr. WZ Johannes Hospital, Kupang 85112, Indonesia; graciella1602@yahoo.com
[7] Department of Microbiology, Faculty of Medicine, Universitas Hasanuddin/Hasanuddin University Hospital, Makassar 90245, Indonesia; dr.munawirmuhammad@yahoo.co.id
[8] Department of Microbiology, Faculty of Medicine, Universitas Indonesia/Cipto Mangunkusumo Hospital, Jakarta 10430, Indonesia; delly.c.lestari@gmail.com
[9] Department of Clinical Pathology, Faculty of Medicine, Universitas Airlangga/Dr. Soetomo Hospital, Surabaya 60286, Indonesia; dr_aryati@yahoo.com
[10] Department of Clinical Pathology, Faculty of Medicine, Universitas Padjadjaran/Hasan Sadikin Hospital, Bandung 40161, Indonesia; idaparwati2008@gmail.com
[11] Department of Clinical Pathology, Faculty of Medicine, Universitas Indonesia/Cipto Mangunkusumo Hospital, Jakarta 10430, Indonesia; tonnyloho@yahoo.com
[12] Department of Clinical Pathology, Faculty of Medicine, Universitas Lambung Mangkurat/Ulin Hospital, Banjarmasin 70233, Indonesia; indahhariadi@gmail.com
[13] Laboratory of Clinical Pathology, Dr. Zainoel Abidin Hospital, Banda Aceh 24415, Indonesia; vividahril@yahoo.com
[14] Department of Clinical Pathology, Faculty of Medicine, Universitas Sumatera Utara/H. Adam Malik Hospital, North Sumatera 20136, Indonesia; loesnihari@yahoo.co.id
[15] Laboratory of Microbiology, Eka Hospital, Pekanbaru 28293, Indonesia; dewianggrainiyovi@gmail.com
[16] Department of Microbiology, Faculty of Medicine, Universitas Brawijaya/Saiful Anwar Hospital, Malang 65112, Indonesia; siwi_fk@ub.ac.id
[17] Lao-Oxford-Mahosot Hospital-Wellcome Trust Research Unit, Microbiology Laboratory, Mahosot Hospital, Vientiane, Laos; david.d@tropmedres.ac
[18] Centre for Tropical Medicine and Global Health, Nuffield Department of Clinical Medicine, Old Road Campus, University of Oxford, Oxford OX3 7FZ, UK; direk@tropmedres.ac
[19] Faculty of Infectious and Tropical Diseases, London School of Hygiene and Tropical Medicine, London WC1E 7HT, UK
[20] Tropical and Emerging Infectious Diseases Division, Menzies School of Health Research, Casuarina, Northern Territory 0811, Australia; bart.currie@menzies.edu.au
[21] Mahidol-Oxford Tropical Medicine Research Unit, Faculty of Tropical Medicine, Mahidol University, Bangkok 10400, Thailand
[22] Department of Microbiology, Faculty of Medicine, Universitas Gadjah Mada/Sardjito Hospital, Yogyakarta 55281, Indonesia

23   Department of Microbiology, Faculty of Medicine, Universitas Udayana/Sanglah Hospital,
      Bali 80113, Indonesia; nyomansribudayanti@gmail.com
24   Primate Research Center, Bogor Agricultural University, Bogor 16151, Indonesia; atie@indo.net.id
*   Correspondence: pattauran@yahoo.com ; Tel.: +62-812-812-4114
†   These authors contributed equally to this work.

Received: 29 January 2018; Accepted: 7 March 2018; Published: 13 March 2018

Abstract: A recent modeling study estimated that there could be as many as 20,000 human melioidosis cases per year in Indonesia, with around 10,000 potential deaths annually. Nonetheless, the true burden of melioidosis in Indonesia is still unknown. The Indonesia Melioidosis Network was formed during the first melioidosis workshop in 2017. Here, we reviewed 101 melioidosis cases (99 human and two animal cases) previously reported and described an additional 45 human melioidosis cases. All 146 culture-confirmed cases were found in Sumatra (n = 15), Java (n = 104), Kalimantan (n = 15), Sulawesi (n = 11) and Nusa Tenggara (n = 1). Misidentification of *Burkholderia pseudomallei* was not uncommon, and most cases were only recently identified. We also evaluated clinical manifestations and outcome of recent culture-confirmed cases between 2012 and 2017 (n = 42). Overall, 15 (36%) cases were children (age <15 years) and 27 (64%) were adults (age ≥15 years). The overall mortality was 43% (18/42). We conducted a survey and found that 57% (327/548) of healthcare workers had never heard of melioidosis. In conclusion, melioidosis is endemic throughout Indonesia and associated with high mortality. We propose that top priorities are increasing awareness of melioidosis amongst all healthcare workers, increasing the use of bacterial culture, and ensuring accurate identification of *B. pseudomallei*and diagnosis of melioidosis.

Keywords: *Burkholderia pseudomallei*; melioidosis; Indonesia

---

1. Introduction

Melioidosis in Indonesia was first diagnosed in Cikande, on Java island, in 1929 [1]. From then to 1960, a few additional cases were reported in Jakarta, Bogor and Surabaya, on Java island [2–5]. More recent reports concerned four culture-confirmed melioidosis cases among tsunami survivors in Banda Aceh, Sumatra, in 2005 [6], 51 culture-confirmed melioidosis patients in Malang, Java from 2011 to 2013 [7], and three culture-confirmed melioidosis patients in Makassar and Luwu Timur, Sulawesi, in 2013 [8]. Nonetheless, the reported cases are likely to be the tip of the iceberg and the true burden of melioidosis in Indonesia is still unclear.

A recent modeling study estimated the annual number of human melioidosis cases in Indonesia at 20,038, with 10,224 deaths annually if mortality was 51% [9]. This alarming estimate is possible, considering that, in Indonesia with a total population of about 260 million, about 1.6 million die every year, and about 350,000 and 150,000 of those who die are estimated to have communicable diseases and diabetes, respectively, defined as the primary causes of death using International Classification of Diseases (ICD) principles and Global Burden of Disease (GBD) analysis [10]. If melioidosis was an undiagnosed contributory cause in only 2% of these, this would account for 10,000 deaths [9]. The under-diagnosis and under-reporting of melioidosis worldwide are considered to be due to a lack of diagnostic microbiology laboratories serving the poor rural populations that are at greatest risk of infection, and a lack of awareness of the disease amongst physicians and laboratory staff [9,11]. Even good microbiological laboratories may initially miss the diagnosis and discard *B. pseudomallei* as a contaminant, especially in non-endemic areas [9,12]. Recent evidence suggests that, in Indonesia, where melioidosis is possibly highly endemic countrywide [9], capacity and utilization of bacterial cultures is limited [13], that misidentification of *B. pseudomallei* as another species or a contaminant is common, and that awareness of the disease among physicians and laboratory staff is very low [6–8].

Under a collaboration between Primate Research Center, Bogor Agricultural University and Health Security Partners (HSP), a workshop on 'Melioidosis: Detection, Diagnosis, Treatment and Prevention Using a One-Health Approach' was held in Bogor, Indonesia, from 14 to 16 August 2017. A total of four doctors, 12 veterinarians, seven microbiologists, one clinical pathologist and 16 other healthcare providers from 33 institutions attended, and the potential burden and challenges of melioidosis were discussed among participants. The Indonesia Melioidosis Network was formed during the meeting. In addition, the Indonesian Association of Clinical Microbiologists (PAMKI) held a session on 'Epidemiology and Clinical Aspect of Melioidosis' during their Annual Scientific Meeting in Padang, from 12 to 14 October 2017, and more evidence of melioidosis in Indonesia was additionally reported at this meeting.

Here, we review the known and additional evidence of melioidosis in Indonesia, present the results of a surveillance study showing awareness and knowledge of the disease and the organism among healthcare providers in Indonesia, and discuss the needs and future challenges to save lives from melioidosis in Indonesia.

2. Melioidosis Cases and Presence of *B. pseudomallei* in Indonesia

We performed (1) a retrospective review of published or reported melioidosis cases in Indonesia, (2) a retrospective study to identify unpublished culture-confirmed melioidosis cases in hospitals in which the microbiology laboratories had isolated *B. pseudomallei* from clinical specimens, and (3) a retrospective study to evaluate clinical manifestations of recent culture-confirmed patients from 2012 to 2017.

Firstly, we searched PubMed and SCOPUS for indigenous cases of melioidosis reported in Indonesia between 1 January 1921 and 30 November 2017, using the MeSH terms 'melioidosis' or '*pseudomallei*'. We also searched bibliographies from selected studies for secondary references. Our search included literature in English, Dutch, German and Indonesian.

In addition to the 64 melioidosis cases previously reviewed [8], we found an additional 35 culture-confirmed human melioidosis cases and two animal cases (Table 1 and Figure 1). Prior to 1960, two additional cases were reported in Cimahi [14] and Salatiga [15] on Java island. We found that an additional report by Verbunt et al. in 1937 [16] was the same case described by Sudibyo [4]. All other cases were recently reported. The first animal case was reported in 2014, being a 3-year-old cynomolgus monkey (*Macaca fascicularis*) raised at Primate Research Center, Bogor [17]. At the 15th Asia-Pacific Congress on Clinical Microbiology and Infection in 2014, a human melioidosis case was reported from Medan, Sumatra [18]. At the first National Melioidosis Workshop in 2017, a human melioidosis case from Yogyakarta, Java [19], 13 cases from Abdul Wahab Sjahranie Hospital, Samarinda, East Kalimantan, eight cases from Dr. Wahidin Sudirohusodo Hospital, Makassar, South Sulawesi, and one case from Prof. Dr. WZ Johannes Hospital, Kupang, East Nusa Tenggara, were reported [20]. At the PAMKI meeting 2017, nine melioidosis cases presenting at Eka Hospital, Pekanbaru, Sumatra [21], and the second animal case from Samboja, Kalimantan [22] were reported. The animal was a Bornean orangutan (*Pongo pygmaeus*) of unknown age from the Borneo Orangutan Survival Foundation in Samboja, East Kalimantan. Both animal cases died shortly after clinical presentation, and the diagnosis was made post-mortem [17,22].

Secondly, to evaluate whether melioidosis had been diagnosed by routine microbiological laboratories in Indonesia but had not been reported, at the first National Melioidosis Workshop and at the PAMKI meeting, we requested participants to review the microbiology laboratory results in their hospitals to determine whether *B. pseudomallei* had been identified. To avoid duplication, cases that had already been reported (Table 1) were not included.

We received information of an additional 45 melioidosis cases (Table 2). A total of 18 and five culture-confirmed melioidosis cases were observed at Sardjito Hospital, Yogyakarta, and at Tarakan Hospital, Jakarta, respectively, from 2012 to 2017. In addition, *B. pseudomallei* was isolated from clinical specimens at Dr. Zainoel Abidin Hospital, Banda Aceh (*n* = 1), Cipto Mangunkusumo Hospital, Jakarta

(n = 4), a private laboratory (Granostic), Surabaya (n = 8), Ulin Hospital, Banjarmasin (n = 1) and Hasan Sadikin Hospital, Bandung (n = 8).

Figure 1 shows the locations of all 146 cases (144 human cases and two animal cases) noted in this article (Tables 1 and 2). Locations were towns where the cases were living or likely to have acquired melioidosis, where such information was available. In the event that the patients' home addresses were not available, the address of the hospitals where the patients presented were used.

Thirdly, we also requested permission to analyze anonymous information of patients diagnosed from 2012 to 2017 to describe clinical manifestations and outcome of recent cases of melioidosis in Indonesia (Table 3). The retrospective study was approved by the education and research departments of five participating hospitals. Overall, we obtained anonymous data of 45 human cases available from Yogyakarta (n = 18), Samarinda (n = 13), Makassar (n = 8), Jakarta (n = 5) and Kupang (n = 1). We excluded three cases with incomplete data.

Of 42 patients included in the analysis, five (12%) were neonates (age <1 month). One and four neonatal cases were observed in Jakarta and Yogyakarta, respectively. All five neonatal cases were blood culture-positive for *B. pseudomallei*, and three of them died. Another seven cases were found in infants (age 1 month to <2 years) and three cases in children (age 2 to <15 years). Thus, of the total, 15 (36%) cases were children (age <15 years) and 27 (64%) were adults (age ≥15 years). Diabetes was the most commonly identified risk factor amongst adults (Table 3), 60% of the cases (25/42) were blood culture-positive for *B. pseudomallei*, and the overall mortality was 43% (18/42).

Specimens, diagnostic methods, and antibiotic susceptibility results of those 42 cases with complete clinical data are described in Table 4. Of the 42 cases, only 15 (36%) had antibiotic susceptibility test (AST) results available. We were informed that AST was often not routinely performed for *B. pseudomallei* because the laboratory staff did not know the correct standard operating procedures, quality control and guidelines on how to handle and perform AST on *B. pseudomallei*. As some AST results were not typical for *B. pseudomallei*, including those previously reported from Malang [7], we note that the AST results may be inaccurate or some isolates might not actually be *B. pseudomallei*. As isolates are not routinely kept in Indonesia, a retrospective study for further evaluation is not possible.

Nonetheless, a total of 10 isolates (five from Samarinda and five from Makassar) reported as *B. pseudomallei* were sent to the Indonesia Research Partnership on Infectious Disease (INA-RESPOND) reference laboratory at Tangerang Regional General Hospital for further characterisation. In addition, 16S rRNA gene sequencing [23] and a PCR assay targeting the type III secretion system of *B. pseudomallei* [24] were performed. Nine of ten isolates were confirmed as *B. pseudomallei* by PCR. One isolate from Makassar was later identified as *Burkholderia stabilis* using 16s sequence analysis. The patient was a 77 year-old male presenting with an acute ischaemic stroke. The positive blood culture was obtained 19 days after hospital admission due to a lack of clinical improvement of alteration of consciousness, and the patient had no other signs and symptoms of sepsis, suggesting that *B. stabilis* was probably a contaminant. This case was not included in the list of melioidosis cases described above. This also supports our hypothesis that some isolates reported as *B. pseudomallei* might be other bacteria, and that training for *B. pseudomallei* identification is critically needed, country-wide.

Details of these nine confirmed isolates and associated clinical manifestations are described in Table 5. Further studies on the nine isolates, including AST, multilocus-sequence typing and whole genome sequence typing, are in progress.

Table 1. Previously reported indigenous human and animal melioidosis cases in Indonesia (n = 101 cases).

Year Presented (References)	Locations	Age(Years)/Gender, Nationality	Clinical Characteristics	Diagnostic Method	Outcome
1929 [1]	Cikande, Java	50/M, Indonesian	Chronic painless nodules in the left thigh	Culture of pus (biochemistry, phenotypic tests and virulence in animal model)	Died
1934 [2]	Jakarta, Java	38/M, Indonesian	Severe sepsis with pulmonary, splenic and prostatic abscesses	Culture of pus (biochemistry, phenotypic tests and virulence in animal model)	Died
1935 [3]	Surabaya, Java	25/F, Indonesian	Abscess in the right gluteal region	Culture of pus (biochemistry, phenotypic tests and virulence in animal model)	Fully recovered
1936 [4,6]	Bogor, Java	60/M, Indonesian	Skin lesion with ulcers on right lower leg after trauma	Culture of pus (biochemistry and phenotypic tests)	Fully recovered
1937 [4]	Jakarta, Java	55/M, Indonesian	Abscess left foot, originated from minor trauma while farming	Culture of pus (biochemistry and phenotypic tests)	Fully recovered
1938 [14] *	Cimahi, Java	48/Unknown, European	Pneumonia and splenic abscess	Culture of pus (biochemistry, phenotypic tests and virulence in animal model)	Died
1950 [5]	Surabaya, Java	28/F, European	Pain in the lower abdomen and high fever	Culture of abscess from the right ovary (biochemistry and phenotypic tests)	Fully recovered
1958 [15] *	Salatiga, Java	Unknown	Diarrhoea	Culture of stool (biochemistry and phenotypic tests)	Died
2005 [6]	Banda Aceh, Sumatra	4 patients; 15/F, 18 mo/M, 10/F and 13/F	Pneumonia	Culture of sputum (API20NE)	Fully recovered (n = 1) or reported as improving (n = 3)
2011–2013 [ ]	Malang, Java	51 patients (unknown age and sex)	Unknown	Culture of sputum, blood, pus and urine (VITEK2)	Unknown
2012 [17] *	Bogor, Java	3/Unknown, cynomolgus monkey	General weakness, decreased appetite, dehydration and cough	Culture of pus (VITEK2)	Died
2013–2014 [5]	Luwu Timur (n = 1) and Makassar (n = 2), Sulawesi	3 patients; 41/M, 45/F and 26/M, Indonesian	Sepsis (n = 1), neck abscess, sepsis and pneumonia (n = 1), and abscess behind the left ear lobe (n = 1)	Culture of blood (n = 1) and pus (n = 2) (VITEK2)	Died (n = 2) or lost to follow-up (n = 1)
2013 [19] *	Yogyakarta, Java	53/F, Indonesian	Neck abscess, pain and dyspnoea.	Culture of pus (Microbact)	Fully recovered
2014 [18] *	Medan, Sumatra	13/M, Indonesian	Fever, dry cough, weight loss and abdominal abscesses	Culture of pus (VITEK2)	Fully recovered
2017 [22] *	Samboja, Kalimantan	Unknown age and sex, Borneo orangutan	Loss of appetite, malaise, less active and apparent fever.	Culture of lung, spleen, and livertissue (VITEK2)	Died
2010–2017 [21] *	Pekanbaru, Sumatra	9 patients (mean age 52 years; range 34–67 years), all males and all Indonesian	Pneumonia, sepsis, abscess, cellulitis, osteomyelitis, pericarditis, seizure and decreased consciousness, and chronic suppurative otitis media with intratemporal complication.	Culture of sputum (n = 4), blood (n = 3) and pus (n = 3) (VITEK2)	Unknown
2014–2017 [20] *	Samarinda, Kalimantan (n = 13), Makassar, Sulawesi (n = 8) and Kupang, Nusa Tenggara (n = 1)	22 patients (median age 53.5 years; range 4–69 years), 15 males and 7 females, and all Indonesian	Sepsis, pneumonia, alteration of consciousness, and localized abscesses	Culture of blood (n = 11), pus (n = 7), tissue (n = 2) and urine (n = 2) (VITEK2) (PCR assay targeting type III secretion system in 9 cases)	Died (n = 9), Fully recovered (n = 9), and Unknown (n = 4)

* Not included in the recent review of melioidosis in Indonesia, published in 2015 [8].

Table 2. Newly reported indigenous melioidosis human cases in Indonesia (*n* = 45 cases).

Year Presented	Locations	Age(years)/Gender, Nationality	Clinical Characteristics	Diagnostic Method	Outcome
2010	Ulin Hospital, Banjarmasin, Kalimantan	Unknown/M	Unknown	Culture of blood (VITEK2)	Died
2010–2017	Private laboratory, Surabaya, Java	8 patients (unknown)	Unknown	Culture of sputum (*n* = 4), blood (*n* = 2), urine (*n* = 1) and nasopharyngeal swab (*n* = 1) (VITEK2)	Unknown
2012–2016	Hasan Sadikin Hospital, Bandung, Java	8 patients (unknown)	Unknown	Culture of blood (*n* = 5), body fluid (*n* = 3; unknown type of body fluid), pus (*n* = 1) (VITEK2)	Unknown
2012–2017	Cipto Mangunkusumo Hospital, Jakarta, Java	4 patients (unknown)	Unknown	Culture of blood (*n* = 1), pus (*n* = 1), sputum (*n* = 1), cerebrospinal fluid (*n* = 1) (VITEK2)	Unknown
2012–2017	Tarakan Hospital, Jakarta, Java	5 patients, 1 mo/M, 3 mo/M, 10 do/M, 2 mo/M and 59/M	Pneumonia (2), diarrhoea (1), alteration of consciousness (2)	Culture of blood (*n* = 4) and sputum (*n* = 1) (Microgen)	Died (*n* = 2), Fully recovered (*n* = 3)
2012–2017	Sardjito Hospital, Yogyakarta, Java	18 patients (median age 7.5 years; range 1 day–78 years), 13 males and 5 females, and all Indonesian	Sepsis, pneumonia, alteration of conscious, localized abscesses and urinary tract infection.	Culture of blood (*n* = 11), pus (*n* = 3), and urine (*n* = 5) (VITEK2)	Died (*n* = 7), Fully recovered (*n* = 11)
2017	Zainoel Abidin Hospital, Banda Aceh, Sumatra	33/M	Unknown	Culture of endotracheal secretion (Vitek2)	Unknown

Table 3. Demographic data, clinical presentations, risk factors and outcomes of 42 culture-confirmed melioidosis cases with available clinical data from 2012 to 2017.

Characteristics	Total Patients (*n* = 42)	Pediatric Patients (*n* = 15)	Adult Patients (*n* = 27)
Demographic information			
Median age (IQR and range)	41.5y (8.8m–56y, 1d–78y)	2m (10d–9.5m, 1d–11y)	55y (47–59.5y, 21–78y)
Male sex	32 (76%)	10 (67%)	22 (82%)
Organ involvement *			
Bacteraemia	25 (60%)	14 (93%)	11 (41%)
Pneumonia	11 (25%)	3 (20%)	8 (30%)
Skin and Soft tissue	9 (21%)	1 (7%)	8 (30%)
Genitourinary	7 (17%)	0 (0%)	7 (26%)
Osteomyelitis	1 (3%)	0 (0%)	1 (4%)
Neurological	1 (3%)	0 (0%)	1 (4%)

Table 3. *Cont.*

Characteristics	Total Patients (n = 42)	Pediatric Patients (n = 15)	Adult Patients (n = 27)
Known risk factors **			
Diabetes mellitus	15 (36%)	0 (0%)	15 (56%)
Chronic kidney disease	5 (12%)	0 (0%)	5 (19%)
Chronic liver disease	2 (5%)	0 (0%)	2 (7%)
Malignancy	2 (5%)	0 (0%)	2 (7%)
Alcohol abuse	1 (2%)	0 (0%)	1 (4%)
Chronic lung disease	1 (2%)	0 (0%)	1 (4%)
Malnutrition	1 (2%)	1 (7%)	0 (0%)
None known	21 (50%)	14 (93%)	7 (26%)
Outcomes			
Full recovery	23 (55%)	8 (53%)	15 (56%)
Died	18 (43%)	7 (47%)	11 (41%)
Unknown	1 (2%)	0 (0%)	1 (4%)

* Bacteraemia was defined as blood culture positive for *B. pseudomallei*. Pneumonia was defined as a clinical diagnosis of pneumonia made by attending physicians (*n* = 7), having productive cough at clinical presentation (*n* = 5) or sputum culture positive for *B. pseudomallei* (*n* = 1). Skin and soft tissue involvement was defined as infections of non-skeletal tissue surrounding or supporting organs and other structures including subcutaneous tissue, muscle and lymph nodes (*n* = 9) or pus culture positive for *B. pseudomallei* (*n* = 8). Genitourinary involvement was defined as urine culture positive for *B. pseudomallei* (*n* = 7). Osteomyelitis was defined as infection of bone (*n* = 1) or pus from bone culture positive for *B. pseudomallei* (*n* = 1); Neurological involvement was defined in a case presenting with sepsis and left hemiplegia. ** Risk factors were defined based on diagnoses made by attending physicians. Six adult patients had two known risk factors. IQR: Interquartile range.

Table 4. Specimens, diagnostic method and reported but unverified antibiotic susceptibility test results in 42 culture-confirmed melioidosis cases with available clinical data from 2012 to 2017.

Characteristics	Total (*n* = 42)
Specimens *	
Blood	25 (60%)
Pus	8 (19%)
Urine	7 (17%)
Tissue **	2 (5%)
Sputum	1 (2%)
Diagnostic method	
Vitek 2 identification system	37 (88%)
Microgen	5 (12%)
Antibiotic susceptibility test	
Not done	27 (64%)
Done ***	
Gentamicin (S)	0/13 (0%)
Amoxicillin-clavulanic acid (S)	2/5 (40%)
Ceftazidime (S)	12/14 (86%)
Doxycycline (S)	7/9 (78%)
Meropenem (S)	14/15 (93%)
Imipenem (S)	2/2 (100%)
Trimethoprim-sulfamethoxazole (S)	6/7 (86%)

* One adult patient had two culture-positive specimens. ** Tibial tissue (1), scrotal tissue (1). *** Data are number of isolates demonstrating susceptibility to the antimicrobial over the total number of isolates tested (%). Data are from the microbiology laboratories that had isolated *B. pseudomallei* from clinical specimens. Some AST results were not typical for *B. pseudomallei*, including resistance to amoxicillin-clavulanic acid, ceftazidime, doxycycline, meropenem and trimethoprim-sulfamethoxazole. We note that the AST results may be inaccurate or some isolates might not actually be *B. pseudomallei*.

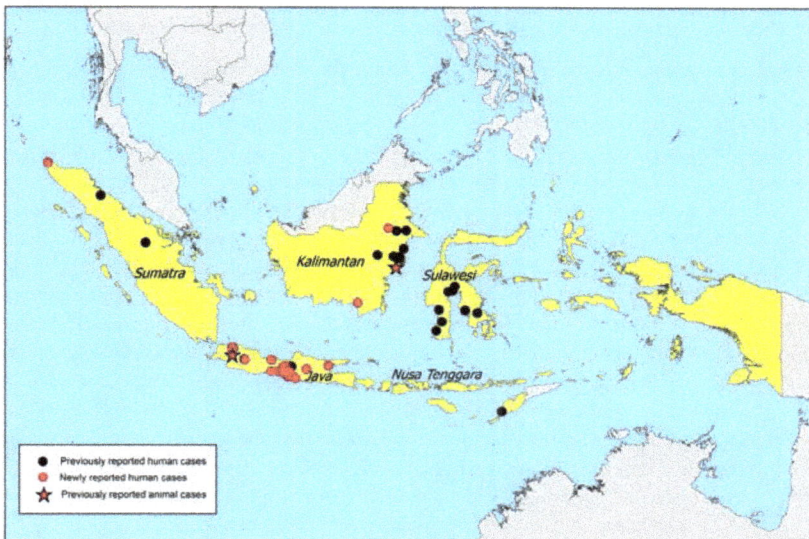

Figure 1. Location of 146 melioidosis cases. Black dots represent locations of 99 previously-reported human cases, red stars represent locations of two previously-reported animal cases and red dots represent locations of 45 newly-reported human cases. An interactive map is available at melioidosis.info website [25].

Table 5. Demographics of nine patients with *B. pseudomallei* confirmed with PCR assays *.

Bacterial Strain	Year of Isolation/ Location of Isolation	Strain Source/Clinical Manifestations	Outcome
HBPMS00001	2015/Konawe, Southeast Sulawesi	Tibial tissue of 55-year old male patient presenting with open wounds with purulent discharge from legs, cough and fatigue	Fully recovered
HBPSK00002	2016/Samarinda, East Kalimantan	Pus of 55-year-old female patient with unknown clinical characteristics	Unknown
HBPMS00003	2016/Kolaka, Southeast Sulawesi	Blood of 56-year-old female patient presenting with decreased consciousness, generalized seizure, focal seizure of hand, headache, fever, swollen knee.	Died
HBPMS00004	2016/Luwu Utara, South Sulawesi	Pus of 39-year-old female patient presenting with lump on neck and weight loss.	Fully recovered
HBPMS00005	2016/Pinrang, South Sulawesi	Blood of 53-year-old male patient presenting with decreased consciuousness, fever, productive cough, shortness of breath, nausea, vomiting, abdominal pain and bloating. Icteric sclera and skin. Left leg swollen, pain and tenderness.	Died
HBPSK00001	2016/Kutai Timur, East Kalimantan	Blood of 4-year-old female patient presenting with fever, petechiae, poor appetite, anaemia	Died
HBPSK00003	2016/Kutai Timur, East Kalimantan	Pus of 37-year-old female patient presenting with skin ulcer on neck, fever	Fully recovered
HBPSK00004	2017/Kutai Kartanegara, East Kalimantan	Blood of 61-year-old male patient presenting with right hemiplegia, fever, decreased consciousness.	Died
HBPSK00005	2016/Samarinda, East Kalimantan	Urine of 44-year-old male patient presenting with fever, abscess on knee	Fully recovered

* 16S rRNA gene sequencing [23] and a PCR assay targeting the type III secretion system of *B. pseudomallei* [24].

3. Current Recommendations and Availability of Measures against Melioidosis

Currently, there are no national guidelines for diagnosis, treatment and prevention of melioidosis in Indonesia. In response to the evidence of the emergence of melioidosis in Indonesia, the international consensus guidelines for diagnosis [11] and treatment [26] of melioidosis have been recommended by the Indonesian Melioidosis Network.

At the first melioidosis workshop, it was recommended that the top priority was to provide education about melioidosis to all clinicians including general practitioners, internists, paediatricians, surgeons, and neurologists, at the hospitals where melioidosis cases have been found (Tables 1 and 2). This could be done by clinical pathologists or microbiologists at case reviews or local meetings in each hospital. Clinicians should be advised to consider melioidosis in any patients presenting with a fever, and communication between clinicians and laboratory staff is recommended if melioidosis is highly suspected; for example, diabetic patients presenting with community-acquired sepsis. Abdul Wahab Sjahranie Hospital, Samarinda has already introduced these steps since September 2016, and the clinicians' response has been positive, with communication between clinicians and laboratory staff occurring for suspected cases and for specimens collected. Two melioidosis cases were diagnosed in 2017 after the implementation of the measures described above. It is important for melioidosis to be included in the curriculum of all medical schools in Indonesia in the future as meliodosis is not currently included in the curricula of any of the medical schools in the country.

Secondly, a simple and easy-to-perform laboratory algorithm for the identification of *B. pseudomallei* from clinical samples, such as that described by Trinh et al. [27], should be implemented in all microbiological laboratories in Indonesia. Future plans include the delivery of a workshop on how to prepare Ashdown agar, identification of *B. pseudomallei*, antibiotic susceptibility testing, and biosafety issues at a national meeting for laboratory staff. Again, in the longer term, these should be included routinely in training programmes for laboratory technicians. Although Vitek 2 is the most common method used for identification of Gram-negative bacilli in Indonesia, there have been some problems with its use for the identification of *B. pseudomallei*, which may have led to under-reporting [28–30]. The BD Phoenix is also used for identification of isolates in some large hospitals in Indonesia. However,

B. pseudomallei is not in the Phoenix database [31], and misidentification of all *B. pseudomallei* isolates as *B. cepacia* is probably occurring in those institutions [31]. These issues will need to be urgently addressed. Microbiology laboratories in Indonesia that need confirmatory tests for isolates suspected as *B. pseudomallei,* can send them to the INA-RESPOND reference laboratory for confirmation by PCR.

4. Surveillance Systems and Reporting of Melioidosis in Indonesia

Melioidosis is not currently a notifiable disease in Indonesia. We are initially considering the establishment of an online system to enable reporting of melioidosis cases from all microbiology hospital laboratories in Indonesia, particularly from those in the Indonesia Melioidosis Network. The system could be similar to ProMED-mail [32] or that of the International Melioidosis Society [25] but specific to Indonesia. The other option would be to use either of these currently running systems. The appropriate surveillance system will be discussed further at the next meeting of the Indonesia Melioidosis Network.

The aim of reporting is to understand the distribution, morbidity and mortality of culture-confirmed melioidosis cases in Indonesia. We are certain that the 146 culture-confirmed melioidosis cases observed to date are just the tip of the iceberg, and continuing and enhancing the reporting system will provide a better understanding of the true burden and distribution of the disease. The results of this surveillance system should be used to encourage health policy makers and the infectious diseases network in Indonesia to give melioidosis the priority it deserves.

5. Awareness of Melioidosis in Indonesia

A questionnaire was developed to evaluate medical practitioners' knowledge and awareness of melioidosis. From 21 August to 4 October 2017, an online questionnaire using Google forms was distributed by the WhatsApp application to multiple formal and informal networks of medical researchers in Indonesia. To reduce response bias, we embedded questions about awareness of melioidosis amongst those on other infectious diseases, including dengue and typhoid. Approval for the study was obtained from the Faculty Medicine Hasanuddin University Ethics Committee, Makassar, Indonesia.

A total of 568 participants completed the questionnaire. The median age of participants was 33 years (IQR 29–36; range 20–65 years), and 196 (34%) were male. Their occupations were general practitioner ($n = 373$, 66%), clinical pathologist ($n = 75$, 13%), internist ($n = 45$, 8%), pulmonologist ($n = 14$, 2%), paediatrician ($n = 9$, 2%), obstetrician ($n = 9$, 2%), neurologist ($n = 8$, 1%), ophthalmologist ($n = 8$, 1%), anaesthesiologist ($n = 5$, 1%), surgeon ($n = 5$, 1%), cardiologist, ($n = 4$, 1%) and others ($n = 13$, 2%). Participants were from Sulawesi ($n = 231$, 41%), Java ($n = 213$, 38%), Kalimantan ($n = 50$, 9%), Sumatra ($n = 28$, 5%), Maluku ($n = 16$, 3%), Papua ($n = 16$, 3%), Nusa Tenggara ($n = 7$, 1%) and Bali ($n = 6$, 1%).

A total of 323 (57%) participants reported that they had never heard of melioidosis, while all participants reported that they had heard of dengue and typhoid. Only 44% of participants ($n = 249$) accurately answered that melioidosis was caused by a bacterium, while 184, 21 and 114 answered that melioidosis was caused by a parasite, a virus and 'I don't know', respectively. 98% ($n = 555$) and 95% ($n = 539$) accurately answered that dengue and typhoid were caused by a virus and a bacterium, respectively. Only 153 participants (27%) accurately answered that the recommended diagnostic tests for melioidosis included blood or urine culture ($n = 151$ and 60, respectively), 285 (50%) answered 'I don't know' how to diagnose melioidosis, and the remaining participants answered inaccurately that the recommended diagnostic tests for melioidosis were stool exam ($n = 19$, 3%) or did not include bacterial culture ($n = 111$, 20%). Only 101 participants (18%) accurately answered that the recommended treatment for melioidosis included ceftazidime ($n = 101$), 231 (41%) answered 'I don't know' how to treat melioidosis, and the remaining participants answered inaccurately that the recommended treatments for melioidosis were chloramphenicol ($n = 56$, 10%), fluoroquinolones ($n = 14$, 2%), antivirals ($n = 24$, 4%), supportive treatment without appropriate antibiotics ($n = 137$,

24%), or fluid management without appropriate antibiotics (*n* = 5, 1%). Eighty-seven percent of the participants stated that MoH should promote education about melioidosis to healthcare workers (*n* = 492) and that MoH should promote awareness of melioidosis to lay people (*n* = 495).

The results of this online questionnaire shows that knowledge about melioidosis is limited among healthcare workers in Indonesia. Education about melioidosis for medical students should be initiated immediately countrywide, and melioidosis should be included in continuing medical education in Indonesia.

Limitations of this online questionnaire include the uneven distribution of participants, and that awareness and knowledge might be underestimated by the biased sampling or overestimated because the study was conducted after the first melioidosis workshop.

6. Current and Future Challenges

We consider that increasing awareness of melioidosis amongst all healthcare workers is the top priority; however, support from all stakeholders is needed. Awareness amongst veterinary professionals also needs to be improved as infections with *B. pseudomallei* have been identified in domestic animals and also certain wildlife including non-human primates (NHP) [33–37].

The second challenge is to increase the use of bacterial culture in Indonesia. In this respect, the under-diagnosis of melioidosis is just a reflection of a generalized limited capacity and under-utilization of diagnostic microbiology in the country. Diagnostic microbiology services in Indonesia face multiple challenges, including: (1) the size and configuration of the Indonesian archipelago, which makes the provision of equitable microbiology services to all parts of the country difficult; (2) the limited number of trained laboratory staff relative to the total population of Indonesia; and (3) historical limitations in the financial and regulatory support from government to develop microbiology services. To overcome these problems, the Indonesian government has established a new national regulation, which includes the provision of microbiology services as one of the requirements for hospital accreditation. This new national regulation has been being implemented gradually in all government hospitals since 2018. We hope that, over the next few years, Indonesia will be able to increase its microbiological capacity considerably.

To improve diagnosis of melioidosis, not only does the capacity of clinical microbiology laboratories need to be expanded [13], but all healthcare workers should also be informed about the importance of bacterial culture in patients presenting with sepsis [38]. Recent evidence suggests that bacterial culture is under-utilized in Indonesia compared to the country's health expenditure, and this could be related to the reimbursement system for bacterial culture, local customs and practice of clinicians, and a lack of support from related stakeholders and organizations [13].

The third challenge is biosafety and biosecurity, as *B. pseudomallei* is classified as a Tier 1 (top tier) Select Agent in the United States that can affect both humans and animals and possibly cause occupational infections [39]. Biosafety guidance for laboratories is needed. All laboratories where melioidosis cases have been found should be evaluated for their facilities, safe practices, and biosecurity with additional training and resources provided if necessary.

Drug availability is not a challenge in Indonesia. Ceftazidime and carbapenems are widely available throughout the country, and may be used and reimbursed within Indonesia's universal health system if the diagnosis can be made.

Future challenges, after diagnosis of melioidosis is improved and if the burden of melioidosis is shown to be as high as expected [9], are to prevent melioidosis by reducing exposure, for example by wearing protective gear such as rubber boots and gloves during exposure to soil. Preventive measures are most important for people with the following conditions: diabetes, heavy alcohol consumption, kidney disease, lung disease, cancer, receiving immunosuppressive therapy and cuts or sores on the skin. Indonesia is an agricultural country, in which the majority of the population are rice farmers, and more than 10 million people are diabetics. It is known that changing behaviour is complex, and a multifaceted intervention is required. In Thailand, there are numerous barriers to adoption of behaviours recommended for melioidosis prevention [40]. Developing an effective prevention programme to reduce people's exposure to *B. pseudomallei* in the environment and to educate them to seek medical attention if melioidosis is suspected, will be a formidable challenge in an Indonesian context.

Acknowledgments: We thank all doctors, microbiologists, clinical pathologists, laboratory staff and healthcare workers who participated in this study. We thank Rene Niehus, Joost Wiersinga and Emma Birnie for German and Dutch translation. We thank Prasad Kuduvalli, the Health Security Partners (HSP) team and Primate Research Center, Bogor Agricultural University, Bogor, for convening the first melioidosis workshop and supporting the Indonesia Melioidosis Network. We thank International Melioidosis Society (IMS) for supporting the Indonesia Melioidosis Network. We thank the Indonesian Association of Clinical Microbiologists (PAMKI) for the support. We thank the Indonesia Research Partnership on Infectious Disease (INA-RESPOND) for molecular diagnostic tests. We also thank Prapass Wannapinij for figure assistance.

Author Contributions: The Indonesia Melioidosis Network conceived the study. P.M.T. collected and analyzed the data, and wrote the first draft of the paper. D.A.B.D., B.J.C. and D.L. assisted with the literature review, participated in workshops, and edited the manuscript. S.W., F.S., and A.D. collected and analyzed the data. M.G., M.M., A.A., I.P., T.L., D.I.N.P. and V.K.M. collected the data. D.C.L., M.A., A.T.A., N.N.S.B. and D.I. contributed to the data and participated in workshop. R.L., D.A. and S.I.R. contributed to the data. W.N.W. and U.A. performed molecular diagnostic tests. All authors contributed to the data of melioidosis in Indonesia and reviewed the manuscript.

Conflicts of Interest: The authors declare no conflict of interest. The sponsors had no role in the design of the studies; in the collection, analyses, or interpretation of data; in the writing of the manuscript, and in the decision to publish the results.

References

1. De Soekarnen, M.C.E.; van de Walle, N. Melioidosis op Java. *Geneeskd. Tijdschr. Ned. Indie* **1932**, *72*, 1618–1635.
2. Pet, M.A.; Fossen, A. Melioidosis der inwendige organen (melioidosis of internal organs). *Geneeskd. Tijdschr. Ned. Indie* **1934**, *74*, 976–981.
3. Bezemer, F. Melioidosis op Celebes. *Geneeskd. Tijdschr. Ned. Indie* **1935**, *75*, 1577–1579.
4. Sudibyo, R.M.S. Twee gevallen van huidmelioidosis. *Geneeskd. Tijdschr. Ned. Indie* **1938**, *78*, 1424–1444.
5. Dunlop, S.J. Rapid recovery in a case of melioidosis. *Doc. Med. Geogr. Trop.* **1952**, *4*, 296–300. [PubMed]
6. Athan, E.; Allworth, A.M.; Engler, C.; Bastian, I.; Cheng, A.C. Melioidosis in tsunami survivors. *Emerg. Infect. Dis.* **2005**, *11*, 1638–1639. [CrossRef] [PubMed]
7. Irmawanti-Rahayu, S.; Noorhamdani, A.S.; Santoso, S. Resistance pattern of *Burkholderia pseudomallei* from clinical isolates at Dr. Saifulanwar General Hospital, Malang-Indonesia. *J. Clin. Microbiol. Infect. Dis.* **2014**, *1*, 17–20.
8. Tauran, P.M.; Sennang, N.; Rusli, B.; Wiersinga, W.J.; Dance, D.; Arif, M.; Limmathurotsakul, D. Emergence of melioidosis in Indonesia. *Am. J. Trop. Med. Hyg.* **2015**, *93*, 1160–1163. [CrossRef] [PubMed]
9. Limmathurotsakul, D.; Golding, N.; Dance, D.A.B.; Messina, J.P.; Pigott, D.M.; Moyes, C.L.; Rolim, D.B.; Bertherat, E.; Day, N.P.J.; Peacock, S.J.; et al. Predicted global distribution of *Burkholderia pseudomallei* and burden of melioidosis. *Nat. Microbiol.* **2016**, *1*, 15008. [CrossRef] [PubMed]
10. Steel, N. Global, regional, and national age-sex specific mortality for 264 causes of death, 1980–2016: A systematic analysis for the Global Burden of Disease Study 2016. *Lancet* **2017**, *390*, 1151–1210. [CrossRef]
11. Hoffmaster, A.R.; AuCoin, D.; Baccam, P.; Baggett, H.C.; Baird, R.; Bhengsri, S.; Blaney, D.D.; Brett, P.J.; Brooks, T.J.; Brown, K.A.; et al. Melioidosis diagnostic workshop, 2013. *Emerg. Infect. Dis.* **2015**, *21*. [CrossRef]
12. Doker, T.J.; Quinn, C.L.; Salehi, E.D.; Sherwood, J.J.; Benoit, T.J.; Glass Elrod, M.; Gee, J.E.; Shadomy, S.V.; Bower, W.A.; Hoffmaster, A.R.; et al. Fatal *Burkholderia pseudomallei* infection initially reported as a *Bacillus* species, Ohio, 2013. *Am. J. Trop. Med. Hyg.* **2014**, *91*, 743–746. [CrossRef] [PubMed]
13. Teerawattanasook, N.; Tauran, P.M.; Teparrukkul, P.; Wuthiekanun, V.; Dance, D.A.B.; Arif, M.; Limmathurotsakul, D. Capacity and utilization of blood culture in two referral hospitals in Indonesia and Thailand. *Am. J. Trop. Med. Hyg.* **2017**, *97*, 1257–1261. [CrossRef] [PubMed]
14. Bonne, C.J.; Hennemann, J.P.; Schijveschuurder, W. Een merkwaardig geval van bronchostenose als gevolg van melioidosis. *Geneeskd. Tijdschr. Ned. Indie* **1939**, *79*, 877–884.
15. Brockelmann, C.H. Melioidosis in Java. *Z. Tropenmed. Parasitol.* **1961**, *12*, 451–460. [PubMed]
16. Verbunt, J.A. Decollatio cutis torpida. Melioidosis. *Geneeskd. Tijdschr. Ned. Indie* **1937**, *77*, 1318–1319.

17. Prabandari, S.; Arifin, E.; Rosmanah, L.; Kartika, D.; Narani, A.; Iskandriati, D.; Pamungkas, J. Fatal *Burkholderia* (*Pseudomonas*) *pseudomallei* septicemia in a cynomolgus monkey (*Macaca fascicularis*) at facility of Primate Research Center, Bogor Agricultural University. In Proceedings of the Kyoto University and Bogor Agricultural University International Symposium, Bogor, Indonesia, 18–21 August 2014.

18. Pasaribu, A.P.; Pasaribu, S. A case of multiple abdominal abscesses due to melioidosis: First case reported from North Sumatera, Indonesia. In Proceedings of the 15th Asia-Pacific Congress on Clinical Microbiology and Infection, Kuala Lumpur, Malaysia, 26–29 November 2014.

19. Aman, A.T.; Paramita, D.; Heryono, F.; Mawarti, Y. A Melioidosis case (sub-mandibular abscess) in Yogyakarta. In Proceedings of the Workshop on Melioidosis: Detection, Diagnosis, Treatment and Prevention Using a One Health Approach, Bogor, West Java, Indonesia, 14–16 August 2017.

20. Tauran, P.M.; Wahyunie, S.; Graciella, M. Indonesian melioidosis cases: Kalimantan, Sulawesi and Nusa Tenggara. In Proceedings of the Workshop on Melioidosis: Detection, Diagnosis, Treatment and Prevention Using A One Health Approach, Bogor, West Java, Indonesia, 14–16 August 2017.

21. Anggraini, D. Cases of melioidosis in private hospital in Pekanbaru. In Proceedings of the Annual Scientific Meeting (ASM) PAMKI, From Basic Microbiology to Clinical Applied, Approaches to New Technologies in Microbial Diagnostic, Padang, West Sumatra, Indonesia, 12–14 October 2017.

22. Lestari, D.C.; Ibrahim, F.; Karuniawati, A.; Pratamiutaminingsih, A.; Chrisnawaty, D. Melioidosis Confirmed from Non-human Primate Specimens. In Proceedings of the Annual Scientific Meeting (ASM) PAMKI, From Basic Microbiology to Clinical Applied, Approaches to New Technologies in Microbial Diagnostic, Padang, West Sumatra, Indonesia, 12–14 October 2017.

23. Thaipadungpanit, J.; Chierakul, W.; Wuthiekanun, V.; Limmathurotsakul, D.; Amornchai, P.; Boonslip, S.; Smythe, L.D.; Limpaiboon, R.; Hoffmaster, A.R.; Day, N.P.; et al. Diagnostic accuracy of real-time PCR assays targeting 16S rRNA and lipL32 genes for human leptospirosis in Thailand: A case-control study. *PLoS ONE* **2011**, *6*, e16236. [CrossRef]

24. Novak, R.T.; Glass, M.B.; Gee, J.E.; Gal, D.; Mayo, M.J.; Currie, B.J.; Wilkins, P.P. Development and evaluation of a real-time PCR assay targeting the type III secretion system of *Burkholderia pseudomallei*. *J. Clin. Microbiol.* **2006**, *44*, 85–90. [CrossRef] [PubMed]

25. MORU. The Map of Melioidosis Cases. Available online: http://www.melioidosis.info/ (accessed on 9 March 2018).

26. Lipsitz, R.; Garges, S.; Aurigemma, R.; Baccam, P.; Blaney, D.D.; Cheng, A.C.; Currie, B.J.; Dance, D.; Gee, J.E.; Larsen, J.; et al. Workshop on treatment of and postexposure prophylaxis for *Burkholderia pseudomallei* and *B. mallei* infection, 2010. *Emerg. Infect. Dis.* **2012**, *18*, e2. [CrossRef] [PubMed]

27. Trinh, T.T.; Hoang, T.S.; Tran, D.A.; Trinh, V.T.; Gohler, A.; Nguyen, T.T.; Hoang, S.N.; Krumkamp, R.; Nguyen, L.T.N.; May, J.; et al. A simple laboratory algorithm for diagnosis of melioidosis in resource-constrained areas: A study from north-central Vietnam. *Clin. Microbiol. Infect.* **2018**, *24*, 84. [CrossRef] [PubMed]

28. Deepaka, R.N.; Crawleyb, B.; Phangc, E. *Burkholderia pseudomallei* identification: A comparison between the API 20NE and Vitek 2 GN systems. *Trans. R. Soc. Trop. Med. Hyg.* **2008**, *102*, S42–S44. [CrossRef]

29. Zong, Z.; Wang, X.; Deng, Y.; Zhou, T. Misidentification of *Burkholderia pseudomallei* as *Burkholderia cepacia* by the VITEK 2 system. *J. Med. Microbiol.* **2012**, *61*, 1483–1484. [CrossRef] [PubMed]

30. Jun, J.-B.; Lee, T.; Jeong, J.; Chun, J.-H.; Shin, Y.-W.; Jung, J. Accidental occupational exposure to *Burkholderia pseudomallei* in South Korea did not result in melioidosis. *Infect. Control Hosp. Epidemiol.* **2017**, *38*, 886–888. [CrossRef] [PubMed]

31. Koh, T.H.; Yong Ng, L.S.; Foon Ho, J.L.; Sng, L.H.; Wang, G.C.Y.; Valentine Tzer Pin Lin, R. Automated identification systems and *Burkholderiapseudomallei*. *J. Clin. Microbiol.* **2003**, *41*, 1809. [CrossRef] [PubMed]

32. ISID. The Program for Monitoring Emerging Diseases. Available online: https://www.promedmail.org/ (accessed on 9 March 2018).

33. Choy, J.L.; Mayo, M.; Janmaat, A.; Currie, B.J. Animal melioidosis in Australia. *Acta Trop.* **2000**, *74*, 153–158. [CrossRef]

34. Limmathurotsakul, D.; Thammasart, S.; Warrasuth, N.; Thapanagulsak, P.; Jatapai, A.; Pengreungrojanachai, V.; Anun, S.; Joraka, W.; Thongkamkoon, P.; Saiyen, P.; et al. Melioidosis in animals, Thailand, 2006–2010. *Emerg. Infect. Dis.* **2012**, *18*, 325–327. [CrossRef] [PubMed]

35. Johnson, C.H.; Skinner, B.L.; Dietz, S.M.; Blaney, D.; Engel, R.M.; Lathrop, G.W.; Hoffmaster, A.R.; Gee, J.E.; Elrod, M.G.; Powell, N.; et al. Natural infection of *Burkholderia pseudomallei* in an imported pigtail macaque (*Macaca nemestrina*) and management of the exposed colony. *Comp. Med.* **2013**, *63*, 528–535. [PubMed]

36. Hicks, C.L.; Kinoshita, R.; Ladds, P.W. Pathology of melioidosis in captive marine mammals. *Aust. Vet. J.* **2000**, *78*, 193–195. [CrossRef] [PubMed]

37. Sprague, L.D.; Neubauer, H. Melioidosis in animals: A review on epizootiology, diagnosis and clinical presentation. *J. Vet. Med. B Infect. Dis. Vet. Public Health* **2004**, *51*, 305–320. [CrossRef] [PubMed]

38. Dellinger, R.P.; Levy, M.M.; Rhodes, A.; Annane, D.; Gerlach, H.; Opal, S.M.; Sevransky, J.E.; Sprung, C.L.; Douglas, I.S.; Jaeschke, R.; et al. Surviving sepsis campaign: International guidelines for management of severe sepsis and septic shock: 2012. *Crit. Care Med.* **2013**, *41*, 580–637. [CrossRef] [PubMed]

39. Benoit, T.J.; Blaney, D.D.; Gee, J.E.; Elrod, M.G.; Hoffmaster, A.R.; Doker, T.J.; Bower, W.A.; Walke, H.T. *Melioidosis Cases and Selected Reports of Occupational Exposures to Burkholderi apseudomallei—United States, 2008–2013*; Centers for Disease Control and Prevention: Atlanta, GA, USA, 2015.

40. Suntornsut, P.; Wongsuwan, N.; Malasit, M.; Kitphati, R.; Michie, S.; Peacock, S.J.; Limmathurotsakul, D. Barriers and recommended interventions to prevent melioidosis in northeast Thailand: A Focus group study using the behaviour change wheel. *PLoS Negl. Trop. Dis.* **2016**, *10*, e0004823. [CrossRef] [PubMed]

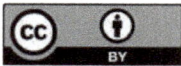

Tropical Medicine and Infectious Disease

MDPI

Review

Melioidosis in the Lao People's Democratic Republic

David A.B. Dance [1,2,3,*] , Manophab Luangraj [1] , Sayaphet Rattanavong [1],
Noikaseumsy Sithivong [4], Oulayphone Vongnalaysane [5], Manivanh Vongsouvath [1]
and Paul N. Newton [1,2,3]

[1]   Lao-Oxford-Mahosot Hospital-Wellcome Trust Research Unit, Microbiology Laboratory, Mahosot Hospital,
      Vientiane, Laos; manophab.l@tropmedres.ac (M.L.); Sayaphet@tropmedres.ac (S.R.);
      Manivanh@tropmedres.ac (M.V.); Paul.Newton@tropmedres.ac (P.N.N.)
[2]   Centre for Tropical Medicine and Global Health, Nuffield Department of Clinical Medicine,
      Old Road Campus, University of Oxford, Oxford OX3 7FZ, UK
[3]   Faculty of Infectious and Tropical Diseases, London School of Hygiene and Tropical Medicine,
      London WC1E 7HT, UK
[4]   National Centre for Laboratory and Epidemiology, Vientiane, Laos; noikaseumsy@gmail.com
[5]   Microbiology Laboratory, Khammouan Provincial Hospital, Thakhek, Laos; bacterialkm@gmail.com
[*]   Correspondence: david.d@tropmedres.ac; Tel.: +856-2077475588

Received: 29 January 2018; Accepted: 13 February 2018; Published: 19 February 2018

Abstract: Melioidosis is clearly highly endemic in Laos, although the disease has only been diagnosed regularly in humans (1359 cases) since 1999, and only a single animal case has been microbiologically confirmed. *Burkholderia pseudomallei* is extensively and abundantly present in soil and surface water in central and southern Laos, but the true distribution of the disease across the country remains to be determined. Surveillance is almost non-existent and diagnostic microbiology services are not yet well established, whilst awareness of melioidosis is low amongst policy-makers, healthcare providers, and the public. It is hoped that this situation will improve over the next decade as the country rapidly develops, especially as this is likely to be accompanied by a further increase in the prevalence of diabetes, meaning that more people in this predominantly agricultural population will be at risk of contracting melioidosis.

Keywords: melioidosis; *Burkholderia pseudomallei*; Laos; Lao PDR

1. History

The Lao People's Democratic Republic (Laos) is a land-locked country in Southeast Asia with a population of approximately 6.5 million people, the majority of whom are subsistence farmers, although the country is developing rapidly. Melioidosis was not recognized in Laos until 1999 [1]. Given that Laos is adjacent to highly endemic parts of Thailand, it is likely that the bacterium that causes it has long been present in the environment but that it was not recognized due to a lack of laboratory facilities and awareness amongst healthcare staff. In fact, the detection of *Burkholderia pseudomallei* in the Lao environment preceded the detection of cases of human melioidosis, although this was not reported until later [2]. An even earlier case was almost certainly acquired in Laos during military action in 1954, although the diagnosis was made in a hospital in Vietnam [3].

2. Review of Melioidosis Cases and Presence of *B. pseudomallei*

2.1. Human

Diagnostic microbiology services for human infectious disease have been relatively underdeveloped in Laos compared withmost neighbouring countries such as Thailand, China, and Vietnam. The confirmation of melioidosis as an important public health problem in Laos followed the establishment of a research collaboration between the Microbiology Laboratory of Mahosot Hospital, one of the main central referral hospitals in the capital, Vientiane, and the Mahidol-Oxford-Research Unit in Thailand, which had been working on melioidosis in Ubon Ratchathani since 1986. This led to the creation of the Lao-Oxford-Mahosot Hospital-Wellcome Trust Research Unit (LOMWRU), which has supported the provision of diagnostic services for melioidosis, including the use of selective culture media and reagents (Ashdown's agar and broth, latex agglutination and API 20NE) and collated data on culture-positive cases since 1999. Between 2000 and 2004, LOMWRU found *B. pseudomallei* in 14 patients with bacteraemia, representing 3% of positive blood cultures [4]. Since then, the number of cases diagnosed has increased each year, reflecting greater awareness of the disease amongst healthcare workers as well as the growing numbers of Lao people with underlying diseases that predispose to melioidosis such as diabetes, which was estimated to have a prevalence of 5.6% of the Lao population in 2016 [5].

In addition to receiving clinical samples from Mahosot Hospital itself, samples are sent to Mahosot Microbiology Laboratory from other hospitals in and around Vientiane and from other provinces, particularly associated with studies of the aetiology of fever in Luangnamtha, Salavan, and latterly Xiangkhouang provinces. In total, the LOMWRU/Mahosot Microbiology Laboratory has diagnosed 1232 cases of culture-positive melioidosis between 1999 and 2017. The majority came from Vientiane Capital and Vientiane Province, which represent the main catchment areas for Mahosot Hospital; however, since Mahosot Hospital acts as a central referral hospital for parts of Laos and accepts samples from other hospitals for the investigation of possible melioidosis, cases have been seen originating from every province in Laos except Luangnamtha. Details of these cases will be reported elsewhere.

In addition, support was provided by the Centre d'Infectiologie Christophe Mérieux du Laos (CICML) to establish a diagnostic microbiology laboratory in Khammouan Provincial Hospital in Thakhek in 2009, and staff were trained in the recognition of *B. pseudomallei* and invited to refer any isolates whose identity was uncertain to LOMWRU. Between 2010 and 2017, 79 patients were confirmed with melioidosis, all of whom came from Khammouan Province.

Between 2011 and 2016, the European Union provided €3,000,000 to support the further development of diagnostic capacity in Laos (https://ec.europa.eu/europeaid/case-studies/eu-support-epidemiology-and-laboratory-capacity-laos_en). Laboratory staff in Champasak, Savannakhet, Luangphrabang, Oudomxai, and Luangnamtha were trained in the identification of *B. pseudomallei* and asked to refer suspect isolates to the National Centre for Laboratory and Epidemiology (NCLE) in Vientiane for confirmation. Between 2012 and 2017, this resulted in the identification of a further 48 cases of culture-positive melioidosis.

The data from these three sources have been combined in Table 1, and Figure 1 presents a map showing the distribution of cases and laboratories capable of confirming the diagnosis. An additional 19 Lao patients diagnosed in Thailand [6] and two additional travel-associated cases [7,8] have not been included in the table. Undoubtedly, these figures only represent the 'tip of the iceberg' in Laos, and the distribution of cases across the country is subject to considerable sampling bias. There are still large areas of the country that do not have access to good diagnostic laboratories. Awareness of melioidosis amongst both physicians and laboratory staff remains low, and, even where laboratories do exist, the use of diagnostic microbiology has not yet been fully assimilated into routine clinical practice. The fact that patients usually have to pay for diagnostic tests acts as a further disincentive to investigating the aetiology of infection.

Table 1. Cases of culture-positive melioidosis diagnosed in Laos [1,2].

Province	1999	2000	2001	2002	2003	2004	2005	2006	2007	2008	2009	2010	2011	2012	2013	2014	2015	2016	2017	TOTAL
Attapeu									1	1					2	3			1	9
Bokeo												1								1
Bolikhamxai [1]					1	2	3	3	3	3	2	3	2	4	8	8	7	7	12	68
Champasak [1]			1	1				1			2				1	4		3	1	14
Houaphan												1	1	1		1			1	5
Khammouan [1]							1	3		2		10	12	19	12	10	6	8	17	100
Luangnamtha																				0
Luangphrabang																1	2			3
Oudomxai												1							1	2
Phongsali																1				1
Salavan										2	6	4	4	3	3	11	9	4	15	61
Savannakhet [1]												1	1		1	3	6	1	2	15
Vientiane Province [1]		1	1	1	1	7	7	9	15	11	19	33	10	13	28	32	33	30	36	287
Vientiane Capital [1]		2	6	4	5	25	20	27	51	31	22	58	41	57	66	65	81	108	73	742
Xaignaburi								1	1	1		2		1		1		4	4	16
Xekong										1										1
Xaisomboun [3]	1										1	2			2	2	3	2	2	17
Xiangkhouang [1]													1		1	1		1	1	5
Unknown [1]						1	2										2	5	1	12
TOTAL	1	3	8	6	9	35	33	44	72	54	50	118	72	98	124	144	149	173	167	1359

[1] Pooled data from LOMWRU, Thakhek Hospital and NCLE. [2] Data reflect patient's home village (where known) but not necessarily place of acquisition of melioidosis. [3] Province established in 2014.

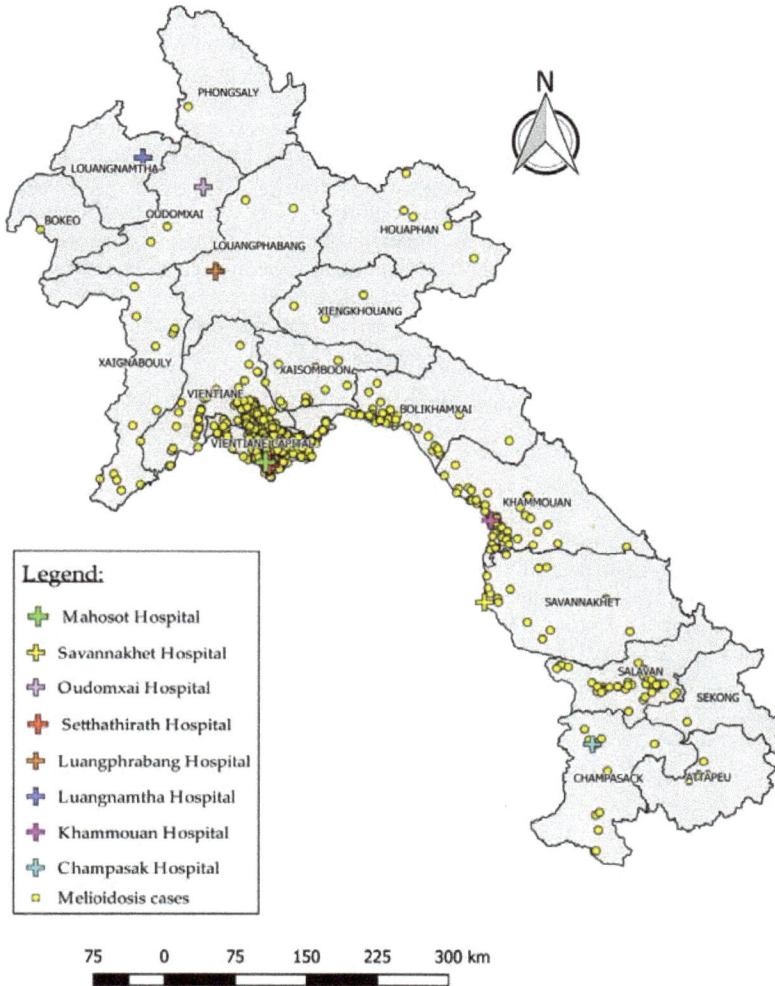

Figure 1. Location of homes of 1310 cases of melioidosis and hospital laboratories capable of making a diagnosis of melioidosis in Laos (data only available for 1310 of 1359 cases).

2.2. Animal

Animal meliodosis is undoubtedly present in Laos, although to date only a single case, in a goat, has been confirmed by the LOMWRU laboratory (Newton, P.N.; Vongsouvath, M. (LOMWRU, Vientiane, Lao PDR). Unpublished observations, 2003). Animal surveillance in Laos is limited. Furtherstudies of melioidosis in animals are just beginning to be initiated.

2.3. Environment

Several studies have demonstrated that *B. pseudomallei* is widespread in the environment, at least in central and southern Laos, although the country has not been extensively and systematically sampled to determine the true nationwide distribution of the organism. *B. pseudomallei* was first isolated in 36% of 110 soil samples collected in and around Vientiane in 1998 [2]. A subsequent study found the organism to be abundantly present in soil in Salavan, but not in a transect from eastern Vientiane to Xiangkhouang [9]. A single isolate from soil in Luangnamtha was reported in this study, although subsequent studies of this isolate have shown that it was actually *Burkholderia cepacia* that cross-reacted in a *B. pseudomallei*-specific latex agglutination test (Dance, D.A.B. (LOMWRU, Vientiane, Lao PDR). Unpublished observations, 2011). *B. pseudomallei* was later confirmed to be present in both soil and surface water in Salavan, including the Sedone river [10]. However, these earlier studies were undertaken using culture alone, which may have underestimated the presence of *B. pseudomallei* [11]. *B. pseudomallei* was also found to be readily isolated from a rice paddy in Vientiane about 56 km from Vientiane's capital [12]. More recently, a nationwide study of the presence of *B. pseudomallei* in the Mekong and its tributaries in Laos demonstrated its presence in 9% of the rivers in the dry season and in 57% of the rivers in the rainy season, mainly in turbid river water with associated *B. pseudomallei*-positive sediments, and exclusively in the south and centre of the country, suggesting that rivers may be useful in assessing the distribution and aquatic dispersal of *B. pseudomallei* [13].

3. Current Recommendations and Availability of Measures against Melioidosis

3.1. Surveillance Systems and Reporting

3.1.1. Human

Melioidosis is not statutorily notifiable in Laos and there is no formal surveillance system for human melioidosis. Data are currently only collated by researchers with an interest in the disease as above. Informally, both LOMWRU and the Thakhek laboratories send monthly anonymized reports of episodes of bacteraemia (and other *B. pseudomallei* isolates in the case of the Thakhek laboratory) to the Ministry of Health and other relevant organisations.

3.1.2. Animal

There is no surveillance system for animal melioidosis in Laos.

3.2. Guidelines

Melioidosis was included in a manual on diagnosis and treatment of infectious diseases produced (in Lao/English and Lao/French editions) by the Institut de la Francophonie pour la Médecine Tropicale du Laos in 2002 (updated in 2004) that was approved by the Minister of Health. Melioidosis was also included in the 'National Treatment Guideline' (fourth edition) in Lao that was issued in 2012. Both of these were distributed to district and provincial hospitals with the aim of improving the quality of management of infections, including melioidosis, but it is not known how widely available they are and whether they are followed. Neither is available online or outside Laos. The recommendations are also not entirely consistent with current international consensus guidelines on melioidosis treatment [14]. In addition, advice about clinical and epidemiological clues to the diagnosis, which samples to submit, and how to treat patients, have been distributed to users of the Mahosot Microbiology Laboratory through the Mahosot Microbiology Review, an internally distributed newsletter which is available both in English and Lao languages. Diagnostic guidance is contained in a laboratory user manual for the Mahosot laboratory, which is to be issued shortly, and plans are in place to include revised treatment guidelines in updated national antibiotic guidelines that are under development.

4. Awareness of Melioidosis

Awareness of the disease amongst health professionals has gradually increased in the area in and around Vientiane since the establishment of LOMWRU but is otherwise patchy, although some clinicians in provinces of relatively high incidence (e.g., Salavan and Savannakhet) regularly consider the diagnosis and manage patients accordingly. The disease is not yet considered a priority by the

Trop. Med. Infect. Dis. **2018**, 3, 21

Ministry of Public Health. Although no formal surveys have been conducted, awareness amongst the public is likely to be even lower than that in Thailand [15].

5. Major Achievements

Activities relating to melioidosis in Laos are at a very early stage. A case series of the first 1088 patients with melioidosis is in preparation and it is planned that a national workshop, analogous to those that have taken place in neighbouring countries such as Cambodia, will be held in the near future. It is hoped that this will lead to the establishment of a national network of clinicians and researchers with an interest in the disease.

6. Current and Future Challenges

Based on the experience at Mahosot Hospital, it is likely that there are still hundreds of people dying of undiagnosed melioidosis in Laos each year, and this is likely to increase as diabetes becomes more common, as it has in neighbouring countries [16]. The biggest challenges facing those who wish to reduce this burden are the relative under-development of diagnostic microbiology services across the country, the lack of a 'culture of culture' amongst clinicians, and a lack of awareness of the disease amongst policy-makers, healthcare providers, and the public. It is hoped that significant progress can be made in these areas over the next decade.

Acknowledgments: The work of LOMWRU is supported by Wellcome (core grant number 106698/Z/14/Z). We are grateful to the doctors, nursing staff, and the staff of the microbiology laboratories of all the hospitals who have provided samples and data, and the Directors of Mahosot Hospital, the Minister of Health and the Director of the Curative Department, Ministry of Health, for their support of these studies.

Author Contributions: D.A.B.D. co-ordinated the review and wrote the first draft. M.L. collated the Mahosot clinical data, populated the table, and prepared the map. N.S. provided NCLE data and O.V. provided the Thakhek data. S.R. participated in most of the environmental studies cited and assisted in the production of the table and map. P.N.N. and M.V. oversaw the routine and research activities relating to melioidosis in LOMWRU and the Mahosot Microbiology Laboratory respectively. All authors reviewed, edited, and approved the final manuscript.

Conflicts of Interest: The authors declare no conflict of interest. The funding sponsors had no role in the design of the study, in the collection, analyses, or interpretation of data, or in the writing of the manuscript.

References

1. Phetsouvanh, R.; Phongmany, S.; Newton, P.; Mayxay, M.; Ramsay, A.; Wuthiekanun, V.; White, N.J. Melioidosis and Pandora's box in the Lao People's Democratic Republic. *Clin. Infect. Dis.* **2001**, *32*, 653–654. [CrossRef] [PubMed]
2. Wuthiekanun, V.; Mayxay, M.; Chierakul, W.; Phetsouvanh, R.; Cheng, A.C.; White, N.J.; Day, N.P.; Peacock, S.J. Detection of *Burkholderia pseudomallei* in soil within the Lao People's Democratic Republic. *J. Clin. Microbiol.* **2005**, *43*, 923–924. [CrossRef] [PubMed]
3. Besseige; Cornet; Trapet; Rigaud; Maury. A propos de deux cas de mélioïdose. *Bull. Soc. Pathol. Exot. Filiales* **1959**, *52*, 437–447. [PubMed]
4. Phetsouvanh, R.; Phongmany, S.; Soukaloun, D.; Rasachak, B.; Soukhaseum, V.; Soukhaseum, S.; Frichithavong, K.; Khounnorath, S.; Pengdee, B.; Phiasakha, K.; et al. Causes of community-acquired bacteremia and patterns of antimicrobial resistance in Vientiane, Laos. *Am. J. Trop. Med. Hyg.* **2006**, *75*, 978–985. [PubMed]
5. Diabetes country profiles-Lao People's Democratic Republic. Available online: http://www.who.int/diabetes/country-profiles/en/ (accessed on 10 December 2017).
6. Tanwisaid, K. The melioidosis cases report of Lao People's Democratic Republic patients in Nakhon Phanom Hospital, northeastern Thailand. *J. Health Sci.* **2008**, *17*, 1193–1197.
7. Badran, S.; Pedersen, T.I.; Roed, C.; Lunding, S.; Birk, N.; Vestergaard, H.; Roder, B.; Lillelund, H.K.; Kurtzhals, J.A.; Kemp, M.; et al. Imported melioidosis in Danish travellers: A diagnostic challenge. *Scand. J. Infect. Dis.* **2010**, *42*, 445–449. [CrossRef] [PubMed]

8. Tamtami, N.A.; Khamis, F.; Al-Jardani, A. Imported case of melioidosis in Oman: Case report. *Oman Med. J.* **2017**, *32*, 62–65. [CrossRef] [PubMed]

9. Rattanavong, S.; Wuthiekanun, V.; Langla, S.; Amornchai, P.; Sirisouk, J.; Phetsouvanh, R.; Moore, C.E.; Peacock, S.J.; Buisson, Y.; Newton, P.N. Randomized soil survey of the distribution of *Burkholderia pseudomallei* in rice fields in Laos. *Appl. Environ. Microbiol.* **2011**, *77*, 532–536. [CrossRef] [PubMed]

10. Vongphayloth, K.; Rattanavong, S.; Moore, C.E.; Phetsouvanh, R.; Wuthiekanun, V.; Sengdouangphachanh, A.; Phouminh, P.; Newton, P.N.; Buisson, Y. *Burkholderia pseudomallei* detection in surface water in southern Laos using Moore's swabs. *Am. J. Trop. Med. Hyg.* **2012**, *86*, 872–877. [CrossRef] [PubMed]

11. Knappik, M.; Dance, D.A.B.; Rattanavong, S.; Pierret, A.; Ribolzi, O.; Davong, V.; Silisouk, J.; Vongsouvath, M.; Newton, P.N.; Dittrich, S. Evaluation of molecular methods to improve the detection of *Burkholderia pseudomallei* in soil and water samples from Laos. *Appl. Environ. Microbiol.* **2015**, *81*, 3722–3727. [CrossRef] [PubMed]

12. Manivanh, L.; Pierret, A.; Rattanavong, S.; Kounnavongsa, O.; Buisson, Y.; Elliott, I.; Maeght, J.L.; Xayyathip, K.; Silisouk, J.; Vongsouvath, M.; et al. *Burkholderia pseudomallei* in a lowland rice paddy: Seasonal changes and influence of soil depth and physico-chemical properties. *Sci. Rep.* **2017**, *7*, 3031. [CrossRef] [PubMed]

13. Zimmermann, R.; Ribolzi, O.; Pierret, A.; Rattanavong, S.; Robinson, M.; Newton, P.N.; Davong, V.; Auda, Y.; Zopfi, J.; Dance, D.A.B. Rivers as transport vehicles and potential sentinels for *Burkholderia pseudomallei* in Laos. *Sci. Rep.* **2018**, submitted.

14. Lipsitz, R.; Garges, S.; Aurigemma, R.; Baccam, P.; Blaney, D.D.; Cheng, A.C.; Currie, B.J.; Dance, D.; Gee, J.E.; Larsen, J.; et al. Workshop on treatment of and postexposure prophylaxis for *Burkholderia pseudomallei* and *B. mallei* infection, 2010. *Emerg. Infect. Dis.* **2012**, *18*, e2. [CrossRef] [PubMed]

15. Chansrichavala, P.; Wongsuwan, N.; Suddee, S.; Malasit, M.; Hongsuwan, M.; Wannapinij, P.; Kitphati, R.; Day, N.P.; Michie, S.; Peacock, S.J.; et al. Public awareness of melioidosis in Thailand and potential use of video clips as educational tools. *PLoS ONE* **2015**, *10*, e0121311. [CrossRef] [PubMed]

16. Reutrakul, S.; Deerochanawong, C. Diabetes in Thailand: status and policy. *Curr. Diabetes Rep.* **2016**, *16*, 28. [CrossRef] [PubMed]

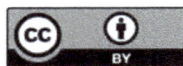

*Tropical Medicine and
Infectious Disease*

MDPI

Review

Melioidosis in Malaysia: Incidence, Clinical Challenges, and Advances in Understanding Pathogenesis

Sheila Nathan [1,*] , Sylvia Chieng [1] , Paul Vijay Kingsley [2], Anand Mohan [3] ,
Yuwana Podin [4], Mong-How Ooi [4,5], Vanitha Mariappan [6], Kumutha Malar Vellasamy [6],
Jamuna Vadivelu [6], Sylvia Daim [7] and Soon-Hin How [8,*]

[1] School of Biosciences and Biotechnology, Faculty of Science and Technology,
    Universiti Kebangsaan Malaysia, Bangi 43600, Malaysia; sylvia@ukm.edu.my
[2] Emergency Department, Pantai Hospital Ipoh, 31400 Ipoh, Malaysia; paulkvijay@gmail.com
[3] Department of Paediatrics, Bintulu Hospital, Bintulu 97000, Malaysia; anand_bintulu@yahoo.com
[4] Institute of Health and Community Medicine, Universiti Malaysia Sarawak,
    Kota Samarahan 94300, Malaysia; pyuwana@unimas.my (Y.P.); monghowooi@gmail.com (M.-H.O.)
[5] Department of Paediatrics, Sarawak General Hospital, Kuching 93586, Malaysia
[6] Department of Medical Microbiology, Faculty of Medicine, University of Malaya,
    Kuala Lumpur 50603, Malaysia; vanitha.ma@gmail.com (V.M.); kumuthamalar@um.edu.my (K.M.V.);
    jamuna@ummc.edu.my (J.V.)
[7] Department of Pathobiology and Medical Diagnostics, Faculty of Medicine and Health Science,
    Universiti Malaysia Sabah, Kota Kinabalu 88400, Malaysia; sylviadaim@ums.edu.my
[8] Department of Internal Medicine, Kulliyyah of Medicine, International Islamic University Malaysia,
    Kuantan 25200, Malaysia
* Correspondence: sheila@ukm.edu.my (S.N.); how_sh@yahoo.com (S.-H.H.);
    Tel.: +60-389213862 (S.N.); +60-199171970 (S.-H.H.)

Received: 9 January 2018; Accepted: 18 February 2018; Published: 27 February 2018

Abstract: Malaysia is an endemic hot spot for melioidosis; however, a comprehensive picture of the burden of disease, clinical presentations, and challenges faced in diagnosis and treatment of melioidosis is not available. This review provides a nonexhaustive overview of epidemiological data, clinical studies, risk factors, and mortality rates from available literature and case reports. Clinical patterns of melioidosis are generally consistent with those from South and Southeast Asia in terms of common primary presentations with diabetes as a major risk factor. Early diagnosis and appropriate management of Malaysian patients is a key limiting factor, which needs to be addressed to reduce serious complications and high mortality and recurrence rates. Promoting awareness among the local healthcare personnel is crucial to improving diagnostics and early treatment, as well as educating the Malaysian public on disease symptoms and risk factors. A further matter of urgency is the need to make this a notifiable disease and the establishment of a national melioidosis registry. We also highlight local studies on the causative agent, *Burkholderia pseudomallei*, with regards to bacteriology and identification of virulence factors as well as findings from host–pathogen interaction studies. Collectively, these studies have uncovered new correlations and insights for further understanding of the disease.

Keywords: melioidosis; *Burkholderia pseudomallei*; Malaysia; epidemiology; bacteriology

1. Introduction

1.1. Historical Background

Melioidosis was first documented in what was then known as Malaya in an outbreak in 1913 involving laboratory guinea pigs and rabbits at the Institute for Medical Research, Kuala Lumpur [1]. Since then, melioidosis has been recognized as an endemic disease in Malaysia. Stanton et al. also described two of the earliest human cases in Kuala Lumpur who presented with symptoms consistent with melioidosis and whose autopsy swabs grew *Bacillus whitmori* [2]. In 1932, Stanton and Fletcher described a total of 39 cases of melioidosis in Kuala Lumpur [3]. There was a long hiatus in documented melioidosis cases in the Malayan Peninsula, possibly due to World War II and post-World War II insurgencies that plagued the Indo-China region through the 1950s and 1960s. In 1957, Malaya gained independence from the United Kingdom and the Malaysian Federation was subsequently formed with the union of Malaya, Singapore, Sabah, and Sarawak in 1963. With the stabilized geopolitical climate, interest in melioidosis was reignited with environmental surveillance and serosurveillance conducted in several states by the United States of America Medical Research Unit (USAMRU) in the 1960s [4–7]. In the nationwide serosurveillance study, participants from Kedah and Sabah (Figure 1) recorded the highest seroprevalence against *B. pseudomallei* [5], while *B. pseudomallei* was isolated from soil and water from several states in Peninsular Malaysia and Sabah [4,6,7]. In 1970, Thin et al. described ten cases of melioidosis involving military personnel presenting at military hospitals in Malacca (Melaka) and Singapore over a three-year period [3].

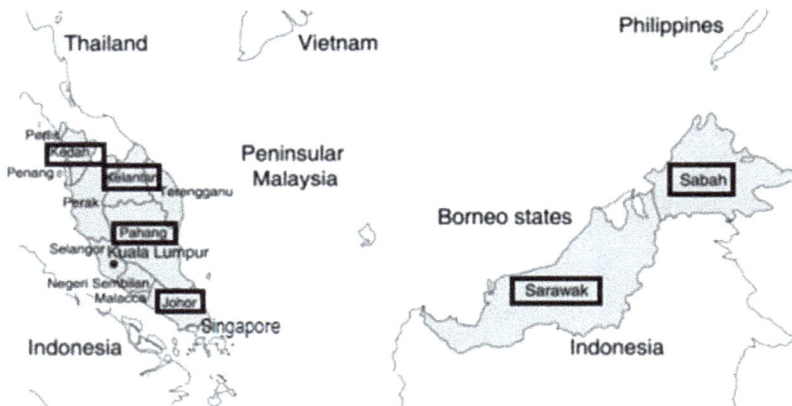

Figure 1. A map of Malaysia indicating the major states with reported cases of melioidosis (black boxes) presented in this review. The majority of case reports are from hospitals and medical centers in Pahang and Sabah due to the diligence of the state health authorities in initiating state-level registries for melioidosis.

Cases of animal melioidosis are not rare, nor are they unfamiliar to veterinarians in Malaysia. Recorded reports of animal melioidosis date back to almost 100 years ago, beginning with the 1921 seminal work of Stanton and Fletcher [8]. Since then, melioidosis has been reported in local goats, sheep, cattle, pigs, deer, monkeys, horses, cats, dogs, and rabbits [9–13]. In addition, a number of State Veterinary Services Departments in Malaysia keep records of animal melioidosis cases for surveillance and control purposes, mainly as a means to mitigate loss of animals of economic importance, especially ruminant livestock. Fatal melioidosis was also reported among orangutans at the Sepilok Rehabilitation Centre in Sandakan, Sabah in 1965 and 1968, where *B. pseudomallei* was successfully isolated from the Centre [14]. Primates are indeed susceptible to *B. pseudomallei* infection, as reported in Johor and Kuala Lumpur in the 1960s, involving pig-tailed macaques, a spider monkey, and a gibbon [10]. The variety of animals reported to be affected by melioidosis and the many locations from which the animal cases came, suggest a wide distribution of *B. pseudomallei* in the environment in Malaysia. Although direct zoonotic transmission of melioidosis appears rare in the country, with only one published report available thus far of a case of transmission from sheep to human [15], the risk may be underestimated. Furthermore, the risk of indirect zoonotic transmission, which could potentially occur via environment contaminated with *B. pseudomallei* shed from infected animals, has not been properly assessed. For the better management and control of human melioidosis in the country, cases of animal melioidosis should not be taken lightly.

Research led by Malaysian clinicians and microbiologists on melioidosis started to gain momentum in the late 1980s and early 1990s with numerous publications—in particular, clinical reports and reviews [16–19]. The research interest subsequently expanded to include molecular microbiology, genomics, and pathogenesis [20–28], with the availability of better facilities, funding, and trained local experts.

1.2. Modes of Transmission

The *B. pseudomallei* natural environmental habitat in endemic areas is soil and water. Most cases of melioidosis occur in persons with regular contact with contaminated soil or water, via penetrating wounds or pre-existing skin abrasions [29]. Inhalation via contaminated dust or water as in severe wet weather conditions is the next most common route of entry and is characterized by pneumonia and more severe infection [30]. Heavy rains precipitate flooding, which facilitates churning of *B. pseudomallei* to the surface soil, aerosolizing the bacteria and increasing exposure potential. Zueter et al. [31] in their case series from Kelantan observed that the highest frequency of admissions occurred during the rainy season from November to February. Hassan et al. [32] found that cases and deaths from melioidosis in the Alor Setar region of Kedah increased linearly with mean monthly rainfall. Pagalavan [33] reported a case after a near-drowning episode, where the patient most probably acquired the infection through aspiration.

2. Burden of Disease and Epidemiology

Melioidosis is not a notifiable disease in Malaysia; therefore, the true incidence of melioidosis in Malaysia is unknown, although more than a thousand cases have been reported throughout Malaysia [34]. Incidence may vary between states, and even within the same state, there may be various hotspots [35]. States that are active in agriculture generally report a higher incidence of melioidosis. Pahang, the largest state in Peninsular Malaysia, where agriculture is the main economic activity, recorded incidences of culture-confirmed adult melioidosis of 6.1 per 100,000 population per year from 2000–2003 [36]. The state of Kedah, which is situated at the Malaysia–Thailand border and is the largest rice producer in Malaysia, reported an incidence of 16.35 per 100,000 population a year [32]. Table 1, Table 2 and Table 4 present selected results from six studies pertaining to Malaysia. Four of these studies used data from systematic compilation of cases from hospital laboratories [18,31,33,36], the fifth used data from a registry [32], and the sixth is a synthesis of published case reports from Malaysia providing more detailed information on individual cases [37]. Table 3 presents results from four studies on paediatric melioidosis in Malaysia.

Table 1. Demographic and risk factors from previously published case series or reports from Malaysia.

	Laboratory or Registry Data					Case Reports
	Zueter et al. [31] (n = 158)	Hassan et al. [32] (n = 145)	How et al. [30] (n = 135)	Pagalavan [33] (n = 44)	Puthucheary et al. [18] (n = 50)	Kingsley et al. [37] (n = 67)
Geographic area	Kubang Kerian, Kelantan	Alor Setar, Kedah	Kuantan, Pahang	Johor Bahru	Kuala Lumpur	Entire country
Data source	1 hospital laboratory	1 hospital-based registry	2 hospital laboratories	1 hospital laboratory	1 hospital laboratory	Published papers
Time period	2001–2015	2005–2008	2000–2003	1999–2003	1976–1991	1975–2015
Inclusion criteria	Confirmed cases	Confirmed cases	Adults (>18 years)	Confirmed cases	Bacteraemia	Confirmed cases
Demographic factors						
Age, median (years)	46 *	50	51	50 *	44 *	44
Male/female ratio	2.8:1	3.0:1	3.6:1	6.3:1	3.2:1	5.1:1
Malay ethnicity %	Most	89	83	71	18	36 †
Risk factors						
Frequency						
At least one %	84	78	85	-	76	58
More than one %	-	-	8.1	-	22	36
None reported %	16	22	15	-	24	42
Environmental exposure						
Farming/fishing/forestry %	-	19	25	13	2.0	12
Construction/trucking %	-	5.5	-	3.0	18	13
Search/rescue + co-inf. with leptospirosis %	-	-	-	-	-	6.0
Drowning %	-	-	-	3.0	-	-
Motor vehicle accident	-	-	1.5	-	-	-
Comorbid conditions						
Diabetes mellitus %	75	57	74	75	38	54
Chronic renal disease %	11	9.7	9.7	19	10	6.0
Tuberculosis %	-	-	-	-	16	9.0
Immune disorders/steroid therapy %	9.5	6.2	2.9	3.0	4.0	6.0
Solid tumors %	4.4	-	0.7	0.7	10	1.5
Hematological malignancies %	-	-	-	-	8.0	-
Chronic lung disease %	-	2.8	3.0	-	-	7.0
Chronic heart disease %	-	-	-	-	-	10
Smoking %	-	-	-	-	-	-
Chronic alcoholism %	-	-	-	0.7	2.0	3.0
Hemolytic anemia %	-	-	-	0.7	2.0	-
Malnutrition/anemia %	-	-	-	-	8.0	-

* Derived; % calculated as percentage of total number of cases; - Not reported; † Computed as a % of those with known race.

Table 2. Clinical manifestations from previously published case series or reports from Malaysia.

| | Laboratory or Registry Data | | | | | Case Reports |
	Zueter et al. [31] (n = 158)	Hassan et al. [32] (n = 145)	How et al. [36] (n = 135)	Pagalavan [33] (n = 44)	Puthucheary et al. [18] (n = 50)	Kingsley et al. [37] (n = 67)
Clinical presentations						
Acute pulmonary %	41	-	41	63	58	33
Acute blood stream %	-	-	19	13	24	61
Disseminated %	29	-	16	-	30	37
Localized %	-	-	-	-	10	9.0
Primary diagnostic groups						
Pulmonary %	41	42	41	56	58	36
Soft tissue abscess/skin %	28	17	-	19	24	36
Bone and joint %	13	4.8	-	6.3	12	6.0
Genitourinary %	3.2	-	-	-	10	7.5
Neurologic %	5.7	4.8	-	-	6.0	7.5
No clinical focus %	22	-	19	13	24	7.5
Primary or secondary foci						
Liver abscess %	12	8.3	3.0	4.5	4.0	18
Splenic abscess %	9.5	10	3.0	9.1	2.0	12
Prostate abscess % †	2.6	0.9	-	-	-	13
Parotid abscess %	2.5	-	-	-	-	1.5
Mycotic pseudoaneurysm %	-	-	-	-	-	7.5
Heart valve vegetation %	-	-	-	3.0	-	-
Pericardial effusion %	-	-	-	-	2.0	1.0
Bacteraemia %	77	52	94	59	100	61
Septic shock %	34	-	-	-	16	19

% Calculated as percentage of total number of cases; - Not reported; † Computed for males.

2.1. Demography and Risk Factors

Melioidosis may occur at any age, including newborns. The peak incidence in the Malaysian case series is between 40 and 60 years of age (median, 44–51 years) (Table 1), the age range during which most co-morbid conditions develop. A preponderance of the disease among males was noted; the gender difference may be due to a higher potential for males to be involved in soil-related occupations and activities facilitating exposure. In four of five case series, most cases were reported in persons of Malay ethnicity, possibly reflecting the higher proportion of Malay rice paddy farmers and agriculture employees with potential for exposure to contaminated water and/or soil [36] or the predominant Malay ethnic composition of certain states [31–33].

Most cases (58–85%) had at least one risk factor reiterating *B. pseudomallei*'s classification as an opportunistic pathogen and that susceptibility of the host is a vital factor in the acquisition of infection. More than one risk factor was reported in 8.1–36% of cases. No risk factor was reported in 15–42% of cases, possibly reflecting under-reporting, unknown residual factors, and high bacterial load or inhalation route in some cases (Table 1). Data on environmental risk factors was sparse in all of the Malaysian case series, underscoring the need to acquire this important information to assist in the education and prevention of melioidosis. Workers in the agricultural and construction sectors, military personnel, eco-tourists, and persons involved in rescue operations are groups known to be at high risk because of their contact with contaminated soil or water [38–40]. Employment in the farming/fishing/forestry industry was reported in 2–25% of cases followed by 3–18% for the construction/trucking industry. Four cases were involved in rescue operations in the recreational forests of Pahang; all of the four cases had co-infection with leptospirosis and three of the four had a fatal outcome [37,40].

Several underlying medical conditions or drug therapy that may impair host defense predispose individuals to melioidosis [41,42]. As reported in other endemic areas of the world, type 2 diabetes mellitus is the most common co-morbid condition associated with melioidosis in Malaysia; 38–75% of melioidosis patients were either newly diagnosed or had pre-existing type 2 diabetes mellitus (Table 1). Other co-morbid conditions associated with melioidosis include chronic renal disease (6–19%), tuberculosis (9–16%), immune disorders/steroid therapy (2.9–9.5%), solid tumors (0.7–10%), haematological malignancies (0.7–8%), chronic lung disease (2.8–3.0%), chronic heart disease (7.0%), smoking (10%), chronic alcoholism (0.7–2.0%), hemolytic anaemia (0.7–2.0%), and malnutrition/anaemia (8%).

2.2. Clinical Presentation

Melioidosis presents as a febrile illness with protean clinical manifestations, ranging from acute fulminant pneumonia and/or septicemia mimicking other community-acquired infections, to a chronic infection that may mimic tuberculosis or malignancy. The disease is characterized by abscess formation in multiple organs and is referred to as 'the great mimicker' because of its similarity to other infections that obscure its correct diagnosis [38]. The pitfalls and optimal approaches to diagnosis have been previously reviewed by Kingsley et al. [43] and are highlighted in a latter section.

In the Malaysian case series, more than 90% of cases were of acute onset [31,37], presenting as acute respiratory infection, acute bacteraemia, or soft tissue infection with fever almost always present. Soft tissue infections include infections of nonskeletal tissue surrounding or supporting organs and other structures including subcutaneous tissue, muscle, lymph nodes, blood vessels, and soft tissue organs (namely, the liver or spleen). Less than 10% of cases were chronic in onset (symptoms more than two months), presenting as chronic pneumonia, chronic skin ulcers/abscesses, and disseminated infection progressing to sepsis, while subclinical infections have also been documented. The major reasons for emergency hospital admissions were acute pulmonary infection progressing to acute respiratory failure, acute bacteraemia progressing to septic shock, severe soft tissue infection, or pyrexia of unknown origin [31,37,43].

The clinical spectrum of melioidosis may be classified into four non-mutually exclusive categories (Table 2): (1) Acute pulmonary infection presenting as pneumonia is the most common clinical presentation, reported in 33–63% of the Malaysian case series. The infection may be primarily acquired via inhalation or alternatively via hematogenous spread following inoculation. (2) Acute blood stream infection was reported in 19–61% of Malaysian case series; patients with co-morbid disease such as diabetes are more likely to present with this form of the disease. Patients may present with a history of fever (median, 6 days; range, 3 days–several months), respiratory distress, abdominal discomfort, muscle tenderness, and disorientation. The clinical picture may vary from a simple bacteraemia with no evident focus of infection, to fulminant septic shock and multiorgan abscesses with 16–34% of cases presenting with septic shock. (3) Disseminated infection, occurring in 16–37% of cases, presents with symptoms of fever, weight loss, abdominal pain, muscle and joint pain, headache, and seizures, and with clinical signs of abscess formation in multiple organs with or without bacteraemia. (4) Acute localized infection, occurring in about 10% of cases, may present as skin ulcers, subcutaneous tissue abscesses, parotid abscess, or ocular infection. The infection may remain localized or may rapidly progress through the blood stream to more widespread infection.

The lungs were the most common site of primary infection followed by soft tissue and bone/joint infection (Table 2). Genitourinary and neurological infections were less frequent. Mortality occurring within 24–48 h of admission precluded a complete workup to identify the site of infection. Pulmonary melioidosis (41–58%) has been observed for both acute and chronic forms of lung involvement. The chronic form of lung involvement mimics tuberculosis where patients present with symptoms of fever and cough with purulent sputum and about one-third of patients possibly having haemoptysis. Pleural involvement occurred in 9–33% of cases and thoracic empyema was occasionally seen. Soft tissue and skin infection (17–36%) is the second most common primary site of presentation. Soft tissue involvement manifests as subcutaneous, intramuscular, and deep-seated abscesses with no particular preference for specific anatomical sites. *B. pseudomallei* could occasionally be isolated from aspiration of abscesses/skin pustules or skin biopsies. Bone and joint infections (6.0–13%) present mainly as septic arthritis, most commonly affecting the knee, followed by the ankle, wrist, and elbow joints, whilst osteomyelitis was less common. Genitourinary infections (3.2–10%) presented as prostatic abscesses, pyelonephritis, perinephric abscesses, or scrotal abscesses. Meanwhile, neurologic melioidosis (4.8–7.5%) presented mainly as pyemic such as brain abscesses, subdural empyema, epidural abscesses, etc. [37]. Hassan et al. [32] and Puthucheary et al. [18] also reported only brain abscesses in their case series whilst meningoencephalitis was uncommon. A similar pattern of pyemic lesions of neurological melioidosis was noted among three cases reported from a registry in Sarawak [44]. The clinical scenario of no identified focus of infection (7.5–24%) was more likely to occur in bacteraemic than nonbacteraemic patients [37].

Besides the primary infection, it was not uncommon for secondary foci of infection to occur. Overall, 49% of cases had secondary foci of infection. Secondary subcutaneous tissue abscesses (21%) were most common in all primary diagnostic groups followed by secondary pneumonia [37]. Liver (4.0–18%) and splenic (2.0–12%) abscesses were commonly found in bacteraemic cases (Table 2) with the 'honeycomb' or 'Swiss cheese' appearance of liver and spleen which is characteristic of melioidosis. Case reports noted a frequency of 13% of prostate abscesses in male patients [37], whereas the case series reported a lower proportion (0.9–2.6%) although this could be attributed to the more complete investigational workup available for case reports than case series. Other rare presentations of melioidosis reported in Malaysia include mycotic pseudoaneurysm (7.5%), pericardial effusion (1.0–2.0%), and heart valve vegetation (3.0%). In mycotic pseudoaneurysm, a pulsatile abdominal mass was the predominant clinical sign and fever was a consistent clinical feature. Diagnosis was made on the basis of CT findings; aneurysms were located in the major abdominal arteries and most had surgical intervention [37].

In summary, the clinical patterns of cases reported from Malaysia are consistent for the most part with previous case reports from South and Southeast Asia where pneumonia is the most common primary presentation followed by soft tissue abscesses with diabetes a major risk factor [37]. Concomitantly, symptoms more frequently observed in Malaysian patients included primary neurological infection and internal foci of infection such as abscess of the liver, spleen, and prostate, and mycotic pseudoaneurysms were higher than previously reported in the region [37]. Neurological melioidosis is primarily pyemic in Malaysia; the distinct syndrome of brain stem encephalitis with flaccid paralysis noted in 4% of melioidosis cases in northern Australia [30] was uncommon in Malaysia and was reported in less than 1% of cases [37].

2.3. Paediatric Melioidosis in Malaysia

B. pseudomallei infections are reported less commonly in children than in adults [45]. In Malaysia, paediatric melioidosis has been described in detail in only four studies, reporting between 13 and 42 culture-confirmed cases each (Table 3). These studies, describing children with melioidosis from both Peninsular Malaysia (Pahang [46], Kuala Lumpur [47]) and Malaysian Borneo (Sabah [44], Sarawak [35]), have shown varying incidences and host risk factors for disease. However, all report high rates of disseminated disease and septicaemia with high case fatality rates. The incidence of paediatric melioidosis has been estimated to be 0.6, 0.7, and 4.1 per 100,000 children in Sabah, Pahang, and Sarawak, respectively. Marked regional variations in incidences are known, although the reasons for these variations remain unclear. For example, incidences as high as 20.2 per 100,000 children were reported in some districts in Sarawak, while no cases were documented in other districts [35].

The importance of an underlying medical condition in the predisposition to childhood melioidosis varied between the different studies in Malaysia. In the study from Kuala Lumpur, 69% of children had an underlying medical condition, mainly haematological malignancy [47]. In Sabah, where high rates of β-globin gene deletions are found in the local ethnic population, 41% of children had thalassemia major. Interestingly, this higher incidence of melioidosis among children with transfusion-dependent thalassemia reduced significantly with the institution of iron chelation therapy, indicating that it was the iron overload that was important in the pathogenesis [44]. Other conditions documented in these studies included primary immunodeficiency, renal failure, diabetes mellitus, hypoaldosteronism, albinism, congenital heart disease, and malnutrition. In contrast, no underlying medical conditions were noted in children with melioidosis in Pahang and Sarawak. However, 32% of those in Sarawak were noted to have poor nutritional status and this may also be an important host risk factor.

In contrast to the paediatric melioidosis literature from most endemic regions [48,49], a large proportion of children with melioidosis in Malaysia presented with disseminated or septicaemic disease. This proportion ranged between 44% and 93% in the various studies. Pneumonia was the predominant manifestation in those with disseminated disease, occurring in as many as 76–83% of cases in Sabah [44] and Sarawak [35]. Undifferentiated fever, with no overt focus of infection, was another important manifestation, occurring in over 28% of children with disseminated melioidosis in two of the studies. Septic arthritis and osteomyelitis occurred in almost 10–15% of children in the Bornean studies. Splenic (and, less frequently, liver) abscesses were also common findings; splenic abscesses were noted in >50% of children in Sabah and Sarawak who had abdominal ultrasound imaging. Neurological involvement was less common, documented in a total of nine children overall. As has been reported in other melioidosis endemic regions, neonatal infections also occurred [50].

Localized melioidosis infection in Malaysian children typically involved either lymph nodes (mainly cervical), skin and soft tissue, or the lacrimal glands. Parotid infections were rare, documented in only 3% of children, in stark contrast to the >25% of children who present with this manifestation in Cambodia and Thailand [49,51]. Children with melioidosis in Malaysia had extremely high fatality rates. Overall, between 24–59% of culture-confirmed melioidosis cases had a fatal outcome. Bacteraemia, disseminated disease, and involvement or dysfunction of a high number of organs were associated with poorer outcomes. Case fatality rates invariably exceeded 75% when septicaemic shock was present. In addition, those with underlying medical conditions had higher fatality rates. In contrast, children with localized disease had significantly better outcomes with only one death recorded.

Table 3. Comparison of results from the four largest studies describing melioidosis among children in Malaysia.

	How et al. [46]	Sam et al. [47]	Fong et al. [44]	Mohan et al. [35]
Geographic area	Pahang	Kuala Lumpur	Sabah	Sarawak
Time period	2000–2003	1976–2005	2001–2012	2009–2014
Inclusion criteria	Culture-confirmed, age < 18 years	Culture-confirmed, age < 15 years	Culture-confirmed, age < 15 years	Culture-confirmed, age < 15 years
Number of cases	13	16	27	42
Annual incidence per 100,000 children	0.7	-	0.6	4.1
Age, median (years)	9.5 *	9.7 *	7.0	4.7
Male/female ratio	3.3:1	4.3:1	1.3:1	1.0:1
Underlying medical conditions (%)	0	69	52	0
Localized disease (%)	46	56	7‡	45
Bacteraemia (%)	54	44	74	48
Septicaemic shock (%)	38	-	52	31
Fatality rate (%)	31	33†	59	24

* Mean; † Includes one child who was taken home in an extremely ill state having failed to respond to ceftazidime, and is presumed to have died; ‡ Includes one child who had liver/splenic abscesses but no other focus of infection or bacteraemia.

Table 4. Mortality and culture-confirmed recurrence from previously published case series or reports from Malaysia.

	Laboratory or Registry Data				Case Reports	
	Zueter et al. [31] (*n* = 158)	Hassan et al. [32] (*n* = 145)	How et al. [36] (*n* = 135)	Pagalavan [33] (*n* = 44)	Puthucheary et al. [18] (*n* = 50)	Kingsley et al. [37] (*n* = 67)
Mortality %	33	34	54	48	65	43
Bacteraemic %	-	48	59	-	65	59
Nonbacteraemic %	-	19	-	-	-	0.0
[1] Recurrence %	2.6	-	19	-	4.0	9.0

% Calculated as percentage of total number of cases; - Not reported; [1] Recurrent is defined as melioidosis infection following the completion of their antibiotic therapy, which may be culture-confirmed or based on clinical presentation.

A delay in diagnosis and in initiation of appropriate antimicrobial treatment was observed in most paediatric melioidosis studies in Malaysia. In Sarawak, the diagnosis was initially missed by nearly 90% of primary healthcare providers and the median duration of symptoms was 14 days before these children were finally admitted to hospital. In Sabah, an appropriate antimicrobial was initiated at admission in <50% of children. These delays likely contributed to the high fatality rates observed and highlight the lack of awareness both in the community and in healthcare professionals in Malaysia.

3. Laboratory Diagnosis of Melioidosis in the Malaysian Healthcare System

Melioidosis is a challenging infectious disease to diagnose even for an endemic country like Malaysia. The absence of pathognomonic clinical presentations, coupled with the lack of familiarity with the disease among attending physicians and laboratory personnel, are the main factors contributing to misdiagnoses especially in rural settings. In Malaysian public tertiary hospitals equipped with modern-day microbiology facilities, laboratory diagnosis of melioidosis is typically included in the routine blood culture test that is done as part of the sepsis workup for patients with fever. Although Ashdown's agar is widely used in other melioidosis-endemic countries [52,53], it is not widely used in diagnostic laboratories in Malaysia. Instead, Francis media agar [21], MacConkey agar, blood agar, and chocolate agar are the common media used in public healthcare, where use of different combinations of agar media varies from one hospital to another.

Once isolated from clinical samples, confirmation of *B. pseudomallei* is either by manual (API 20NE biochemical kit, bioMérieux, Marcy-l'Étoile, France) or automated biochemical systems (Vitek 2, bioMérieux, France; BD Phoenix, Becton Dickinson, Franklin Lakes, NJ, USA; MALDI-TOF MS, Bruker, Bremen, Germany) for any bacterial isolates initially confirmed to be nonmotile, Gram-negative, and oxidase-positive bacilli. Nonetheless, there are also pitfalls in biochemical tests where *B. pseudomallei* isolates were misidentified as other *Burkholderia* species, as previously observed by Podin et al. [54]. Two tests recommended in the guidelines of the Melioidosis Diagnostic Workshop 2013 [55] are not currently included in the routine clinical microbiology laboratory identification workflow, due to various reasons such as budgetary constraints and regional variations of *B. pseudomallei* phenotypes: antibiotic susceptibility tests for amoxicillin-clavulanate, colistin, and gentamicin, and the *B. pseudomallei*-specific latex agglutination assay. While highly sensitive, rapid, and specific, the use of *B. pseudomallei*-specific latex agglutination assay is too costly for public hospitals. Although antibiotic susceptibility tests for amoxicillin-clavulanate, colistin, and gentamicin are not done routinely, this diagnostic algorithm is certainly worth adopting in Malaysia as it has been shown to be useful in resource-limited laboratories in north-central Vietnam [56]. However, gentamicin-susceptible isolates need to be assessed with extra care due to the discovery of gentamicin-susceptible strains that are predominantly found in Central Sarawak [26]. On average, about 3–5 days are still needed for most hospital laboratories in Malaysia to diagnose melioidosis: 20–48 h of blood and agar plate culture, followed by 48–72 h of biochemical identification processes.

Serological tests to detect the presence of anti-*B. pseudomallei* antibody titers using either the indirect hemagglutination assay (IHA) or enzyme-linked immunosorbent assay (ELISA) are widely accepted as unreliable for the diagnosis of melioidosis in Malaysia. The current use of IHA and ELISA in the country is limited to contact investigations and interim monitoring of persons found associated with melioidosis-confirmed cases of either humans or animals. Mohd Noor et al. [57] reported the potential application of their optimized in-house IgM ELISA method for diagnosis of acute melioidosis. The robustness of this assay in diagnosing acute melioidosis in public hospital settings remains to be seen and is pending validation. At the institutional level, the Institute for Medical Research, which is the biomedical research arm of the Malaysian Ministry of Health, has since replaced IHA with the optimized in-house IgM ELISA as the method of choice to test for recent exposure to *B. pseudomallei*. Although not standardized at the national level, molecular methods for confirmation of *B. pseudomallei* are also available and doable in Malaysia using either conventional polymerase chain reaction (PCR) or real-time PCR on the type three secretion system (TTSS)-1 and other gene targets with high levels of specificity and sensitivity [58]. If carefully adapted into the existing melioidosis diagnostic workup, these molecular methods may have a shorter diagnostic turnaround time. Nonetheless, bacterial culture cannot be totally abandoned as direct detection of *B. pseudomallei* remains complicated due to presence of inhibitors [59].

4. Mortality and Recurrence

Based on incidence and mortality of melioidosis in Malaysia, it is estimated that more than 2000 patients die of melioidosis per year, which is much higher than death resulting from dengue or tuberculosis infection. Despite advances in treatment, the case fatality ranged from one-third to about half of patients (33–54%) in four of the five Malaysian case series and in the review of case reports that included all cases, irrespective of bacteraemic status (Table 3). However, when stratified by bacteraemic status, the mortality was about threefold higher among bacteraemic cases compared with nonbacteraemic cases (48–65% vs. 19%). This was previously observed by Puthucheary et al. [18] when they reported 65% mortality, selected on the basis of positive bacteraemic status. A study evaluating patients with bacteraemic melioidosis in Kelantan also reported up to 63% mortality [60]. The normal pathological consequence of bacteraemia is septic shock. Septic shock was the strongest predictor for mortality; in most cases, signs of septic shock occurred within 24 h of admission, presenting as acute respiratory distress syndrome. The mortality among cases with septic shock was 100% compared to 30% among cases without septic shock [37]. Zueter et al. [31] also concluded that septic shock [odds ratio (OR) = 16.5, 95% confidence interval (CI = 6.1–44.9)] was the strongest predicting factor for mortality adjusted for other factors.

With regards to other factors contributing to mortality, Zueter et al. [31] found that age >40 years (OR = 6.47, 95% CI = 1.7–23.8) and the presence of at least one co-morbid condition (OR = 3.0, 95% CI = 1.1–8.4) were independent predicting factors. Among co-morbid conditions, diabetes mellitus was the major underlying risk factor for mortality; 69% of patients had diabetes mellitus in the case series by Hassan et al. [32]. With regards to organ involvement, pneumonia and bacteraemia accounted for most deaths. How et al. [36] found that patients with pneumonia, multiple organ involvement, and bacteraemia had a statistically-significant higher mortality than patients with subcutaneous, musculoskeletal, or internal organ involvement without pneumonia; mortality from acute pneumonia was about 65–73% [18,32,36,37]. Hassan et al. [32] reported that patients with soft tissue abscesses were also at risk for mortality and that osteomyelitis/septic arthritis and liver and splenic abscesses were good predictors of mortality among bacteraemic cases. Patients with pneumonia had approximately threefold higher mortality than those with soft tissue abscesses (63% vs. 18%, *p* = 0.003) [37]. Zueter et al. [31] found that 23% of fatal melioidosis cases were directly attributable to lack of prompt acute-phase treatment.

Patients who survive an initial episode of acute melioidosis have a high potential to develop clinical recurrence, possibly due to failure of the host to eliminate the organism during the initial episode of infection (relapse) or due to reinfection. In Malaysia, the reported rate of culture-confirmed clinical recurrence varied from 2.6% to 19% (Table 4). Chaowagul et al. [61] reported a twofold higher recurrence rate of 15–30% per year in northeast Thailand. The lower recurrent infection rate in Malaysia is perhaps an underestimate, reflecting the high proportion of cases lost to follow-up and shorter duration of follow-up. Published data on the recurrence rate in Malaysia did not specifically note the proportion of relapse and reinfection because serotyping is not routinely performed for clinical isolates.

Similar to tuberculosis, melioidosis infection may be dormant with prolonged latency [11]. Factors contributing to dormancy include survival of *B. pseudomallei* in protected environments, such as phagocytic cells or enclosed abscesses, or the ability of the organism to form a protective covering in infected tissues where antimicrobials cannot penetrate [11]. Reactivation from a latent focus and recurrence into a fulminating form may occur when host defense is compromised as in diabetes mellitus [62]. Risk factors for recurrence amongst Malaysian patients included severity of disease (positive blood culture, multifocal disease), incomplete or inadequate treatment with amoxicillin-clavulanate during the intensive phase of treatment, and improper eradication therapy—amoxicillin-clavulanate, oral quinolones, or doxycycline monotherapy—and nonadherence or duration less than 12 weeks [11]. The most important factor predisposing to relapse is nonadherence to eradication therapy (oral antimicrobial therapy) or inadequate antibiotic therapy. Recurrence was noted to occur in immunocompromised patients despite the full course of microbial therapy. Zueter et al. [31] reported that incomplete treatment, or missed or delayed diagnosis, contributed to the occurrence of recurrent infection among four patients in their case series, all of whom died during the recurring episodes. How et al. [36] reported that patients who did not receive specific therapy and those who received specific therapy for less than two weeks had a 40% and 25% higher risk of relapse, respectively.

5. Molecular Pathogenesis of *B. pseudomallei*

5.1. B. Pseudomallei Bacteriology

B. pseudomallei is intrinsically resistant to a diverse group of antibiotics including penicillins, rifamycins, aminoglycosides, and many third-generation cephalosporins. It is also relatively resistant to quinolones and macrolides, limiting options for therapeutic treatment of melioidosis [11]. Among 81 *B. pseudomallei* isolates from Malaysia tested against nine different antimicrobial agents, susceptibility to ceftazidime, amoxicillin-clavulanic acid, meropenem, imipenem, and trimethroprim-sulfamethoxazole was noted [63]. Despite the high percentage of susceptibility reported, it was interesting to note that the overall results highlighted the emergence of multidrug-resistant isolates. Of the 81 isolates, six were found to carry *bpeB*, *amrB*, *penA*, and BPSS1119 genes, believed to be associated with multidrug resistance. Although the majority of *B. pseudomallei* in Malaysia is gentamicin resistant, more than 80% of *B. pseudomallei* from Central Sarawak of Malaysian Borneo were found to be susceptible to aminoglycosides and macrolides, attributed to a novel nonsynonymous mutation within the *amrB* gene of the AmrAB-OprA efflux pump [26]. Unaltered virulence was observed for these gentamicin-sensitive isolates, suggesting that the loss of aminoglycoside and macrolide resistance has little consequence for virulence and might even enhance environmental survival of these isolates. Thus far, this intriguing phenomenon has not been observed in other parts of Malaysia. A recent study by Zueter et al. [64] on genotyping of 83 clinical *B. pseudomallei* isolates from Peninsular Malaysia revealed 32 different sequence types (STs), of which 13 were novel. All non-novel STs were previously identified in other Asian countries [65,66], suggesting that Malaysian isolates may not be distinct from those of Southeast Asian countries. A lack of relationship between *B. pseudomallei* STs and clinical melioidosis presentation agrees with previous studies indicating an absence of association between any ST and disease outcome, but host and environmental factors are possible reasons for the diverse nature of the clinical presentation of melioidosis [67,68].

5.2. Host–B. pseudomallei Interaction and Identification of Potential Virulence Factors

Host–pathogen interaction studies on *B. pseudomallei* have been actively undertaken in Malaysia, facilitated by the availability of various established host model systems, such as in vitro cell-based models and in vivo models (vertebrate and invertebrate). Findings from these studies have contributed new knowledge to the field of melioidosis pathogenesis and the identification of new potential virulence factors as well as mechanisms of immune response subversion.

Chin et al. [69] investigated the host transcriptional response in a murine acute-phase melioidosis model through microarray-based expression profiling, and highlighted the vital link between innate and adaptive immunity during *B. pseudomallei* infection. They demonstrated that TLR2 was induced to initiate an inflammatory response, followed by an increase in transcripts associated with cell death, caspase activation, and peptidoglysis that ultimately promote tissue injury in the host [69]. In addition, suboptimal activation and function of the downstream complement system correlated with uncontrolled spread of bacteria, eventually leading to death of the infected host. In a parallel study on a diabetic model of acute melioidosis, Chin et al. [70] suggested that the presence of elevated glucose levels impaired the host innate immune system by delaying the identification and recognition of *B. pseudomallei* surface structures. Subsequently, this resulted in delayed activation of various inflammatory and immune responses, as well as the general 'alarm signal' of infection, which may contribute to the increased susceptibility of individuals with pre-existing diabetes to melioidosis [70].

Utilizing the invertebrate model *Caenorhabditis elegans*, the team at Universiti Kebangsaan Malaysia demonstrated that direct prolonged interaction between *C. elegans* and *B. pseudomallei* is required for a complete lethal effect, suggesting that live or proliferating bacteria continuously produce toxins in order to mediate the full killing effect [71,72]. To explore the possibility of toxin-mediated killing, Ooi et al. [72] demonstrated over-expression of the *C. elegans* ABC transporter gene, *pgp-5*, upon *B. pseudomallei* infection, suggesting that the host actively thwarted the pathogenic assaults during infection. A genome-wide transcriptome analysis of infected *C. elegans* revealed a previously-undescribed mechanism by which *B. pseudomallei* suppressed host immunity by specifically targeting an intestinal transcription factor, GATA/ELT-2, thus reducing its availability and consequently inhibiting the expression of GATA transcriptional targets, which include host defense effectors [73].

Chieng et al. [74] conducted a study to understand *B. pseudomallei* adaptation to the intracellular environment of macrophage cells and demonstrated that the bacterium adapted rapidly within macrophages through regulation of its metabolism and growth rates. Of note, the type VI secretion system was induced throughout the infection, highlighting its major role in ensuring pathogen survival and replication in the cell cytosol. However, expression of many known virulence factors was suppressed, suggesting possible host immune system avoidance by intracellular *B. pseudomallei* [74]. In a separate study by the group from University Malaya, Vellasamy et al. [27] investigated the host immune response to *B. pseudomallei* infection in lung epithelial cells. They demonstrated the over-expression of several host carbohydrate metabolic pathways and suppression of the alternate complement, coagulation, lysosome, and phagosome pathways, suggesting bacterial adaptation and evasion of the host innate immune response. Overall, new knowledge from host–pathogen interaction studies of *B. pseudomallei* has revealed mechanisms by which the host responds and some of the mechanisms by which the pathogens avoid host defenses, thereby surviving and growing in host cells. This information should contribute to the identification of new therapeutic targets and vaccine candidates.

The ability of *B. pseudomallei* to adhere, invade, survive, and replicate within mammalian host cells is among the key factors in its pathogenesis [28]. A cohort of Malaysian human, animal, and environmental *B. pseudomallei* isolates was characterized by various biochemical assays to determine the secretion of selected virulence determinants [75,76]. A proteome analysis of *B. pseudomallei* culture supernatant identified metabolic enzymes, transcription/translation regulators, potential virulence factors, chaperones, transport regulators, and hypothetical proteins, several of which were immunoreactive [77]. This study was extended to further evaluate the role of the cell invasion protein, BipC, in pathogenesis of *B. pseudomallei*. BipC, an immunoreactive protein, is involved in actin binding to facilitate internalization of *B. pseudomallei* into host cells, as a bipC mutant was impaired in adherence, invasion, and intracellular survival in epithelial cells, and BipC protein is required for full virulence in a murine model of melioidosis [78,79]. Recently, Vadivelu et al. [80] showed that *B. pseudomallei* localized within the nuclear compartment of host cells, suggesting that the nucleus may play a role as an occult or transient niche for persistence of intracellular pathogens, potentially leading to recurrent episodes or recrudescence of infection.

B. pseudomallei is also known to form biofilm, an important aspect in bacterial pathogenesis due to its ability to promote bacterial survival or spread within the host and protection from antibiotics [81]. Small colony variants (SCVs) of *B. pseudomallei*, which displayed significantly greater capacity to form biofilms, were shown to be less lethal in a *C. elegans* infection model compared to the K96243 isolate, reflecting the SCV ability to persist in the infected host. Recently, Chin et al. [82] noted that genes involved in surface-associated motility, surface composition, and cell wall biogenesis were over-expressed in a high biofilm producer and are probably required for the initial attachment of biofilms. Up-regulation of genes related to the two component signal transduction systems and a denitrification enzyme pathway suggest that the *B. pseudomallei* high biofilm producer is able to sense the surrounding environmental conditions and regulate the production of extracellular polymeric substance matrix, a hallmark of microbial biofilm formation [82].

Overall, in vivo and in vitro studies using experimental melioidosis animal and cell culture models have aided in revealing a variety of bacterial factors that may contribute to survival, pathogenicity and long-term persistence of *B. pseudomallei* within the host.

6. Challenges and Future Perspectives

A major challenge in the war against melioidosis in Malaysia is the lack of awareness among healthcare personnel and the general public as well as difficulties and limitations of fast and effective diagnosis. Melioidosis molecular diagnostic methods are confined to only a small number of laboratories in research and academic institutions in Malaysia, and are more often employed for research purposes. Two factors have probably prevented the widespread application of molecular methods for routine clinical diagnosis of melioidosis: (1) the seemingly lower demand for these methods compared to those for other infectious diseases such as dengue and tuberculosis, and (2) the unanalyzed cost effectiveness of these molecular methods on melioidosis treatment and management in the country.

Until an effective, portable, and simple diagnostic device is developed for melioidosis, the diagnosis challenge for Malaysia is at least twofold. Awareness about melioidosis among physicians, healthcare personnel, and the general public should be enhanced with periodic and continuous health promotion, education, and/or training. In addition, a diagnostic workflow that is more rapid than the existing one and preferably more robust needs to be developed, validated, and adopted in as many of the public hospitals as possible. In the currently available healthcare services and infrastructure, it is probably more feasible and pragmatic if more people are sufficiently trained to suspect melioidosis, such that patients insist on seeking early medical treatment, while physicians and healthcare personnel are able to initiate empirical treatment and concurrently submit patient samples to the nearest available laboratory for definitive diagnosis in a timely manner. The successful diagnosis of melioidosis, and for many other diseases, requires—at the minimum—the tripartite interaction and cooperation among patients, physicians, and laboratory personnel in Malaysia.

Prevention of infection in areas where the disease is endemic can be difficult since contact with contaminated soil is common. In endemic areas, persons with open skin wounds and those with diabetes or other comorbid conditions should be educated to avoid contact with soil and standing water, as they are at increased risk for acquiring melioidosis. Wearing boots during agricultural work can prevent infection through the feet and lower legs. Post-exposure antimicrobial prophylaxis (PEP) is suggested for at-risk rescue operations workers [83]. In healthcare settings, using standard contact precautions (mask, gloves, gown, and hand washing) is considered sufficient protection.

In some states of Malaysia, the incidence of melioidosis is more frequent, with a large number of people being diagnosed each year. In the state of Pahang, the incidence and mortality rates are relatively high. To tackle this, the Medical Department of the International Islamic University Malaysia (IIUM) with the assistance of the State Health Department, started the Pahang Melioidosis Registry. The aim of this registry is to create awareness among doctors in Pahang on diagnosis and treatment of melioidosis and to reduce patient mortality [84]. In 2014, the Sabah Health Department published a guideline for clinical and public health management of melioidosis in Sabah. The Sabah Melioidosis Registry keeps an account of all cases and local authorities are making efforts to spread awareness about early symptoms and disease management [85].

Melioidosis continues to pose a potential threat, especially in Southeast Asian countries. The relatively low case fatality rate in Malaysia's neighbor, Singapore, is likely to be related to increased

Trop. Med. Infect. Dis. **2018**, *3*, 25

awareness amongst healthcare personnel, resulting in early diagnosis and treatment, optimal antibiotic therapy, and improved supportive management. In Malaysia, there remain many problems in the clinical management of this disease, particularly for patients from rural areas of the country as well as young children. How these issues negatively impact the productivity and socio-economy of the country remains uninvestigated. Low-cost, practical, accurate, and fast detection kits are not available in the market yet. The emergence of intrinsically antibiotic-resistant strains of *B. pseudomallei* and co-infection with leptospirosis are also challenges that have to be addressed quickly. Recently, a network of microbiologists, molecular biologists, and clinicians has been established and is referred to as the Malaysian Melioidosis Network. The aims of the network are primarily (1) to foster cooperation between the bench-scientists and healthcare personnel; (2) to work closely with the Ministry of Health Malaysia and provide informed advice on public awareness, improved diagnostics, and emergence of antimicrobial resistance; and (3) to campaign for melioidosis to be classified as a notifiable disease with well-curated incidence data made available. These efforts are currently ongoing.

Acknowledgments: The authors would like to acknowledge sources of funding from the Ministry of Health Malaysia, the Ministry of Science, Technology and Innovation Malaysia (06-05-16-MB003 and 02-05-20-SF0006 awarded to SN), the Ministry of Higher Education Malaysia (RACE/b(2)/1246/2015(02) awarded to YP, UM.C/625/1/HIR/060 (J-20004-73594) awarded to VM, KMV and JV)) and the authors' respective institutions (UKM-DIP-2015-022 awarded to SN) for financial support. No funds are available to cover the costs to publish in open access.

Author Contributions: S.N., S.C., P.V.K., A.M., Y.P., M-H.O., V.M., K.M.V., J.V., S.D. and S-H.H. contributed to the drafting of the manuscript; S.N., Y.P. and S.C. wrote the paper.

Conflicts of Interest: The authors declare no conflict of interest. The funding sponsors had no role in the writing of the manuscript, and in the decision to publish the review.

References

1. Stanton, A.T.; Fletcher, W. Melioidosis: A disease of rodents communicable to man. *Lancet* **1925**, *205*, 10–13. [CrossRef]
2. Stanton, A.T.; Flectcher, W.; Kanagarayer, K. Two cases of melioidosis. *J. Hyg. (London)* **1924**, *23*, 268–276. [CrossRef]
3. Thin, R.N.T.; Brown, M.; Stewart, J.B.; Garrett, C.J. Melioidosis: A report of ten cases. *QJM Int. J. Med.* **1970**, *39*, 115–127.
4. Strauss, J.M.; Jason, S.; Mariappan, M. *Pseudomonas pseudomallei* in soil and surface water of Sabah, Malaysia. *Med. J. Malays.* **1967**, *22*, 31–32.
5. Strauss, J.M.; Alexander, A.D.; Rapmund, G.; Gan, E.; Dorsey, A.E. Melioidosis in Malaysia: III. Antibodies to *Pseudomonas pseudomallei* in the human population. *Am. J. Trop. Med. Hyg.* **1969**, *18*, 703–707. [CrossRef] [PubMed]
6. Strauss, J.; Ellison, D.; Gan, E.; Jason, S.; Marcarelli, J.L.; Rapmund, G. Melioidosis in Malaysia. IV. Intensive ecological study of Carey Island, Selangor, for *Pseudomonas pseudomallei*. *Med. J. Malays.* **1969**, *24*, 94–100.
7. Strauss, J.M.; Groves, M.G.; Mariappan, M.; Ellison, D.W. Melioidosis in Malaysia. II. Distribution of *Pseudomonas pseudomallei* in soil and surface water. *Am. J. Trop. Med. Hyg.* **1969**, *18*, 698–702. [CrossRef] [PubMed]
8. Stanton, A.T.; Fletcher, W. *Melioidosis*; John Bale and Danielson Ltd.: London, UK, 1932; Volume 21.
9. Mustaffa Babjee, A.; Nor Aidah, A.R. Melioidosis in animals. In *Melioidosis: Prevailing Problems and Future Directions*; Puthucheary, S.D., Malik, Y.A., Eds.; SP-Muda Printing: Kuala Lumpur, Malaysia, 1994.
10. Vellayan, S. Melioidosis in zoo animals in Malaysia. In *Melioidosis: Prevailing Problems and Future Directions*; Puthucheary, S.D., Malik, Y.A., Eds.; SP-Muda Printing: Kuala Lumpur, Malaysia, 1994.
11. Puthucheary, S.D. Melioidosis in Malaysia. *Med. J. Malays.* **2009**, *64*, 266–274.
12. Naama, T.; Norazura, A.H.; Chin, S.W.; Mazlan, L.; Nurul Fatiha, A.S.; Masrin, A.; Naheed, M.H.; Ramlan, M. Melioidosis in various animal species diagnosed in the Veterinary Research Institute from 2007 to 2011. In Proceedings of the International Conference on One Health and 24th VAM Congress, Putrajaya, Malaysia, 21–23 September 2012; pp. 129–130.

13. Lim, M.L.; Ismail, S.S.; Rahman, N.; Watanabe, M. Melioidosis: A localised osteomyelitis in a cat. *J. Vet. Malaya* **2015**, *27*, 24–26.

14. De Silva, G.S. Notes on the orang-utan rehabilitation project in Sabah. *Malays. Nat. J.* **1971**, *24*, 40–77.

15. Idris, A.; Rachmat, R.F.N.; Ali, S.M.M. Melioidosis: A case of sheep to human transmission. *J. Vet. Malays.* **1998**, *10*, 77–79.

16. Puthucheary, S.D.; Lin, H.P.; Yap, P.K. Acute septicaemic melioidosis: A report of seven cases. *Trop. Geogr. Med.* **1981**, *33*, 19–22. [PubMed]

17. Yee, K.C.; Lee, M.K.; Chua, C.T.; Puthucheary, S.D. Melioidosis, the great mimicker: A report of 10 cases from Malaysia. *J. Trop. Med. Hyg.* **1988**, *91*, 249–254. [PubMed]

18. Puthucheary, S.D.; Parasakthi, N.; Lee, M.K. Septicaemic melioidosis: A review of 50 cases from Malaysia. *Trans. R. Soc. Trop. Med. Hyg.* **1992**, *86*, 683–685. [CrossRef]

19. Noordin, K.; Abdullah, M.M.; Natarjan, C.; Wahab, Y.A.; Abdullah, K. Pseudoaneurysm of the renal artery associated with melioidosis. *Br. J. Urol.* **1995**, *75*, 680–681. [PubMed]

20. Nathan, S.A.; Puthucheary, S.D. An electronmicroscopic study of the interaction of *Burkholderia pseudomallei* and human macrophages. *Malays. J. Pathol.* **2005**, *27*, 3–7. [PubMed]

21. Francis, A.; Aiyar, S.; Yean, C.Y.; Naing, L.; Ravichandran, M. An improved selective and differential medium for the isolation of *Burkholderia pseudomallei* from clinical specimens. *Diagn. Microbiol. Infect. Dis.* **2006**, *55*, 95–99. [CrossRef] [PubMed]

22. Su, Y.C.; Wan, K.L.; Mohamed, R.; Nathan, S. A genome level survey of *Burkholderia pseudomallei* immunome expressed during human infection. *Microbes Infect.* **2008**, *10*, 1335–1345. [CrossRef] [PubMed]

23. Chua, K.H.; See, K.H.; Thong, K.L.; Puthucheary, S.D. DNA fingerprinting of human isolates of *Burkholderia pseudomallei* from different geographical regions of Malaysia. *Trop. Biomed.* **2010**, *27*, 517–524. [PubMed]

24. Puthucheary, S.D.; Puah, S.M.; Chai, H.C.; Thong, K.L.; Chua, K.H. Molecular investigation of virulence determinants between a virulent clinical strain and an attenuated strain of *Burkholderia pseudomallei*. *J. Mol. Microbiol. Biotechnol.* **2012**, *22*, 198–204. [CrossRef] [PubMed]

25. Wong, Y.C.; Pain, A.; Nathan, S. High-throughput sequencing of large-scale transposon mutants: A genetic tool to identify essential genes of *Burkholderia pseudomallei*. In Proceedings of the 7th World Melioidosis Congress, Bangkok, Thailand, 18–20 September 2013; p. 179.

26. Podin, Y.; Sarovich, D.S.; Price, E.P.; Kaestli, M.; Mayo, M.; Hii, K.; HieUng, N.; Wong, S.; Wong, I.; Wong, J.; et al. *Burkholderia pseudomallei* isolates from Sarawak, Malaysian Borneo, are predominantly susceptible to aminoglycosides and macrolides. *Antimicrob. Agents Chemother.* **2014**, *58*, 162–166. [CrossRef] [PubMed]

27. Vellasamy, K.M.; Mariappan, V.; Shankar, E.M.; Vadivelu, J. *Burkholderia pseudomallei* differentially regulates host innate immune response genes for intracellular survival in lung epithelial cells. *PLoS Negl. Trop. Dis.* **2016**, *10*. [CrossRef] [PubMed]

28. Mariappan, V.; Vellasamy, K.M.; Vadivelu, J. Host-adaptation of *Burkholderia pseudomallei* alters metabolism and virulence: A global proteome analysis. *Sci. Rep.* **2017**, *7*. [CrossRef] [PubMed]

29. Currie, B.J.; Fisher, D.A.; Howard, D.M.; Burrow, J.N.; Lo, D.; Selva-Nayagam, S.; Anstey, N.M.; Huffam, S.E.; Snelling, P.L.; Marks, P.J.; et al. Endemic melioidosis in tropical northern Australia: A 10-year prospective study and review of the literature. *Clin. Infect. Dis.* **2000**, *31*, 981–986. [CrossRef] [PubMed]

30. Cheng, A.; Currie, B. Melioidosis: Epidemiology, pathophysiology, and management. *Clin. Microbiol. Rev.* **2005**, *18*, 383–416. [CrossRef] [PubMed]

31. Zueter, A.R.; Yean, C.Y.; Abumarzouq, M.; Rahman, Z.A.; Deris, Z.Z.; Harun, A. The epidemiology and clinical spectrum of melioidosis in a teaching hospital in a north-eastern state of Malaysia: A fifteen-year review. *BMC Infect. Dis.* **2016**, *16*. [CrossRef] [PubMed]

32. Hassan, M.R.A.; Pani, S.P.; Peng, N.P.; Voralu, K.; Vijayalakshmi, N.; Mehanderkar, R.; Aziz, N.A.; Michael, E. Incidence, risk factors and clinical epidemiology of melioidosis: A complex socio-ecological emerging infectious disease in the Alor Setar region of Kedah, Malaysia. *BMC Infect. Dis.* **2010**, *10*. [CrossRef] [PubMed]

33. Pagalavan, L. Melioidosis: The Johor Bahru experience. *Med. J. Malays.* **2005**, *60*, 599–605.

34. Melioidosis—Databases. Available online: http://www.melioidosis.info/info.aspx?pageID=107 (accessed on 2 November 2017).

35. Mohan, A.; Podin, Y.; Tai, N.; Chieng, C.-H.; Rigas, V.; Machunter, B.; Mayo, M.; Wong, D.; Chien, S.-L.; Tan, L.-S.; et al. Pediatric melioidosis in Sarawak, Malaysia: Epidemiological, clinical and microbiological characteristics. *PLoS Negl. Trop. Dis.* **2017**, *11*, e0005650. [CrossRef] [PubMed]

36. How, S.H.; Ng, K.H.; Jamalludin, A.R.; Shah, A.; Rathor, Y. Melioidosis in Pahang, Malaysia. *Med. J. Malays.* **2005**, *60*, 606–613.

37. Kingsley, P.V.; Leader, M.; Nagodawithana, N.S.; Tipre, M.; Sathiakumar, N. Melioidosis in Malaysia: A review of case reports. *PLoS Negl. Trop. Dis.* **2016**, *10*, e0005182. [CrossRef] [PubMed]

38. Chandni, R. Melioidosis: The great mimicker. In *Medicine Update*; The Association of Physicians of India: Mumbai, India, 2013; pp. 14–18.

39. Pruekprasert, P.; Jitsurong, S. Case report: Septicemic melioidosis following near drowning. *Southeast Asian J. Trop. Med. Public Health* **1991**, *22*, 276–278. [PubMed]

40. Sapian, M.; Khairi, M.T.; How, S.H.; Rajalingam, R.; Sahhir, K.; Norazah, A.; Khebir, V.; Jamalludin, A.R. Outbreak of melioidosis and leptospirosis co-infection following a rescue operation. *Med. J. Malays.* **2012**, *67*, 293–297.

41. Currie, B.J.; Ward, L.; Cheng, A.C. The epidemiology and clinical spectrum of melioidosis: 540 cases from the 20-year Darwin prospective study. *PLoS Negl. Trop. Dis.* **2010**, *4*, e900. [CrossRef] [PubMed]

42. Limmathurotsakul, D.; Wongratanacheewin, S.; Teerawattanasook, N.; Wongsuvan, G.; Chaisuksant, S.; Chetchotisakd, P.; Chaowagul, W.; Day, N.P.J.; Peacock, S.J. Increasing incidence of human melioidosis in northeast Thailand. *Am. J. Trop. Med. Hyg.* **2010**, *82*, 1113–1117. [CrossRef] [PubMed]

43. Kingsley, P.V.; Arunkumar, G.; Tipre, M.; Leader, M.; Sathiakumar, N. Pitfalls and optimal approaches to diagnose melioidosis. *Asian Pac. J. Trop. Med.* **2016**, *9*, 515–524. [CrossRef] [PubMed]

44. Fong, S.M.; Wong, K.J.; Fukushima, M.; Yeo, T.W. Thalassemia major is a major risk factor for pediatric melioidosis in Kota Kinabalu, Sabah, Malaysia. *Clin. Infect. Dis.* **2015**, *60*, 1802–1807. [CrossRef] [PubMed]

45. Sanderson, C.; Currie, B.J. Melioidosis: A pediatric disease. *Pediatr. Infect. Dis. J.* **2014**, *33*, 770–771. [CrossRef] [PubMed]

46. How, H.S.; Ng, K.H.; Yeo, H.B.; Tee, H.P.; Shah, A. Pediatric melioidosis in Pahang, Malaysia. *J. Microbiol. Immunol. Infect.* **2005**, *38*, 314–319. [PubMed]

47. Sam, I.C.; Puthucheary, S.D. Melioidosis in children from Kuala Lumpur, Malaysia. *Ann. Trop. Paediatr.* **2006**, *26*, 219–224. [CrossRef] [PubMed]

48. McLeod, C.; Morris, P.S.; Bauert, P.A.; Kilburn, C.J.; Ward, L.M.; Baird, R.W.; Currie, B.J. Clinical presentation and medical management of melioidosis in children: A 24-year prospective study in the Northern Territory of Australia and review of the literature. *Clin. Infect. Dis.* **2015**, *60*, 21–26. [CrossRef] [PubMed]

49. Turner, P.; Kloprogge, S.; Miliya, T.; Soeng, S.; Tan, P.; Sar, P.; Yos, P.; Moore, C.E.; Wuthiekanun, V.; Limmathurotsakul, D.; et al. A retrospective analysis of melioidosis in Cambodian children, 2009–2013. *BMC Infect. Dis.* **2016**, *16*. [CrossRef] [PubMed]

50. Thatrimontrichai, A.; Maneenil, G. Neonatal melioidosis: Systematic review of the literature. *Pediatr. Infect. Dis. J.* **2012**, *31*, 1195–1197. [CrossRef] [PubMed]

51. Lumbiganon, P.; Viengnondha, S. Clinical manifestations of melioidosis in children. *Pediatr. Infect. Dis. J.* **1995**, *14*, 136–140. [CrossRef] [PubMed]

52. Ashdown, L.R. An improved screening technique for isolation of *Pseudomonas pseudomallei* from clinical specimens. *Pathology* **1979**, *11*, 293–297. [CrossRef] [PubMed]

53. Wiersinga, W.J.; Currie, B.J.; Peacock, S.J. Melioidosis. *N. Engl. J. Med.* **2012**, *367*, 1035–1044. [CrossRef] [PubMed]

54. Podin, Y.; Kaestli, M.; McMahon, N.; Hennessy, J.; Ngian, H.U.; Wong, J.S.; Mohana, A.; Wong, S.C.; William, T.; Mayo, M.; et al. Reliability of automated biochemical identification of *Burkholderia pseudomallei* is regionally dependent. *J. Clin. Microbiol.* **2013**, *51*, 3076–3078. [CrossRef] [PubMed]

55. Hoffmaster, A.R.; Aucoin, D.; Baccam, P.; Baggett, H.C.; Baird, R.; Bhengsri, S.; Blaney, D.D.; Brett, P.J.; Brooks, T.J. G.; Brown, K.A.; et al. Melioidosis diagnostic workshop, 2013. *Emerg. Infect. Dis.* **2015**, *21*, 1–9.

56. Trinh, T.T.; Hoang, T.S.; Tran, D.A.; Trinh, V.T.; Göhler, A.; Nguyen, T.T.; Hoang, S.N.; Krumkamp, R.; Nguyen, L.T.N.; May, J.; et al. A simple laboratory algorithm for diagnosis of melioidosis in resource-constrained areas: A study from north-central Vietnam. *Clin. Microbiol. Infect.* **2017**. [CrossRef] [PubMed]

57. Mohd Noor, A.; Ahmad, N.; Rozita, W.; Mahiyuddin, W. The optimization of IgM in-house ELISA for the laboratory diagnosis of melioidosis in Malaysia. *Int. J. Pathol. Clin. Res.* **2015**, *1*. [CrossRef]

58. Novak, R.T.; Glass, M.B.; Gee, J.E.; Gal, D.; Mayo, M.J.; Currie, B.J.; Wilkins, P.P. Development and evaluation of a real-time PCR assay targeting the type III secretion system of *Burkholderia pseudomallei*. *J. Clin. Microbiol.* **2006**, *44*, 85–90. [CrossRef] [PubMed]

59. Richardson, L.J.; Kaestli, M.; Mayo, M.; Bowers, J.R.; Tuanyok, A.; Schupp, J.; Engelthaler, D.; Wagner, D.M.; Keim, P.S.; Currie, B.J. Towards a rapid molecular diagnostic for melioidosis: Comparison of DNA extraction methods from clinical specimens. *J. Microbiol. Methods* **2012**, *88*, 179–181. [CrossRef] [PubMed]

60. Deris, Z.Z.; Hasan, H.; Suraiya, M.N.S. Clinical characteristics and outcomes of bacteraemic melioidosis in a teaching hospital in a northeastern state of Malaysia: A five-year review. *J. Infect. Dev. Ctries.* **2010**, *4*, 430–435. [PubMed]

61. Chaowagul, W.; White, N.J.; Dance, D.A.B.; Wattanagoon, Y.; Naigowit, P.; Davis, T.M.E.; Looareesuwan, S.; Pitakwatchara, N. Melioidosis: A major cause of community-acquired septicemia in northeastern Thailand. *J. Infect. Dis.* **1989**, *159*, 890–899. [CrossRef] [PubMed]

62. Lim, K.S.; Chong, V.H. Radiological manifestations of melioidosis. *Clin. Radiol.* **2010**, *65*, 66–72. [CrossRef] [PubMed]

63. Khosravi, Y.; Vellasamy, K.M.; Mariappan, V.; Ng, S.-L.; Vadivelu, J. Antimicrobial susceptibility and genetic characterisation of *Burkholderia pseudomallei* isolated from Malaysian patients. *Sci. World J.* **2014**, *2014*. [CrossRef] [PubMed]

64. Zueter, A.R.; Rahman, Z.A.; Abumarzouq, M.; Harun, A. Multilocus sequence types of clinical *Burkholderia pseudomallei* isolates from peninsular Malaysia and their associations with disease outcomes. *BMC Infect. Dis.* **2018**, *18*, 5. [CrossRef] [PubMed]

65. Godoy, D.; Randle, G.; Simpson, A.J.; Aanensen, D.M.; Pitt, T.L.; Kinoshita, R.; Spratt, B.G. Multilocus sequence typing and evolutionary relationships among the causative agents of melioidosis and glanders, *Burkholderia pseudomallei* and *Burkholderia mallei*. *J. Clin. Microbiol.* **2003**, *41*, 2068–2079. [CrossRef] [PubMed]

66. McCombie, R.L.; Finkelstein, R.A.; Woods, D.E. Multilocus sequence typing of historical *Burkholderia pseudomallei* isolates collected in Southeast Asia from 1964 to 1967 provides insight into the epidemiology of melioidosis. *J. Clin. Microbiol.* **2006**, *44*, 2951–2962. [CrossRef] [PubMed]

67. Cheng, A.C.; Godoy, D.; Mayo, M.; Gal, D.; Spratt, B.G.; Currie, B.J. Isolates of *Burkholderia pseudomallei* from northern Australia are distinct by multilocus sequence typing, but strain types do not correlate with clinical presentation. *J. Clin. Microbiol.* **2004**, *42*, 5477–5483. [CrossRef] [PubMed]

68. Cheng, A.C.; Day, N.P.J.; Mayo, M.J.; Gal, D.; Currie, B.J. *Burkholderia pseudomallei* strain type, based on pulsed-field gel electrophoresis, does not determine disease presentation in melioidosis. *Microbes Infect.* **2005**, *7*, 104–109. [CrossRef] [PubMed]

69. Chin, C.Y.; Monack, D.M.; Nathan, S. Genome wide transcriptome profiling of a murine acute melioidosis model reveals new insights into how *Burkholderia pseudomallei* overcomes host innate immunity. *BMC Genom.* **2010**, *11*. [CrossRef] [PubMed]

70. Chin, C.Y.; Monack, D.M.; Nathan, S. Delayed activation of host innate immune pathways in streptozotocin-induced diabetic hosts leads to more severe disease during infection with *Burkholderia pseudomallei*. *Immunology* **2012**, *135*, 312–332. [CrossRef] [PubMed]

71. Lee, S.H.; Ooi, S.K.; Mahadi, N.M.; Tan, M.W.; Nathan, S. Complete killing of *Caenorhabditis elegans* by *Burkholderia pseudomallei* is dependent on prolonged direct association with the viable pathogen. *PLoS ONE* **2011**, *6*. [CrossRef]

72. Ooi, S.K.; Lim, T.Y.; Lee, S.H.; Nathan, S. *Burkholderia pseudomallei* kills *Caenorhabditis elegans* through virulence mechanisms distinct from intestinal lumen colonization. *Virulence* **2012**, *3*. [CrossRef] [PubMed]

73. Lee, S.H.; Wong, R.R.; Chin, C.Y.; Lim, T.Y.; Eng, S.A.; Kong, C.; Ijap, N.A.; Lau, M.S.; Lim, M.P.; Gan, Y.H.; et al. *Burkholderia pseudomallei* suppresses *Caenorhabditis elegans* immunity by specific degradation of a GATA transcription factor. *Proc. Natl. Acad. Sci. USA* **2013**, *110*, 15067–15072. [CrossRef] [PubMed]

74. Chieng, S.; Carreto, L.; Nathan, S. *Burkholderia pseudomallei* transcriptional adaptation in macrophages. *BMC Genom.* **2012**, *13*. [CrossRef] [PubMed]

75. Lee, S.H.; Chong, C.E.; Lim, B.S.; Chai, S.J.; Sam, K.K.; Mohamed, R.; Nathan, S. *Burkholderia pseudomallei* animal and human isolates from Malaysia exhibit different phenotypic characteristics. *Diagn. Microbiol. Infect. Dis.* **2007**, *58*, 263–270. [CrossRef] [PubMed]

76. Liew, S.M.; Tay, S.T.; Wongratanacheewin, S.; Puthucheary, S.D. Enzymatic profiling of clinical and environmental isolates of *Burkholderia pseudomallei*. *Trop. Biomed.* **2012**, *29*, 160–168. [PubMed]

77. Vellasamy, K.M.; Mariappan, V.; Hashim, O.; Vadivelu, J. *Burkholderia pseudomallei* host-pathogen interactions: Role of live bacteria and secretory proteins. *Int. J. Infect. Dis.* **2012**, *16*, e275. [CrossRef]

78. Kang, W.T.; Vellasamy, K.M.; Vadivelu, J. Eukaryotic pathways targeted by the type III secretion system effector protein, BipC, involved in the intracellular lifecycle of *Burkholderia pseudomallei*. *Sci. Rep.* **2016**, *6*. [CrossRef] [PubMed]

79. Kang, W.T.; Vellasamy, K.M.; Rajamani, L.; Beuerman, R.W.; Vadivelu, J. *Burkholderia pseudomallei* type III secreted protein BipC: Role in actin modulation and translocation activities required for the bacterial intracellular lifecycle. *PeerJ* **2016**, *4*, e2532. [CrossRef] [PubMed]

80. Vadivelu, J.; Vellasamy, K.M.; Thimma, J.; Mariappan, V.; Kang, W.T.; Choh, L.C.; Shankar, E.M.; Wong, K.T. Survival and intra-nuclear trafficking of *Burkholderia pseudomallei*: Strategies of evasion from immune surveillance? *PLoS Negl. Trop. Dis.* **2017**, *11*. [CrossRef] [PubMed]

81. Ramli, N.S.K.; Eng Guan, C.; Nathan, S.; Vadivelu, J. The effect of environmental conditions on biofilm formation of *Burkholderia pseudomallei* clinical isolates. *PLoS ONE* **2012**, *7*. [CrossRef] [PubMed]

82. Chin, C.Y.; Hara, Y.; Ghazali, A.K.; Yap, S.J.; Kong, C.; Wong, Y.C.; Rozali, N.; Koh, S.F.; Hoh, C.C.; Puthucheary, S.D.; et al. Global transcriptional analysis of *Burkholderia pseudomallei* high and low biofilm producers reveals insights into biofilm production and virulence. *BMC Genom.* **2015**, *16*. [CrossRef] [PubMed]

83. Yew, K.L. Antimicrobial prophylaxis for melioidosis and leptospirosis for at risk rescue workers. *Med. J. Malays.* **2013**, *68*, 88.

84. How, S.H.; Ng, T.H.; Jamalludin, A.R.; Tee, H.P.; Kuan, Y.C.; Alex, F.; Aminudin, C.A.; Sapari, S.; Quazi, M.H. Pahang melioidosis registry. *Med. J. Malays.* **2009**, *64*, 27–30.

85. Suleiman, M.; Flecia, K.; Ponolin, P.; Jasni, G. *Guideline for Clinical and Public Health Management of Melioidosis in Sabah*; Public Health Division, Sabah State Health Department: Kota Kinabalu, Sabah, 2014.

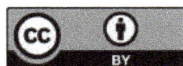

Tropical Medicine and Infectious Disease

MDPI

Review

Melioidosis in Mexico, Central America, and the Caribbean

Javier I. Sanchez-Villamil [1] and Alfredo G. Torres [1,2,*]

1 Department of Microbiology and Immunology, University of Texas Medical Branch, Galveston, TX 77555, USA; jaisanch@utmb.edu
2 Department of Pathology, Sealy Center for Vaccine Development, University of Texas Medical Branch, Galveston, TX 77555, USA
* Correspondence: altorres@utmb.edu; Tel.: +1-409-747-0189

Received: 21 December 2017; Accepted: 21 February 2018; Published: 26 February 2018

Abstract: *Burkholderia pseudomallei* is the causative agent of melioidosis, an endemic disease in tropical areas around the world. Cumulative human cases have demonstrated that melioidosis is prevalent and increasingly recognized in the American continent. Even though the first reports of melioidosis in Mexico, Central America, and the Caribbean Islands date back to the late 1940s, the potential of the disease as a public health concern in the region has not been fully appreciated. Unfortunately, recent studies predicting the global distribution of the disease and the demonstration of melioidosis endemicity in Puerto Rico have not increased recognition of the disease by health professionals in this region. Furthermore, a lack of both diagnostic capacity and awareness of the disease has resulted in a limited number of studies that have attempted to accurately determine its prevalence and geographical distribution. In this review, a summary of reported cases in the countries of this region are presented, as well as recommendations to increase the diagnosis and awareness of the disease as an important public health problem in Mexico, Central America, and the Caribbean islands.

Keywords: *Burkholderia pseudomallei*; melioidosis; Mexico; Central America; Caribbean; epidemiology; awareness

---

1. Introduction

Melioidosis is an emerging, potentially fatal disease caused by *Burkholderia pseudomallei*, which can be acquired through inoculation, inhalation, or ingestion. Inhalation of the bacterium results in the most rapid and fulminant disease, whereas percutaneous inoculation is slower to progress and is often limited to a cutaneous lesion [1,2]. *B. pseudomallei* can also cause asymptomatic infections in healthy individuals, or can induce an acute, chronic, or latent disease. Melioidosis can be confused with pneumonia or tuberculosis, and the bacterium is resistant to a wide variety of antibiotics, while its pathogenic mechanismsare not completely understood. Further, the disease most commonly affects individuals with underlying conditions, including type 2 diabetes, excessive alcohol consumption, and chronic lung disease [1,3,4]. Target organs commonly include the lung, spleen, and prostate, but *B. pseudomallei* has also been shown to establish infections in the bone marrow, central nervous system, kidneys, and the gastrointestinal tract [5].

The magnitude of melioidosis in the Western Hemisphere is not fully understood. However, cases occur sporadically in the Americas, with an increasing number of them observed among people with no travel history to known endemic countries [6]. New endemic foci have been reported in countries such as Mexico, Costa Rica, Guadeloupe, and Puerto Rico. A prior review of melioidosis cases in the Americas described 120 identified human cases that occurred between 1947 and 2015, 95 of which (79%) were likely acquired in the Americas; the mortality rate was 39% [6], indicating that *B. pseudomallei* is widespread in the American continent. Additionally, Limmathurotsakul et al.

predicted that *B. pseudomallei* is present in tropical latitudes, and that the highest risk zones included South and Central America [7]. Mexico had the highest predicted incidence of melioidosis in North America, with 550 cases per 100,000 population each year; while in Central America, El Salvador was predicted to have 114 cases, and, in the Caribbean, 24 cases were predicted for Haiti [7]. In addition to the high prevalence of diabetes (13.1% Mexico, 10.1% Central America, and 11.2% in The Caribbean) [8] and limited access to health care, this study suggested that melioidosis might be endemic in many countries of this region, but be significantly underreported. Given the diagnostic limitations and little or no surveillance, it is likely that *B. pseudomallei* is present in many more tropical countries where it has not yet been identified [9].

Melioidosis requires specific antibiotic treatment, since *B. pseudomallei* has natural resistance to several commonly used antibiotics such as penicillin, ampicillin, first and second generation cephalosporins, gentamicin, tobramycin, and streptomycin [10]. However, it is still important to determine the antimicrobial sensitivity profile to newer antibiotics [11]. Current therapy recommendations are based on the outcome of a number of clinical trials in endemic regions and other clinical observations [12]; however, in non-melioidosis endemic areas, empiric antimicrobial therapy for pneumonia may not include drugs that are active against *B. pseudomallei*. Therefore, melioidosis represents a challenge for clinical and microbiology laboratory staff in regard to diagnosing it accurately, ensuring appropriate therapy, and alerting public health officials to its potential endemicity.

Defining the global distribution and updating the epidemiology of *B. pseudomallei* is important for developing an accurate melioidosis risk map, and expanding the list of countries with sporadic occurrence that may be upgraded to endemic status as a result of the recognition of increasing numbers of indigenous cases and the detection of *B. pseudomallei* in the environment. Further, an accurate disease distribution analysis will help raise awareness among healthcare workers in affected areas. Here, we present an updated review of *B. pseudomallei* cases in this region that were published from 1945 to 2017. We deliberately did not include Canada and the United States of America (USA) as, although there have been two apparent cases of indigenous melioidosis in the continental USA in recent years [13,14], they occurred in a part of the USA that is predicted to not be suitable for the environmental survival of *B. pseudomallei*, and there was no evidence of a local environmental source. We also excluded Canada, since although (similar to the USA) there have been a number of cases imported from other endemic areas [15–18], there is no concrete evidence of indigenous melioidosis in either country.

2. Review of Melioidosis Cases and Presence of *B. pseudomallei* in Each Country

We conducted a search of the literature (PubMed, MEDLINE, and Google Scholar) in order to identify published reports of melioidosis cases originating from Mexico, Central America, and the Caribbean islands. Some keywords used included combinations of '*Burkholderia pseudomallei*', 'melioidosis', 'Mexico', 'Central America', 'Caribbean', '*Pseudomonas pseudomallei*', and '*Malleomyces pseudomallei*'. Thus, we reviewed 37 papers (from 1945 to 2017) and, when available, the following information was collected from each article: year of diagnosis, number of cases, gender, age, travel history, country of diagnosis, diagnostic laboratory results, signs, symptoms, and patient outcomes. ArcGIS online (ESRI, Redlands, CA, USA) was used to generate the map in Figure 1. Reported cases are summarized in Table 1, and are discussed in more detail below.

Table 1. Summary of published melioidosis cases in Mexico, Central America, and the Caribbean.

Year	Number of Cases	Patient (Age and Gender)	Country Where Infection Likely Occurred	Travel History	Country of Diagnosis	Outcome	Ref.
1945 [a]	1	31-year-old male	Panama	Panama	USA	Discharged	[19]
1957 [b]	1	20-year-old male	Panama	Panama	USA	Survived	[20,21]
1958 [a]	1	22-year-old male	Mexico	Mexico, Japan, and Korea	USA	Survived	[22]
Unknown	13	Variable	El Salvador	Residents of El Salvador with unknown travel history	El Salvador	10 survived/3 died	[6,23]
1982 [b]	1	62-year-old female	Puerto Rico	NR	Puerto Rico	Died	[24]
1985 [b]	1	72-year-old male	Mexico	No travel history outside Mexico	USA	Died	[25]
1989	3	Variable	Mexico	Unknown	Mexico	1 survived/2 died	[26]
1994 [c]	1	66-year-old male	Martinique	Travel history to Africa and South America	France	Survived	[27]
1997	1	11-year-old male	Puerto Rico	Travel history to USA for medical care	USA	Died	[28]
1997	1	4-year-old female	Guadeloupe	Resident of France with travel history to Guadeloupe	Guadeloupe	Survived	[29]
1998	1	56-year-old male	Costa Rica	Unknown	Costa Rica	Died	[30]
1998	1	Age of female unknown	Martinique	Unknown travel history	France	Survived	[31]
1999	1	Age of male of unknown	Martinique	Unknown travel history	France	Survived	[31]
2000	1	63-year-old male	Costa Rica	No travel history outside Costa Rica	Costa Rica	Died	[6,32]
2000	1	37-year-old female	El Salvador	Resident of El Salvador	USA	Survived	[6]
2001	1	Unknown age or sex	El Salvador	Resident of El Salvador	USA	Survived	[33]
2003	1	55-year-old female	Puerto Rico	Resident of Puerto Rico with travel to USA	Puerto Rico	Died	[34]
2003	1	47-year-old male	El Salvador	Travel history to El Salvador	USA	Died	[6,35]
2005	2	48-year-old male 80-year-old female	Honduras	Travel history to Honduras	USA	1 survived/1 died	[36]
2006	1	17-year-old male	British Virgin Islands	British Islands and Canada	Canada	Survived	[37]
2009	1	17-year-old male	Dominican Republic	Resident of Dominican Republic with travel history to Argentina	Argentina	Survived	[38]
2009	1	7-year-old female	Aruba	Travel history to Puerto Rico, Portugal, and Australia	USA	Survived	[39]
2009	1	88-year-old male	Puerto Rico	Veteran with service in Panama and Korea	USA	Survived	[6,40]
2009	1	Unknown	Costa Rica	Unknown	USA	Survived	[41]
2009	1	Unknown	Mexico	Unknown	USA	Unknown	[40]
2010	1	30-year-old male	Mexico	Resident of Mexico	USA	Died	[6,40]
2010	1	38-year-old male	Puerto Rico	No travel history outside of Puerto Rico	Puerto Rico	Died	[42]
2010	1	15-year-old female	Guadeloupe	Resident of France with travel history to Guadeloupe	France	Survived	[40,43]

Table 1. *Cont.*

Year	Number of Cases	Patient (Age and Gender)	Country Where Infection Likely Occurred	Travel History	Country of Diagnosis	Outcome	Ref.
2010	1	35-year-old male	Martinique	Resident of Switzerland with travel history to Martinique	Switzerland	Died	[44]
2010	1	42-year-old female	Costa Rica	Costa Rica and Mexico	USA	Survived	[6]
2011	2	22-year-old male 10-year-old female	Mexico	Travel history to Mexico	USA	2 survived	[6]
2011	1	46-year-old female	Aruba	Resident of UK with travel history to Aruba and the Caribbean	USA	Survived	[45]
2011	1	31-year-old male	Panama	No travel history outside Panama	Panama	Survived	[46]
2012	1	60-year-old male	Puerto Rico	Resident of Puerto Rico	USA	Survived	[40,42]
2012	1	71-year-old male	Guatemala	Resident of Guatemala	USA	Survived	[6,40]
2012	1	29-year-old male	Mexico	Travel to Acapulco, Mexico one week before disease	Mexico	Survived	[47]
2013	1	22-year-old female	Guatemala	Resident of Guatemala	USA	Survived	[6]
2013	1	66-year-old male	Mexico	Served in Vietnam war	USA	Survived	[40,48]
2014	1	45-year-old male	Costa Rica	Unknown travel history	Costa Rica	Survived	[49]
2014	1	59-year-old female	Mexico	Travel to Los Cabos, Mexico 7 days before disease	USA	Survived	[50]
2014	1	70-year-old female	Mexico	No travel history outside Mexico	USA	Survived	[51]
2014	1	17-year-old male	Trinidad and Tobago	Travel history to Trinidad and Tobago	Canada	Survived	[18]
2015	1	48-year-old male	Mexico	No travel history outside Mexico	Mexico	Survived	[52]
2017	3	Unknown	Guadeloupe	Unknown	Guadeloupe	2 survived/1 died	[41]
2017	1	Unknown	Puerto Rico	Puerto Rico	USA	Survived	Unpublished data from CDC

[a] The bacterial culture was reported as *Malleomyces pseudomallei*. [b] The bacterial culture was reported as *Pseudomonas pseudomallei*. [c] Bacterial cultures after this year were reported as *Burkholderia pseudomallei*. NR, not reported.

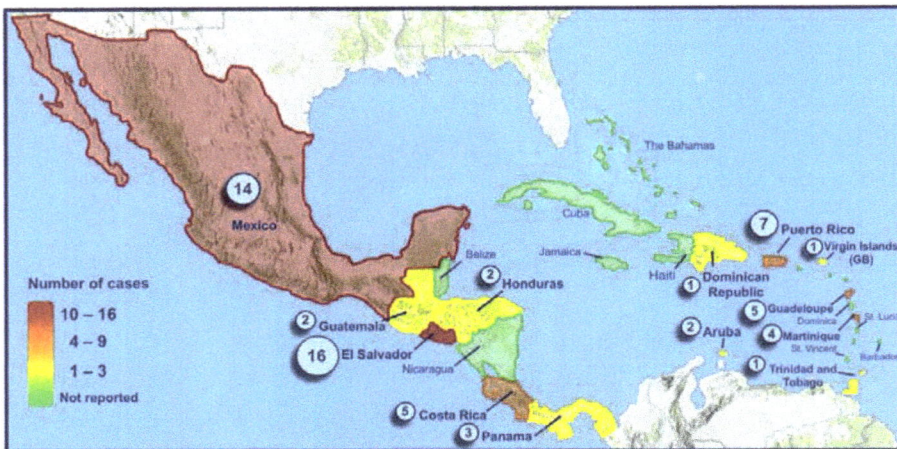

Figure 1. Melioidosis cases reported (1945–2017). Adapted from: Esri, HERE, DeLorme, increment P corp., NPS, NRcan, Ordnance Survey, © OpenStreetMap contributors, USGS, NGA, NASA, CGIAR, N Robinson, NCEAS, NLS, OS, NMA, Geodatastyrelsen, Rijkswaterstaat, GSA, Geoland, FEMA, Intermap, and the GIS user community.

2.1. Mexico

Fourteen cases of melioidosis have been reported that were likely acquired in Mexico (see Table 1). The first case reported dated from 1958, and was of a 22-year-old white man from Oklahoma, USA, with a travel history to border towns in Mexico [22]. He was diagnosed with melioidosis in the USA by complement fixation studies for '*Malleomyces pseudomallei*'. However, no bacteriologic confirmation was obtained on material from the abscesses cavity [22]. The second case, which was diagnosed in the USA, was reported in 1985 [25]. The patient was a 72-year-old Hispanic male, who had lived in the city of Manzanillo all of his life, and who was working as a clerk. He had never traveled outside of Mexico. He died 72 h after admission to the hospital. At autopsy, the lungs showed patchy areas of consolidation, and histological sections revealed suppurative acute bronchopneumonia [25]. The third case was presented in 1989 at a cystic fibrosis conference. Three of 19 sputum samples from patients with cystic fibrosis were positive for '*Pseudomonas pseudomallei*', of which two patients died from pulmonary illness [26]. Years later, in 2009 [40], 2010 [6], and 2013 [40], other cases of melioidosis were reported in Mexico that were diagnosed in USA; however, the documented information regarding signs, symptoms, and travel history is very limited. The only information available from the case reported in 2010 is that it resulted in death [6]. Subsequently, in 2011, two more Mexican patients were diagnosed in the USA, one of whom was a 10-year-old child, and the second was a 22-year-old alcoholic female [6]. In both cases, the patients survived the disease. There is another report of melioidosis diagnosed in Mexico in 2012 in a 29-year-old medical resident with an acute illness (fever, malaise, and dyspnea) with 72 h of disease progression, with a history of recent travel to a tropical Mexican region (Acapulco) one week previously [47]. Computed tomography (CT) showed irregular hyperdense images with ground glass opacities in the lung, and he received treatment with trimethoprim/sulfamethoxazole with adequate progress and cure. Microbiological identification was performed using the VITEK®2 (bioMérieux, Marcy-l'Étoile, France) system that has been reported sometimes to have problems differentiating between *B. pseudomallei* and *B. cepacia* [53]. In this case, the isolate was not confirmed by a reference laboratory, such as the Centers for Disease Control and Prevention (CDC).

Further cases of melioidosis in Mexico have been reported more recently. In 2014, a 59-year-old female with a four-day history of right-sided upper back and anterior chest pain, fever, and shortness of breath was diagnosed in the USA with melioidosis, which was believed to have been contracted in Mexico [50]. She had traveled to Los Cabos, Mexico, one week before hospital admission. A CT scan of the chest showed an irregular mass in the apical segment of the right upper lobe with ground glass opacities, and an enlarged right paratracheal lymph node. The isolate was later confirmed and identified as *B. pseudomallei* by the CDC. It is important to note that the patient had diabetes mellitus and a well-controlled HIV infection, as well as having received a renal transplant. Additionally, she was present when a hurricane hit the zone, and so had multiple risk factors for acquiring the disease. Another important associated risk factor was reported in a 70-year-old smoker from Mexico with no history of travel to any other melioidosis-endemic area [51]. The patient presented with fever, chills, and an enlarging left neck mass. CT revealed a supraclavicular mass that was drained, and the organism grown was confirmed by the CDC as *B. pseudomallei*. The patient reported symptom resolution with a decrease in the size of the supraclavicular mass after antibiotic therapy. In 2015, the first case of melioidosis was reported in a northern state of Mexico (Sonora) in a 48-year-old male who presented with fever and a history of abscess in the right subscapular region with hepatomegaly and splenomegaly, but without pulmonary symptoms [52]. Microbiological identification using the VITEK®2 (bioMérieux) system identified the pathogen as *B. pseudomallei*, and the use of trimethoprim/sulfamethoxazole resolved his symptoms. The recent increasing occurrence of melioidosis in patients with no travel history outside Mexico indicates that *B. pseudomallei* is endemic, mainly in tropical regions of the country. It is likely that, due to the lack of advanced diagnostic methods, melioidosis remains an underdiagnosed disease in this country.

2.2. Central America

Cases have been reported in Central America from Guatemala to Panama, except in Nicaragua and Belize (Figure 1).

2.2.1. Guatemala

Only two cases of melioidosis have been reported in Guatemala between 2012–2013 (Table 1). The first report was from a 71-year-old male with diabetes [6], and the second was from a 22-year-old healthy female. In the former case, the potential risk of exposure was the use of a thermal sulfur hot spring in that country [6]. Both cases survived, and were diagnosed in the United States; however, no more detailed information was available.

2.2.2. El Salvador

Thirteen cases of melioidosis were reported in 1981 by Bloch et al. in residents of El Salvador who had never traveled outside of the country [6,23] (Table 1). However, limited information is available from those cases. A subsequent case of melioidosis was reported in 2000 in a 37-year-old female resident of El Salvador who survived the disease, despite having diabetes mellitus [6]. Additionally, Salvadorian refugees have been diagnosed with melioidosis during immigration health screening. One refugee was diagnosed with melioidosis in the USA in 2001 [33]. In this case, the patient presented with a cerebral abscess, but survived. However, the identity of the bacterium was not confirmed by a reference laboratory. The last documented case was diagnosed in 2003 in a 47-year-old male with diabetes mellitus, who had traveled to El Salvador three weeks earlier [35]. A CT scan indicated the presence of pulmonary abscesses, and the patient died from sepsis and multiorgan system failure [35]. Bacterial isolates were confirmed as *B. pseudomallei*. This case is of importance, because the laboratory workers manipulating the samples were exposed to *B. pseudomallei* cultures without utilizing proper laboratory practices; however, no workers were infected. In response to this incident, laboratory safety recommendations for *B. pseudomallei* were revised [35].

2.2.3. Honduras

Two cases of melioidosis were reported in 2005 in patients who traveled to Honduras a few days before hospital admission (Table 1). A 48-year-old male with diabetes and Guillain–Barré syndrome, with a history of recent travel to Honduras, was diagnosed with pneumonia and perirectal abscess. *B. pseudomallei* was isolated from cultures of blood and abscess fluid. Fortunately, the patient survived the infection [36]. In the same year, an 80-year-old female resident of Honduras was admitted to hospital with a diagnosis of pneumonia after four days of headache, fever, and muscle pain [36]. She died after two days in hospital, and *B. pseudomallei* was identified in a blood culture drawn when she was admitted. Both cases were diagnosed in the USA, and the identification of *B. pseudomallei* was confirmed by real-time PCR [36].

2.2.4. Costa Rica

Melioidosis in Costa Rica was reported in 1998 in a 56-year-old male with diabetes mellitus, presenting with fever and lung infection; he died a few days after hospital admission [30] (Table 1). The isolate from blood and bronchial aspirate was later confirmed and identified as *B. pseudomallei* by VITEK®2 (bioMérieux) [30]. The second case diagnosed was reported in 2000 in a 63-year-old male smoker with diabetes mellitus and a history of working with cattle, [6,32]. The patient developed fever and a cough with yellowish expectoration. A chest roentgenogram revealed an inflammatory infiltrate in the right lung. He died 72 h post-admission. *B. pseudomallei* was identified from a blood sample and bronchial secretions by the National Reference Laboratory (Hospital Nacional de Niños, Costa Rica). Another case was reported in 2009, but no detailed information was provided [41]. In 2010, a 42-year-old female was diagnosed with melioidosis, which was probably acquired while vacationing in Costa Rica [6]. The latter two patients both survived. In 2014, the first case of *B. pseudomallei* infection of the central nervous system was reported in this country [49]. A 45-year-old male with diabetes mellitus presented with headache, fever, photophobia and convulsive crisis. Cerebrospinal fluid and empyema cultures were positive for *B. pseudomallei*, as identified by the VITEK®2 (bioMérieux) system and confirmed by a local reference laboratory (INCIENSA) [49]. The patient survived after 20 weeks of ceftazidime and trimethoprim/sulfamethoxazole treatment.

2.2.5. Panama

The first reports of melioidosis in the Americas, dating from 1945–1957, were acquired in Panama (Table 1). The first of these possible cases of melioidosis was diagnosed in the USA in 1945 in a 31-year-old male who was employed in the Panama Canal Zone from 1927–1928 [19]. The patient was admitted to hospital for the diagnosis and treatment of sinuses and ulcers of the right buttock and thigh that had been present for eight years [19]. The organism was isolated from pus and tissue debris, and was reported as '*Malleomyces pseudomallei*'. It was reported that before the chronic phase of the disease, the patient had suffered from an acute pneumonic phase. A second case of melioidosis, which was probably acquired in Panama, was reported in 1957 [20,21]. The patient was a 20-year-old male who was treated for 'flu-like syndrome'. After three days, he developed genitourinary symptoms, and later became systemically ill. He had pyuria, and a chest roentgenogram showed a small infiltrate in the upper lobe of the left lung. After one month, he developed an acute septic arthritis of the shoulder joint; pus was removed, and *Pseudomonas pseudomallei* was isolated in culture [20]. However, in the two aforementioned cases, the cultures were not available for further studies, and could not be considered as verified cases of melioidosis. Another case of melioidosis in Panama has been reported more recently. In 2011, a 31-year-old male with diabetes mellitus, who developed liver and skin abscesses, was diagnosed with *B. pseudomallei* infection [46]. The patient had no travel history outside the country [46]. Unfortunately, limited information about the methodology that was used for *B. pseudomallei* identification was included.

2.3. Caribbean Islands

2.3.1. Puerto Rico

As of October 2017, there have been seven cases of melioidosis reported or associated with Puerto Rico, based on case reports or submissions to the USA CDC reference laboratory. The earliest case was reported in 1982 in a 62-year-old Puerto Rican woman with systemic lupus erythematosus [24] (Table 1). The patient had a one-week history of fever, chills, generalized weakness, and malaise. She had a history of chronic non-productive cough; additionally, she had never traveled outside the country. The patient died 48 h after admission, and the CDC later confirmed the organism as *Pseudomonas pseudomallei* [24]. The second case reported in Puerto Rico was in 1998 in an 11-year-old male with chronic granulomatous disease [28]. At the time of admission, he presented with fever, right neck pain, and two weeks of productive cough. A chest CT revealed a right hilar mass and right paraesophageal lymphadenopathy, as well as a right supraclavicular mass. The API rapid NFT (non-fermentative) system identified *B. pseudomallei*, and this identification was subsequently confirmed by the CDC. The patient died after a few days of antibiotic therapy [28]. In 2003, a *B. pseudomallei* infection was reported in a 55-year-old female with diabetes mellitus, who had been exposed to flood waters during the rainy season in this country [34]. This report highlighted the role played by flood waters as a risk factor in the epidemiology of melioidosis. In 2009, an 88-year-old male Puerto Rican veteran who had served in Korea and Panama was diagnosed in USA with melioidosis [6,40]. The potential risk of exposure was environmental (digging a ditch), and he survived the disease [6,40]. No additional information was provided. In 2010, a 38-year-old male presented with symptoms of chest pain and shortness of breath; his only relevant medical history was obesity [42]. He died 1 h after arriving at the hospital. A histological analysis demonstrated acute necrotizing pneumonia with pyogranulomatous splenitis, hepatitis, and focal myocarditis. *B. pseudomallei* was identified by the CDC [42]. Doker et al. also reported another confirmed case of melioidosis in 2012 [42]. A 60-year-old male with a three-day history of nausea, anorexia, and abdominal and chest pain, was admitted to an emergency room [42]. He had diabetes mellitus, obesity, alcohol use, and was a smoker.In addition, the patient reported intermittent intravenous use of heroin and cocaine. *B. pseudomallei* was identified and confirmed at the CDC; the patient survived [42]. Thus, the earliest case in Puerto Rico was reported in 1982, followed by one in each of the following years: 1998, 2003, 2009, 2010, 2012, and 2017. Six of the seven clinical cases came from the eastern portion of the island. No information is currently available on the origins of the seventh case, which occurred in the summer of 2017.

Due to the sporadic nature of these reports, surveillance was not considered a priority until the 2012 case, which prompted a closer look at the potential local endemicity of the disease [42]. The study included a serological survey, which found that 6% of the contacts of the 2010 patient and 25% of the contacts of the 2012 patient were seropositive; the study also found an association between seropositivity and a history of skin wounds and/or a history of drug use. Environmental sampling of soil near the 2012 patient's residence yielded two *B. pseudomallei* isolates that were closely related to the isolate from the patient, strongly indicating that this area was the source of his infection [42,54]. The results of this study prompted an extensive environmental survey of soil and water based on potential habitats around the island. Isolates of *B. pseudomallei* were recovered from soil samples in the northern part, indicating that the organism is not geographically restricted to the eastern portion of the island (C.M. Hall, personal communication). This suggests that surveillance around the island may yield more cases. However, the effects of Hurricane Maria in 2017 were still being dealt with at the time of writing this manuscript. It is unknown how long it will take to rebuild the public health infrastructure of the island.

In addition to the presence of *B. pseudomallei* in humans and the environment in Puerto Rico, Hemme et al. found the presence of antibodies against *B. pseudomallei* in one of 24 non-human primates (*Erythrocebus patas*) that were tested [55]. This study suggested probable transmission through contact with contaminated soil and water.

2.3.2. Other Caribbean Islands

Sporadic cases of melioidosis have been associated with other Caribbean islands, and are typically diagnosed in tourists who return to their home countries or residents who seek medical treatment or consultation in countries with laboratory capability to diagnose the disease. Islands that are associated with cases of melioidosis include Aruba [39,45], the British Virgin Islands [37], Guadeloupe [29,43,56], the Dominican Republic [38], Martinique [27,31,44], Trinidad, and Tobago [18]. A case of melioidosis was reported in a child with cystic fibrosis who had travelled to Aruba some three months previously [39]. Interestingly, the occurrence of melioidosis in animals, particularly sheep, goats, and pigs, had previously been reported in the 1950s [57]. Unfortunately, no isolates from the animal melioidosis outbreak were available for confirmation; however, this remains the only reported instance of animal melioidosis in this region.Two cases of melioidosis have been reported from Guadeloupe [29,43] and a report of three further cases from Guadeloupe in 2017 is also in submission [56]. The CDC is also currently investigating two cases of melioidosis in the US Virgin Islands [56]. Based on predicted environmental suitability, it is likely that other Caribbean islands may be endemic for this bacterium [7]. Discussions with various stakeholders in the Caribbean indicate that surveillance for melioidosis is typically not a priority for them [56].

3. Current Challenges in the Diagnosis and Treatment ofMelioidosis in the Region

Melioidosis has generated further interest in view of the detection of *B. pseudomallei* infection in countries that were previously considered non-endemic (Figure 1). These sporadic occurrences over a prolonged period are unlikely to have resulted from repeated importation, and along with a high predicted incidence of the disease in this region [7], suggest that the pathogen is likely to be endemic but underdiagnosed across this region. The high proportion of melioidosis cases in this review that were diagnosed and confirmed outside of the region, mainly in the USA (26 of 63 cases, representing 41.27%), strongly suggests a lack of reliable diagnostic testing within the region. Significant confusion exists regarding the identification and diagnosis of melioidosis in this part of the world. Puerto Rico was the first country in the region where *B. pseudomallei* endemicity was clearly demonstrated [42].However, in Mexico, Central America, and other Caribbean islands, the diagnosis is being made with increasing frequency based on identification with commercial systems such as API 20E, API 20NE, VITEK®1 and 2 (bioMérieux). However, a limitation of these commercially-available systems is that the misidentification of *B. pseudomallei* for *B. cepacia* may occur with VITEK®2 [53]. However, API 20NE and 20E have correctly identified 98% and 99% of *B. pseudomallei* cases, respectively [58].

There is a variety of serological assays (ELISAs, indirect hemagglutination assay, and indirect immunofluorescence assay) available for the identification of *B. pseudomallei* in endemic regions, although their usefulness is limited by high rates of background antibody [59,60]. However, seroprevalence studies would be very valuable to assess the endemicity in this region, because only Puerto Rico has been clearly demonstrated as endemic, using a combined approach of seroepidemiology and environmental detection [42]. Ashdown's selective agar is still considered the gold standard for optimal diagnosis, and is recommended for the isolation of *B. pseudomallei* from clinical specimens from sites with a normal flora. However, it is not always available and is not routinely used in non-endemic areas [61]. *B. pseudomallei* grows on many commercially available culture media (MacConkey, sheep blood and chocolate agar), but it is likely that many laboratories in the region may misidentify the bacterium as *Pseudomonas* species or other *Burkholderia* species, particularly with some commercial systems with poorly ability to identify *B. pseudomallei* [62–64]. Likewise, clinical manifestations of melioidosis do not make the diagnosis any simpler, because the disease is frequently clinically indistinguishable from many infections caused by other bacteria. This indicates that a limited experience and lack of familiarity with *B. pseudomallei* amongst clinicians and laboratory staff, in combination with unreliable diagnostic tests in non-endemic regions, may result in continued misidentification of the pathogen, and therefore underestimation of melioidosis cases in the region.

Pneumonia was the most common clinical presentation associated with the melioidosis cases described here. Chronic melioidosis with cavitary lung lesions and subcutaneous and visceral abscesses were also found in many cases, and the protean nature of melioidosis was evidenced by one case affecting the central nervous system. Therefore, the diagnosis of melioidosis should be considered by physicians in any patients presenting with those signs and symptoms who are returning from or residing in potentially endemic tropical regions. In addition, medical personnel should be aware of the conditions that predispose to melioidosis, including diabetes mellitus, alcoholism, chronic lung disease, cancer, and other immunosuppressive disorders [62], which should increase the chances of making the diagnosis.

The accurate diagnosis of melioidosis is important in order to guide antibiotic treatment and prevent relapse. The recent recommendations for therapy of melioidosis have been comprehensively summarized elsewhere [12,65]. One other issue requiring attention to reduce the risk of melioidosis acquisition in the healthcare setting is the possible accidental exposure of laboratory workers to infection. Sniffing culture plates is an unsafe laboratory procedure that is still performed in some countries of this region, and should be forbidden. Based on anecdotal experience, several clinical laboratorians in Mexico routinely sniff culture plates in order to identify the characteristic smell (referred to as a corn 'tortilla'-like) of *Pseudomonas aeruginosa* colonies (with which *Burkholderia* spp. may be confused), which is a potentially high-risk activity in a laboratory setting. Consequently, physicians should notify laboratory staff when samples are submitted from patients with symptoms, risk factors, or history that is suggestive of melioidosis.

4. Awareness of Melioidosis

Disease awareness and education are important for melioidosis prevention and diagnosis. Consequently, physicians and health care personnel must be made aware of the increasing number of cases of apparently indigenous melioidosis reported in Mexico, Central America, and the Caribbean islands. For example, health departments should raise awareness of melioidosis by distributing printed information, in addition to running training seminars and workshops for healthcare professionals. The future development of practical tools to detect, assess, and notify cases should be evaluated and implemented by health organizations such as PAHO (Pan American Health Organization) and CARPHA (The Caribbean Public Health Agency); it is worth noting that the websites for these agencies do not currently mention melioidosis. Modeling of the predicted distribution and burden of melioidosis showed that the population at risk in this region is about 246 million, in which 2000 could have melioidosis, and 1000 might die each year [7]. If the prediction is correct, melioidosis is more than a sporadic disease in this region.

Unfortunately, public awareness of melioidosis is very low, even in endemic countries such as Thailand [66]. It is evident that people from Mexico, Central America, and the Caribbean Islands are not aware of the disease, and therefore, they do not know anything about how to prevent it. Raising awareness and knowledge about melioidosis among researchers and representatives of the public health sectors will allow the development and implementation of guidelines for prevention, diagnosis, and therapy. Furthermore, health departments should consider making melioidosis a reportable disease, which would help improve surveillance and encourage the redefinition of endemic areas.

5. Future Challenges

Current melioidosis morbidity and mortality in well-known endemic regions have decreased due to better clinical management and advances in diagnostic techniques. However, in Mexico, Central America, and the Caribbean islands, the inadequate diagnosis and treatment of patients with melioidosis is a public health problem that is almost certainly leading to unnecessary deaths. In this context, national reporting systems should be improved in order to inform strategies to prevent, prepare for, detect, and respond to melioidosis cases.

Therefore, (1) timely and accurate diagnosis is needed to ensure effective antibiotic therapy; (2) there is a need to introduce selective media, such as Ashdown agar, in order to improve the yield of *B. pseudomallei* from patients who are suspected to have melioidosis; (3) it is necessary to instruct healthcare professionals about diagnosis, treatment, and preventive measures to combat melioidosis; (4) reporting cases that occur in areas where melioidosis is not currently recognized as endemic will help technicians and clinicians become familiar with this pathogen, and alert public health officials. Finally, recognizing melioidosis as an endemic disease affecting this region will allow the establishment of educational campaigns for professionals and the general public, especially those with risk factors, and the development of guidelines for the prevention and treatment of the disease.

Acknowledgments: This study was supported by NIH NIAID R01 AI12660101 grant awarded to Alfredo Torres. The contents are solely the responsibility of the authors and do not necessarily represent the official views of the NIAID or NIH. The authors would also like to acknowledge Jay E. Gee, Mindy G. Elrod and Alex R. Hoffmaster for their recommendations to the Puerto Rico and the Caribbean Islands sections.

Author Contributions: J.I.S.-V. and A.G.T. compiled and organized the data; J.I.S.-V. and A.G.T. wrote the manuscript.

Conflicts of Interest: The authors declare no conflict of interest.

References

1. Currie, B.J.; Ward, L.; Cheng, A.C. The epidemiology and clinical spectrum of melioidosis: 540 cases from the 20 year darwin prospective study. *PLoS Negl. Trop. Dis.* **2010**, *4*, e900. [CrossRef] [PubMed]
2. Yeager, J.J.; Facemire, P.; Dabisch, P.A.; Robinson, C.G.; Nyakiti, D.; Beck, K.; Baker, R.; Pitt, M.L. Natural history of inhalation melioidosis in rhesus macaques (*Macaca mulatta*) and African green monkeys (*Chlorocebus aethiops*). *Infect. Immun.* **2012**, *80*, 3332–3340. [CrossRef] [PubMed]
3. Churuangsuk, C.; Chusri, S.; Hortiwakul, T.; Charernmak, B.; Silpapojakul, K. Characteristics, clinical outcomes and factors influencing mortality of patients with melioidosis in southern Thailand: A 10-year retrospective study. *Asian Pac. J. Trop. Med.* **2016**, *9*, 256–260. [CrossRef] [PubMed]
4. Suputtamongkol, Y.; Chaowagul, W.; Chetchotisakd, P.; Lertpatanasuwun, N.; Intaranongpai, S.; Ruchutrakool, T.; Budhsarawong, D.; Mootsikapun, P.; Wuthiekanun, V.; Teerawatasook, N.; et al. Risk factors for melioidosis and bacteremic melioidosis. *Clin. Infect. Dis.* **1999**, *29*, 408–413. [CrossRef] [PubMed]
5. Currie, B.J. Melioidosis: Evolving concepts in epidemiology, pathogenesis, and treatment. *Semin. Respir. Crit. Care Med.* **2015**, *36*, 111–125. [CrossRef] [PubMed]
6. Benoit, T.J.; Blaney, D.D.; Doker, T.J.; Gee, J.E.; Elrod, M.G.; Rolim, D.B.; Inglis, T.J.; Hoffmaster, A.R.; Bower, W.A.; Walke, H.T. A review of melioidosis cases in the Americas. *Am. J. Trop. Med. Hyg.* **2015**, *93*, 1134–1139. [CrossRef] [PubMed]
7. Limmathurotsakul, D.; Golding, N.; Dance, D.A.; Messina, J.P.; Pigott, D.M.; Moyes, C.L.; Rolim, D.B.; Bertherat, E.; Day, N.P.; Peacock, S.J.; et al. Predicted global distribution of *Burkholderia pseudomallei* and burden of melioidosis. *Nat. Microbiol.* **2016**, *1*, 15008. [CrossRef] [PubMed]
8. International Diabetes Federation. *IDF Diabetes Atlas*, 8th ed.; International Diabetes Federation: Brussels, Belgium, 2017.
9. Hoffmaster, A.R.; AuCoin, D.; Baccam, P.; Baggett, H.C.; Baird, R.; Bhengsri, S.; Blaney, D.D.; Brett, P.J.; Brooks, T.J.; Brown, K.A.; et al. Melioidosis diagnostic workshop, 2013. *Emerg. Infect. Dis.* **2015**, *21*, e141045.
10. Leelarasamee, A.; Bovornkitti, S. Melioidosis: Review and update. *Rev. Infect. Dis.* **1989**, *11*, 413–425. [CrossRef] [PubMed]
11. Harris, P.; Engler, C.; Norton, R. Comparative in vitro susceptibility of *Burkholderia pseudomallei* to doripenem, ertapenem, tigecycline and moxifloxacin. *Int. J. Antimicrob. Agents* **2011**, *37*, 547–549. [CrossRef] [PubMed]
12. Dance, D. Treatment and prophylaxis of melioidosis. *Int. J. Antimicrob. Agents* **2014**, *43*, 310–318. [CrossRef] [PubMed]

13. Stewart, T.; Engelthaler, D.M.; Blaney, D.D.; Tuanyok, A.; Wangsness, E.; Smith, T.L.; Pearson, T.; Komatsu, K.K.; Keim, P.; Currie, B.J.; et al. Epidemiology and investigation of melioidosis, southern Arizona. *Emerg. Infect. Dis.* **2011**, *17*, 1286–1288. [CrossRef] [PubMed]

14. Doker, T.J.; Quinn, C.L.; Salehi, E.D.; Sherwood, J.J.; Benoit, T.J.; Glass Elrod, M.; Gee, J.E.; Shadomy, S.V.; Bower, W.A.; Hoffmaster, A.R.; et al. Fatal *Burkholderia pseudomallei* infection initially reported as a *Bacillus* species, Ohio, 2013. *Am. J. Trop. Med. Hyg.* **2014**, *91*, 743–746. [CrossRef] [PubMed]

15. Chagla, Z.; Aleksova, N.; Quirt, J.; Emery, J.; Kraeker, C.; Haider, S. Melioidosis in a returned traveller. *Can. J. Infect. Dis. Med. Microbiol.* **2014**, *25*, 225–226. [CrossRef] [PubMed]

16. Germain, M.; Auger, F.; Murray, G. Melioidosis in a traveller—Quebec. *Can. Dis. Wkly. Rep.* **1989**, *15*, 109–111. [PubMed]

17. Turner, M.O.; Lee, V.T.; FitzGerald, J.M. Melioidosis in a diabetic sailor. *Chest* **1994**, *106*, 952–954. [CrossRef] [PubMed]

18. Hogan, C.; Wilmer, A.; Badawi, M.; Hoang, L.; Chapman, M.; Press, N.; Antonation, K.; Corbett, C.; Romney, M.; Murray, M. Melioidosis in Trinidad and Tobago. *Emerg. Infect. Dis.* **2015**, *21*, 902–904. [CrossRef] [PubMed]

19. McDowell, F.; Varney, P.L. Melioidosis, report of first case from the Western Hemisphere. *J. Am. Med. Assoc.* **1947**, *134*, 361. [CrossRef] [PubMed]

20. Joy, R.J.; Scalettar, R.; Sodee, D.B. Optic and peripheral neuritis. Probable effect of prolonged chloramphenicol therapy. *JAMA* **1960**, *173*, 1731–1734. [CrossRef] [PubMed]

21. Biegeleisen, J.Z., Jr.; Mosquera, R.; Cherry, W.B. Case of human melioidosis; clinical, epidemiological and laboratory findings. *Rev. Ecuat. Hig. Med. Trop.* **1964**, *21*, 23–37. [CrossRef] [PubMed]

22. Darby, J.P.; Mendez, E. Chronic melioidosis: Serologic diagnosis and antibiotic treatment. *US Armed Forces Med. J.* **1960**, *11*, 1203–1210.

23. Bloch, M.; Soundy, J.; Guzman, A. Infections from *Pseudomonas* other than *aeruginosa*. *Rev. Inst. Investig. Med. (El Salvador)* **1981**, *10*, 164–189.

24. Christenson-Bravo, B.; Rodríguez, J.E.; Vázquez, G.; Ramírez Ronda, C.H. *Pseudomonas pseudomallei* (melioidosis): Acute septicemia and meningitis in patient with systemic lupus erythematosus. *Bol. Asoc. Med. P. R.* **1986**, *78*, 347–349. [PubMed]

25. Barnes, P.F.; Appleman, M.D.; Cosgrove, M.M. A case of melioidosis originating in North America. *Am. Rev. Respir. Dis.* **1986**, *134*, 170–171. [PubMed]

26. Lezana, J.L.; Novoa, O.; Lezana, M.A. Epidemiology of *Pseudomonas* in Mexican CF patients. In Proceedings of the Cystic Fibrosis Conference, Tarpon Springs, FL, USA, 11–14 October 1989.

27. Olive, C.; Loetitia, G.; Desbois, N.; Roche, B.; Jouannelle, J.; Dodin, A. Septic pyemic form of human melioidosis: A first case in the French Antilles. *Presse. Med.* **1995**, *24*, 1270. [PubMed]

28. Dorman, S.E.; Gill, V.J.; Gallin, J.I.; Holland, S.M. *Burkholderia pseudomallei* infection in a Puerto Rican patient with chronic granulomatous disease: Case report and review of occurrences in the Americas. *Clin. Infect. Dis.* **1998**, *26*, 889–894. [CrossRef] [PubMed]

29. Pérez, J.M.; Petiot, A.; Adjidé, C.; Gerry, F.; Goursaud, R.; Juminer, B. First case report of melioidosis in Guadeloupe, a French West Indies Archipelago. *Clin. Infect. Dis.* **1997**, *25*, 164–165. [CrossRef] [PubMed]

30. Villegas, I.; Herrera, M.L.; Vargas, A.; Duarte, I.; Campos, M. Primer aislamiento de *Burkholderia pseudomallei* en Costa Rica. *Rev. Méd. Hosp. Nac. Niños (Costa Rica)* **1998**, *33*, 1–2.

31. Theodose, R.; Olive, C.; Dubreuil, F.; Dupont-Fontamille, J.; Jean-Baptiste, G.; Jouannelle, J. A propos des trois premiers cas en Martinique d'infection a *Burkholderia pseudomallei*. *Rev. Med. Interne.* **2000**, *21*, 592. [CrossRef]

32. Messino Julio, A.; Villegas Villareal, I. Melioidosis en Costa Rica: Reporte del primer caso. *Acta Med. Costarric.* **2000**, *42*, 131–133.

33. Inglis, T.J.; Rolim, D.B.; Sousa, A.Q. Melioidosis in the Americas. *Am. J. Trop. Med. Hyg.* **2006**, *75*, 947–954. [PubMed]

34. Christenson, B.; Fuxench, Z.; Morales, J.A.; Suárez-Villamil, R.A.; Souchet, L.M. Severe community-acquired pneumonia and sepsis caused by *Burkholderia pseudomallei* associated with flooding in Puerto Rico. *Bol. Asoc. Med. P. R.* **2003**, *95*, 17–20. [PubMed]

35. Centers for Disease, C.; Prevention. Laboratory exposure to *Burkholderia pseudomallei*—Los Angeles, California, 2003. *MMWR Morb. Mortal. Wkly. Rep.* **2004**, *53*, 988–990.

36. CDC. Imported melioidosis—South Florida. *MMWR Morb. Mortal. Wkly. Rep.* **2006**, *55*, 873–876.
37. Corral, D.M.; Coates, A.L.; Yau, Y.C.; Tellier, R.; Glass, M.; Jones, S.M.; Waters, V.J. *Burkholderia pseudomallei* infection in a cystic fibrosis patient from the Caribbean: A case report. *Can. Respir. J.* **2008**, *15*, 237–239. [CrossRef] [PubMed]
38. Almuzara, M.; Barberis, C.; Bravo, M.; Pisarevsky, A.; Petrucci, E.; Famiglietti, A.; Lasala, M.; Vay, C. A case of melioidosis in Argentina. *Medicina (B Aires)* **2011**, *71*, 39–41. [PubMed]
39. O'Sullivan, B.P.; Torres, B.; Conidi, G.; Smole, S.; Gauthier, C.; Stauffer, K.E.; Glass, M.B.; Gee, J.E.; Blaney, D.; Smith, T.L. *Burkholderia pseudomallei* infection in a child with cystic fibrosis: Acquisition in the Western Hemisphere. *Chest* **2011**, *140*, 239–242. [CrossRef] [PubMed]
40. Gee, J.E.; Allender, C.J.; Tuanyok, A.; Elrod, M.G.; Hoffmaster, A.R. *Burkholderia pseudomallei* type G in Western Hemisphere. *Emerg. Infect. Dis.* **2014**, *20*, 682–684. [CrossRef] [PubMed]
41. Blaney, D. Cases Information. Available online: http://www.melioidosis.info/info.Aspx?Pageid=107 (accessed on 1 December 2017).
42. Doker, T.J.; Sharp, T.M.; Rivera-Garcia, B.; Perez-Padilla, J.; Benoit, T.J.; Ellis, E.M.; Elrod, M.G.; Gee, J.E.; Shieh, W.J.; Beesley, C.A.; et al. Contact investigation of melioidosis cases reveals regional endemicity in Puerto Rico. *Clin. Infect. Dis.* **2015**, *60*, 243–250. [CrossRef] [PubMed]
43. Meckenstock, R.; Therby, A.; Marque-Juillet, S.; Monnier, S.; Khau, D.; Pangon, B.; Greder-Belan, A. Cutaneous melioidosis in adolescent returning from Guadeloupe. *Emerg. Infect. Dis.* **2012**, *18*, 359–360. [CrossRef] [PubMed]
44. Gétaz, L.; Abbas, M.; Loutan, L.; Schrenzel, J.; Iten, A.; Simon, F.; Decosterd, A.; Studer, R.; Sudre, P.; Michel, Y.; et al. Fatal acute melioidosis in a tourist returning from Martinique Island, November 2010. *Euro Surveill.* **2011**, *16*, 19758.
45. Mickail, N.; Klein, N.C.; Cunha, B.A.; Schoch, P.A. Melioidosis breast abscesses. *J. Infect.* **2012**, *64*, 434–435. [CrossRef] [PubMed]
46. Adames, E.M.A.; Barrios González, J.A. *Burkholderia pseudomallei* liver and skin abscesses. *Rev. Médico Cient.* **2012**, *25*, 35–43.
47. Martínez-Hernández, L.; González-Híjar, A.; Valdéz-Vázquez, R.; García-López, S.; González-Chon, O. Melioidosis: Reporte de caso y revisión de la literatura. *Neumol. Cir. Torax.* **2013**, *72*, 291–298.
48. Benoit, T.J.; Blaney, D.D.; Gee, J.E.; Elrod, M.G.; Hoffmaster, A.R.; Doker, T.J.; Bower, W.A.; Walke, H.T.; Centers for Disease, C.; Prevention. Melioidosis cases and selected reports of occupational exposures to *Burkholderia pseudomallei*—United States, 2008–2013. *MMWR Surveill. Summ.* **2015**, *64*, 1–9. [PubMed]
49. Villalobos Zúñiga, M.A.; Badilla Baltodano, G. Caso 8-2014: Primer caso de infección del sistema nervioso central por *Burkholderia pseudomallei* en Costa Rica. *Rev. Cl. EMed. UCR* **2014**, *4*, 1–6. [CrossRef]
50. Cheng, J.W.; Hayden, M.K.; Singh, K.; Heimler, I.; Gee, J.E.; Proia, L.; Sha, B.E. *Burkholderia pseudomallei* infection in US traveler returning from Mexico, 2014. *Emerg. Infect. Dis.* **2015**, *21*, 1884–1885. [CrossRef] [PubMed]
51. Truong, K.K.; Moghaddam, S.; Al Saghbini, S.; Saatian, B. Case of a lung mass due to melioidosis in Mexico. *Am. J. Case Rep.* **2015**, *16*, 272–275. [PubMed]
52. Boroel-Cervantes, C.; Ibarra-Valdez, M.; Miranda-Pacheco, S.; Sánchez-Camarena, E.; Wolburgth-Franco, T.; Ortiz-González, A.; Domínguez-Ríos, J.L. Melioidosis: Reporte del primer caso en el estado de Sonora, México. *Rev. Med. Inst. Mex. Seguro. Soc.* **2017**, *55*, 257–259. [PubMed]
53. Podin, Y.; Kaestli, M.; McMahon, N.; Hennessy, J.; Ngian, H.U.; Wong, J.S.; Mohana, A.; Wong, S.C.; William, T.; Mayo, M.; et al. Reliability of automated biochemical identification of *Burkholderia pseudomallei* is regionally dependent. *J. Clin. Microbiol.* **2013**, *51*, 3076–3078. [CrossRef] [PubMed]
54. Gee, J.E.; Gulvik, C.A.; Elrod, M.G.; Batra, D.; Rowe, L.A.; Sheth, M.; Hoffmaster, A.R. Phylogeography of *Burkholderia pseudomallei* isolates, Western Hemisphere. *Emerg. Infect. Dis.* **2017**, *23*, 1133–1138. [CrossRef] [PubMed]
55. Hemme, R.R.; Lopez-Ortiz, R.; Garcia, B.R.; Sharp, T.M.; Galloway, R.L.; Elrod, M.G.; Hunsperger, E.A. Serological evidence of infection with endemic human pathogens among free-ranging old world monkeys in Puerto Rico. *Am. J. Trop. Med. Hyg.* **2016**, *94*, 1095–1099. [CrossRef] [PubMed]
56. Gee, J.E.; Elrod, M.G.; Hoffmaster, A.R.; Bacterial Special Pathogens Branch, Division of High Consequence Pathogens and Pathology, Centers for Disease Control and Prevention, Atlanta, Georgia, USA. Personal communication, 2017.

57. Sutmoller, P.; Kraneveld, F.C.; Van Der Schaaf, A. Melioidosis (*pseudomalleus*) in sheep, goats, and pigs on Aruba (Netherland Antilles). *J. Am. Vet. Med. Assoc.* **1957**, *130*, 415–417. [PubMed]

58. Lowe, P.; Engler, C.; Norton, R. Comparison of automated and nonautomated systems for identification of *Burkholderia pseudomallei*. *J. Clin. Microbiol.* **2002**, *40*, 4625–4627. [CrossRef] [PubMed]

59. Currie, B.J. Melioidosis: An important cause of pneumonia in residents of and travellers returned from endemic regions. *Eur. Respir. J.* **2003**, *22*, 542–550. [CrossRef] [PubMed]

60. Sirisinha, S.; Anuntagool, N.; Dharakul, T.; Ekpo, P.; Wongratanacheewin, S.; Naigowit, P.; Petchclai, B.; Thamlikitkul, V.; Suputtamongkol, Y. Recent developments in laboratory diagnosis of melioidosis. *Acta Trop.* **2000**, *74*, 235–245. [CrossRef]

61. Cheng, A.C.; Wuthiekanun, V.; Limmathurosakul, D.; Wongsuvan, G.; Day, N.P.; Peacock, S.J. Role of selective and nonselective media for isolation of *Burkholderia pseudomallei* from throat swabs of patients with melioidosis. *J. Clin. Microbiol.* **2006**, *44*, 2316. [CrossRef] [PubMed]

62. Wiersinga, W.J.; Currie, B.J.; Peacock, S.J. Melioidosis. *N. Engl. J. Med.* **2012**, *367*, 1035–1044. [CrossRef] [PubMed]

63. Frickmann, H.; Neubauer, H.; Haase, G.; Peltroche-Llacsahuanga, H.; Pérez-Bouza, A.; Racz, P.; Loderstaedt, U.; Hagen, R.M. Fatal urosepsis due to delayed diagnosis of genitourinary melioidosis. *Laboratoriumsmedizin* **2013**, *37*. [CrossRef]

64. Mohanty, S.; Pradhan, G.; Panigrahi, M.K.; Mohapatra, P.R.; Mishra, B. A case of systemic melioidosis: Unravelling the etiology of chronic unexplained fever with multiple presentations. *Pneumonol. Alergol. Pol.* **2016**, *84*, 121–125. [CrossRef] [PubMed]

65. Estes, D.M.; Dow, S.W.; Schweizer, H.P.; Torres, A.G. Present and future therapeutic strategies for melioidosis and glanders. *Expert Rev. Anti. Infect. Ther.* **2010**, *8*, 325–338. [CrossRef] [PubMed]

66. Chansrichavala, P.; Wongsuwan, N.; Suddee, S.; Malasit, M.; Hongsuwan, M.; Wannapinij, P.; Kitphati, R.; Day, N.P.; Michie, S.; Peacock, S.J.; et al. Public awareness of melioidosis in Thailand and potential use of video clips as educational tools. *PLoS ONE* **2015**, *10*, e0121311. [CrossRef] [PubMed]

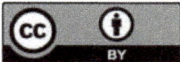

*Tropical Medicine and
Infectious Disease*

MDPI

Review

Melioidosis in Myanmar

Mo Mo Win [1,*], Elizabeth A. Ashley [2,3], Khwar Nyo Zin [4], Myint Thazin Aung [5],
Myo Maung Maung Swe [2], Clare L. Ling [3,6], François Nosten [3,6], Win May Thein [7], Ni Ni Zaw [7],
May Yee Aung [8], Kyaw Myo Tun [9], David A. B. Dance [3,10,11] and Frank M. Smithuis [2,3,12]

[1] Department of Medical Research, Yangon, Myanmar
[2] Myanmar Oxford Clinical Research Unit, Yangon, Myanmar; liz@tropmedres.ac (E.A.A.);
myomgswe@gmail.com (M.M.M.S.); frank.m.smithuis@gmail.com (F.M.S.)
[3] Centre for Tropical Medicine and Global Health, Nuffield Department of Clinical Medicine, Old Road
Campus, University of Oxford, Oxford OX3 7FZ, UK; clare@tropmedres.ac (C.L.L.);
francois@tropmedres.ac (F.N.); david.d@tropmedres.ac (D.A.B.D)
[4] Department of Microbiology, Yangon General Hospital, University of Medicine 1, Yangon, Myanmar;
drknzin@gmail.com
[5] Pathology Department, Microbiology Section, North Okkapala General Hospital, University of Medicine 2,
Yangon, Myanmar; myintthazinaung@gmail.com
[6] Shoklo Malaria Research Unit, Mahidol-Oxford Tropical Medicine Research Unit, Faculty of Tropical
Medicine, Mahidol University, Mae Sot 63110, Thailand
[7] Mandalay General Hospital, University of Medicine, Mandalay, Myanmar;
winmaythein14@gmail.com (W.M.T.); sandblood7@gmail.com (N.N.Z.)
[8] Pathology Department, Microbiology section, Thingungyun Hospital, University of Medicine 1, Yangon,
Myanmar; immyaung@gmail.com
[9] Department of Preventive & Social Medicine, Defence Services Medical Academy, Yangon, Myanmar;
kyaw@dsmrc.net
[10] Lao-Oxford-Mahosot Hospital-Wellcome Trust Research Unit, Microbiology Laboratory, Mahosot Hospital,
Vientiane, Laos
[11] Faculty of Infectious and Tropical Diseases, London School of Hygiene and Tropical Medicine,
London WC1E 7HT, UK
[12] Medical Action Myanmar, Yangon, Myanmar
* Correspondence: drmomowin@gmail.com; Tel.: +95-1-375459 (ext. 508)

Received: 9 February 2018; Accepted: 23 February 2018; Published: 1 March 2018

Abstract: Sporadic cases of melioidosis have been diagnosed in Myanmar since the disease was
first described in Yangon in 1911. Published and unpublished cases are summarized here, along
with results from environmental and serosurveys. A total of 298 cases have been reported from
seven states or regions between 1911 and 2018, with the majority of these occurring before 1949.
Findings from soil surveys confirm the presence of *Burkholderia pseudomallei* in the environment in all
three regions examined. The true epidemiology of the disease in Myanmar is unknown. Important
factors contributing to the current gaps in knowledge are lack of awareness among clinicians and
insufficient laboratory diagnostic capacity in many parts of the country. This is likely to have led to
substantial under-reporting.

Keywords: melioidosis; *Burkholderia pseudomallei*; Myanmar

---

1. Introduction and History of Melioidosis in Myanmar

All historical accounts of melioidosis start with Myanmar (formerly Burma), since the disease
was first recognized in 1911 in Rangoon (now Yangon) General Hospital by Alfred Whitmore, a
British pathologist who worked in Burma between 1906 and 1924 [1]. In 1913, Whitmore reported 38
post-mortem cases of a 'glanders-like disease', the majority of whom were male and bore stigmata of

morphine injection. Krishnaswamy, Whitmore's assistant, reported in 1917 that he had personally seen more than 200 cases in Rangoon over six years, during which the disease accounted for approximately one in every 20 autopsies he had conducted [2]. In the ensuing years, reported case numbers in the country dwindled, and after the end of World War II, the disease disappeared from sight for more than 50 years. This hiatus corresponded firstly with the transition from colonial rule to independence (in 1948) and later with a prolonged period of military rule in Myanmar (1962–2011), during which the country became closed off from the rest of the world, investment in healthcare slowed, and research stagnated. Microbiologists working in larger centres inside Myanmar have reported sporadic cases over the last 20 years, but the true epidemiology of the disease is unknown. Most health facilities in Myanmar do not have the capacity to identify *B. pseudomallei*, and most health staff are not aware of this disease. It is therefore likely that melioidosis is significantly underdiagnosed in Myanmar, and the projected annual number of cases (more than 6000) and deaths (more than 3000) from a recent modelling study could well be an accurate reflection of the true situation [3].

2. Review of Melioidosis Cases and Presence of *B. pseudomallei* in the Country

We searched the PubMed database for cases of melioidosis or evidence of *B. pseudomallei* using the following search terms: ((Myanmar) OR Burma)) AND ((melioid*) OR pseudomallei) OR glanders*)). A separate search was performed for 'Parotid abscess AND Myanmar' (no hits). We also consulted the Myanmar medical literature and the melioidosis global database [4], and contacted consultant microbiologists in the biggest centres in the country (public sector).

2.1. Results

Evidence for the presence of *B. pseudomallei* in Myanmar comes from reports of clinical cases, environmental sampling and serosurveys. Melioidosis has never been diagnosed in animals in Myanmar although, by analogy with neighbouring countries, infections in animals are almost certainly occurring undiagnosed.

2.1.1. Clinical Cases

We found a total of 298 published and unpublished cases of melioidosis in Myanmar since 1913 (Table 1). The vast majority (257) were published before the end of 1948. The next report of a case diagnosed inside the country came about half a century later in 2000 in Mandalay [5]. Of the remaining cases, several were diagnosed outside Myanmar, and the remainder came from a very small number of centres. Eighty-five were known to have been culture-confirmed. The report by Krishnaswamy in which he mentions 200 cases does not state explicitly that these were culture-confirmed; however, given his position as Whitmore's assistant and the descriptions of the first 38 cases in which the diagnosis was confirmed by culture, it is likely that these too were confirmed cases. Of note, only five cases (~2%) were in females and three in children. A total of 276/298 (93%) cases were diagnosed in patients from the Yangon area with six from Kayin state, two from Rakhine state, one from Bago region, two from Ayeyarwady, two from Magway, two from Pyay and four not specified (Table 1 and Figure 1).

Table 1. Cases of melioidosis reported from Myanmar.

Year of Report	First Author	N Cases	N Fatalities	N Culture Confirmed	Location in Myanmar	Remarks
1913	Whitmore [1]	38	38	38	Yangon	Case-series identified post-mortem
1915	Knapp [6]	11	11	1 (remaining NS)	Yangon	Case-series identified post-mortem
1917	Krishnaswamy [2]	~200	~200	NS	Yangon	Cases of 'morphia injector's septicaemia' identified post-mortem
1945	Cox [7]	1	1	1	Not known	US Army soldier
1947	Harries [8]	6	2	5	Between Pyay & Yangon (5), Rakhine (1)	West African soldiers serving in Myanmar
1948	Sen [9]	1	1	1	Yangon	Case identified post-mortem
1979	van der Schaaf [10]	1	1	1	Not known	Ex-Royal Netherlands East Indies Army (KNIL) prisoner of war. Post-mortem identification
1994	Wilairatana [11]	1	0	1	Not known	Myanmar national diagnosed in Bangkok
1999	Kunishima [12,13]	1	0	1	Not known	Returned traveler (diagnosed in Japan)
1999	Lee [14]	1	0	1	Yangon	Returned traveler (diagnosed in Taiwan)
2000	May Kyi Aung [5]	1	0	1	Mandalay	Female
2002	Than Than Aye; referenced in [15]	1	NS	NS	Yangon	Cerebral melioidosis (no information)
2002	Leeuwenburgh [16]	1	0	1	Not known	Returned female traveler (diagnosed in Netherlands)
2004	May Kyi Aung [17]	1	1	1	Yangon	-
2004	Mo Mo Win [18]	1	0	1	Yangon (Hmawbi)	
2004	Su Su Hlaing [19]	1	0	1	Pyay	Concomitant tetanus
2005	Demar [20]	1	0	1	Shwepyitha (Yangon) or Kyunbin(Bago)	Returned traveler (diagnosed in France)
2008	May Kyi Aung [21]	3	NS	3	Yangon	Survey of 133 patients with abscesses in 22 Yangon hospitals
2012	Thae Thae Min [22]	2	0 [1]	2	Magway	Study of 307 patients hospitalised with infectious diseases
2013	Zaw Than Htun [15]	3	NS	3	Yangon (Hmawbi, Thanlyin), Ayeyarwady (Mawkyun)	Includes one female
2014	Chu [23]	2	2	2	Thai-Myanmar border (close to Kayin state) [2]	Two fatal cases (one female)

Table 1. *Cont.*

Year of Report	First Author	N Cases	N Fatalities	N Culture Confirmed	Location in Myanmar	Remarks
2014	Mar Mar Kyi [24]	1	0	1	Taungoo (Bago)	Healthy student with multiple skin abscesses
2015	Mo Mo Win [4]	2	1[3]	2	Yangon	-
2016	Brummaier [25]	1	0	1	Thai-Myanmar border (close to Kayin state)[2]	Ten-year-old boy with subcutaneous abscesses
2016	Mo Mo Win [4]	2	1	2	Yangon	-
2016–2017	Shoklo Malaria Research Unit [4]	3	0	3	Thai-Myanmar border (close to Kayin state)[2]	Includes one child
2017	Mo Mo Win (pers.comm)	7	1	7	Rakhine(1), Ayeyarwady (1), Yangon (5)	Includes one female
2017	Ni Ni Zaw (pers.comm.)	1	NS	1	Mandalay	-
2018	Kyaw Myo Tun (pers.comm.)	1	1	1	Yangon	-
2018	Mo Mo Win (pers.comm)	1	0[4]	1	Yangon	-
	TOTAL	298				

Cases are adult males unless otherwise stated. [1] One patient survived. The other patient was referred to another centre (no outcome recorded). [2] The cases from the Thai-Myanmar border were diagnosed in a migrant population from Myanmar. [3] Second patient's outcome not known. [4] Discharged home in pre-terminal condition at request of family; NS = not stated.

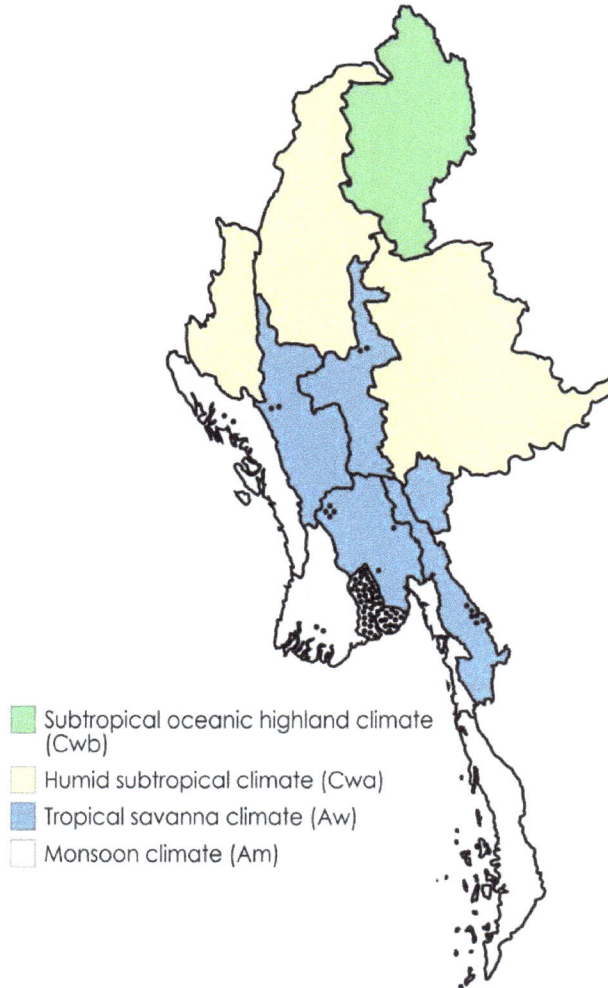

Figure 1. Map of Myanmar showing distribution of reported cases (1912–present) by state or region, categorized by predominant climate type. Each black dot represents a case.

In 2014, the results of all the blood cultures processed by the laboratory of Yangon General Hospital between 2005 and 2013 were published [26]. *B. pseudomallei* was not isolated from any of the 3865 cultures; however, the authors note that bacterial isolation and sub-optimal identification techniques may have been one explanation. In addition, the number of cultures requested was low relative to the number of admissions in this busy hospital, which exceeds 50,000 per year.

2.1.2. Serological Evidence for *B. pseudomallei* in Myanmar

The gold standard for the diagnosis of melioidosis is bacterial isolation. Serology is difficult to interpret in endemic countries due to background positivity rates, but gives some indication of population exposure. A cross-sectional sero-survey of 968 migrant workers from Myanmar was undertaken in Thailand, close to the western border, in 2005 using a haemagglutination assay [27].

The majority of participants (99%) came from Kayin or Mon States and Bago or Yangon Regions. The median [IQR] population IHA titre was 1:20 [1:10 to 1:40], with no regional variation observed. Sixty-nine (7%) participants had a titre ≥1:160, which is a recommended cut-off in Thailand used to support a clinical diagnosis of melioidosis. Only 8% of surveyed adults were agricultural workers. Between 2016 and 2017, blood samples were taken for serological testing using a hemolysin co-regulated protein 1 (Hcp1)-based ELISA from 265 febrile patients presenting to a three outpatient clinics in a large suburb of Yangon as part of a research study [28]. All patients tested negative (optical density cut-off 1.16); median [interquartile range] of 0.02 [0.01–0.04] [29].

2.1.3. Evidence from Environmental Surveys

Myanmar has a variable landscape, ranging from the delta region in the south and west, to the drier central plains, and ending at the Himalayan foothills in the north. Using a mathematical modelling approach and taking into account known cases, climate and soil type, Myanmar has been predicted to provide a very suitable environment for the causative bacterium [3]. Results of a farm survey performed in two townships in Yangon (Thanlyin and Hmawbi) were reported in 2016. From 120 soil samples and 12 water samples collected and processed according to standard microbiological guidelines for the detection of *B. pseudomallei*, there were seven positive results (confirmed by molecular methods) [30]. A national survey is underway by the authors, and preliminary testing has detected the bacterium by culture of soil samples from townships in Yangon, Kayin and Mon Regions, which is in agreement with the provenance of some of the reported clinical cases (Table 2). Full results should be available by the end of 2018.

Table 2. Preliminary results of a soil survey being conducted in Myanmar.

Site Number	State or Region	Township	Total Number of Samples	Number of Positive Samples
1	Yangon	Hmawbi [1]	40	0
2	Yangon	Tontay	10	5
3	Yangon	Thanlyin	20	0
4	Yangon	Kyauktan	20	3
5	Yangon	Thone Gwa	20	0
6	Yangon	Kha Yan	20	0
7	Yangon	Dala	20	0
8	Kayin	Kyain Seikgyi	60	0
9	Kayin	Myawaddy	140	9
10	Kayin	Kawkareik	50	1
11	Kayin	Hpa-an	50	1
12	Mon	Kyaikhto	40	0
13	Mon	Bilin	30	0
14	Mon	Thaton	30	0
15	Mon	Yae	30	0
16	Mon	Thanbyuzayat	40	5
17	Mon	Kyaikmaraw	30	2
18	Mon	Mawlamyaing	20	0
19	Mon	Chaung Sone	20	0
20	Mon	Paung	20	0

[1] Note: an earlier survey found *B. pseudomallei* in Hmawbi (see text).

3. Current Recommendations and Availability of Measures Against Melioidosis

Currently, there is no requirement to notify cases of melioidosis in the country. The Ministry of Health and Sports has set up a national system for communicable disease surveillance and response. This targets epidemic-prone diseases, specific diseases under national surveillance (DUNS), emerging infectious diseases, climate-related communicable diseases, and vaccine-preventable diseases, but not melioidosis [31]. Under-recognition of the disease is very likely due to a lack of awareness among health staff, under-utilisation of microbiology services by clinicians and inability of many laboratories to identify the organism due to poor availability of necessary reagents, as well as a shortage of microbiologists, particularly in rural areas. There are no standard treatment guidelines for melioidosis, and the few patients identified are managed on a case by case basis.

4. Awareness of Melioidosis

With the exception of a few 'enthusiasts', melioidosis is almost entirely unknown among healthcare providers. Raising awareness among health staff, clinicians and laboratory staff is therefore the essential prerequisite to identifying melioidosis patients. When diagnostic and treatment services for suspected melioidosis cases are established, raising awareness among the population working in agriculture should follow in high-risk areas. Microbiology in Myanmar is perceived as a diagnostic rather than a clinical service, and there is limited interaction between microbiologists and clinicians, which means opportunities to raise awareness are missed. This was highlighted in the report by Hlaing et al. in 2004 of melioidosis co-infection in a patient with tetanus. A report that *B. pseudomallei* had been isolated was duly sent to the ward, but went unnoticed for several days and was acted upon only when the patient deteriorated.

5. Current and Future Challenges

The burden of melioidosis in Myanmar needs to be defined. The evidence suggests that the disease is under-recognised and under-reported. While the majority of cases have been reported from Yangon, evidence from a multicentre abscess survey, routine blood culture surveillance data at a large centre and a recent serosurvey suggests it may not be a leading cause of sepsis in the greater Yangon region, despite the fact that it was clearly an important cause of death in the early 20th century [2,21,26]. Reasons for a possible decline in incidence in areas of Yangon where it was common previously are unclear, although the strong link with injection drug use in the early fatal cases raises the possibility of contamination of the morphine, which is likely to have originated from Upper Burma [32]. An alternative explanation is that this group was relatively immunocompromised and more susceptible to infection following exposure in Yangon itself, and that with increasing urbanization, the risk of exposure has fallen. It is probable that there are unrecognised melioidosis 'hot-spots' elsewhere, so accurate data across the whole country are needed. Diabetes mellitus, a well-known risk factor for melioidosis, has moved into the top ten causes of death in the country in the last three years (http://www.healthdata.org/myanmar), which may drive up case numbers in the future. Important contributing factors to the current lack of knowledge are a lack of microbiology laboratory diagnostic capacity, particularly in smaller townships and rural areas, low rates of blood culture requesting, and lack of awareness of the disease among clinicians. Many laboratories at township level have been upgraded as part of the National Health Plan, but are not functional due a shortage of microbiologists. Myanmar has a national reference laboratory (National Health Laboratory), established in 1963, and a system for disease reporting. Addition of *B. pseudomallei* to the list of notifiable pathogens might yield more information on the distribution of cases in the country, but is unlikely to uncover large numbers until the capacity and usage of diagnostic microbiology increase. Environmental surveys may be useful to help target scarce resources to augment case-based surveillance in areas where it is likely to have the highest yield. This should be accompanied by advocacy meetings with state/regional and township health authorities to raise awareness among clinicians and health providers.

Acknowledgments: Thank you to Yoel Lubell, Thomas Althaus and Narisara Chantratita from the Mahidol Oxford Tropical Medicine Research Unit and Faculty of Tropical Medicine, Mahidol University, Thailand, for sharing unpublished serology data. The soil survey was funded by Medical Action Myanmar. MOCRU, LOMWRU and SMRU are part of the MORU Tropical Health Network, funded by the Wellcome Trust of Great Britain.

Author Contributions: M.M.W. and E.A. wrote the first draft. M.M.W., D.A.B.D., M.M.M.S., K.N.Z., M.T.A., F.N., W.M.T., N.N.Z., M.Y.A., K.M.T. and F.S. searched for published cases in the Myanmar literature and/or provided information on unpublished cases, recent environmental surveys and the current situation in Myanmar. All authors reviewed, edited and approved the submitted version.

Conflicts of Interest: The authors declare no conflict of interest. The funding sponsors had no role in the design of the study; in the collection, analyses, or interpretation of data; in the writing of the manuscript, and in the decision to publish the results.

References

1. Whitmore, A. An account of a glanders-like disease occurring in Rangoon. *J. Hyg.* **1913**, *13*, 1–34. [CrossRef] [PubMed]
2. Krishnaswamy, C.S. Morphia injector's septicaemia. *Indian Med. Gaz.* **1917**, *52*, 296–299.
3. Limmathurotsakul, D.; Golding, N.; Dance, D.A.; Messina, J.P.; Pigott, D.M.; Moyes, C.L.; Rolim, D.B.; Bertherat, E.; Day, N.P.; Peacock, S.J.; et al. Predicted global distribution of *Burkholderia pseudomallei* and burden of melioidosis. *Nat. Microbiol.* **2016**, *1*, 15008. [CrossRef] [PubMed]
4. Melioidosis. Info Online Database. 2018. Available online: http://www.melioidosis.info/ (accessed on 25 February 2018).
5. Aung, M.K. Case report: Melioidosis—A hidden disease in Myanmar. *Myanmar J. Curr. Med. Pract.* **2000**, *5*, 57–59.
6. Knapp, H.H.G. Morphine injector's septicaemia ('Whitmore's disease'). *Indian Med. Gaz.* **1915**, *50*, 287–288.
7. Cox, C.D.; Arbogast, J.L. Melioidosis. *Am. J. Clin. Pathol.* **1945**, *15*, 567–570. [CrossRef] [PubMed]
8. Harries, E.J.; Lewis, A.A.; et al. Melioidosis treated with sulphonamides and penicillin. *Lancet* **1948**, *1*, 363–366. [CrossRef]
9. Sen, S. A case of melioidosis. *Indian Med. Gaz.* **1948**, *83*, 186–187.
10. van der Schaaf, A. Veterinary experiences as a Japanese prisoner of war and ex-POW along the Burma railroad from 1942 to January 1946. *Vet. Quart.* **1979**, *1*, 212–228. [CrossRef] [PubMed]
11. Wilairatana, P.; Looareesuwan, S. Melioidotic otitis media. *Southeast Asian J. Trop. Med. Public Health* **1994**, *25*, 776–777. [PubMed]
12. Hadano, Y. Imported melioidosis in Japan: A review of cases. *Infect. Drug Resist.* **2018**, *11*, 163–168. [CrossRef] [PubMed]
13. Kunishima, H.; Seki, R.; Iwabuchi, T.; Nakamura, T.; Ishida, N.; Takagi, T.; Shimada, J. Case of melioidosis associated with acute empyema and cellulitis of the leg. *Nihon Naika Gakkai Zasshi J. Jpn. Soc. Intern. Med.* **1999**, *88*, 1101–1103.
14. Lee, S.C.; Ling, T.S.; Chen, J.C.; Huang, B.Y.; Sheih, W.B. Melioidosis with adrenal gland abscess. *Am. J. Trop. Med. Hyg.* **1999**, *61*, 34–36. [CrossRef] [PubMed]
15. Htun, Z.T.; Hla, T.; Myat, T.W.; Lin, N.; Wah, T.T. Detection of *Burkholderia pseudomallei* in patients with suppurative infections attending Yangon General Hospital and New Yangon General Hospital. *Myanmar Health Sci. Res. J.* **2013**, *25*, 114–119.
16. Leeuwenburgh, I.; Driessen, J.T.; van Keulen, P.H.; Stijnen, P.J.; Verburg, G.P. Melioidosis. *Nederlands Tijdschrift voor Geneeskunde* **2002**, *146*, 723–725. [PubMed]
17. Aung, M.K. Indigenous isolates of *Burkholderia pseudomallei*—The causative agent of melioidosis. *Myanmar J. Curr. Med. Pract.* **2004**, *9*, 13–15.
18. Win, M.M. A case of melioidosis from Yangon General Hospital. *Myanmar J. Curr. Med. Pract.* **2004**, *9*, 5–7.
19. Hlaing, S.S. Isolation of *Pseudomonas pseudomallei* (*Burkholderia pseudomallei*) from a case of tetanus in YGH. *Myanmar J. Curr. Med. Pract.* **2004**, *9*, 8–12.
20. Demar, M.; Ferroni, A.; Dupont, B.; Eliaszewicz, M.; Bouree, P. Suppurative epididymo-orchitis and chronic prostatitis caused by *Burkholderia pseudomallei*: A case report and review. *J. Travel Med.* **2005**, *12*, 108–112. [CrossRef] [PubMed]
21. Aung, M.K.; Mar, T.T. Re-emergence of melioidosis in Myanmar. *Transact. Royal Soc. Trop. Med. Hyg.* **2008**, *102*, S10–S11. [CrossRef]
22. Min, T.T. Characterization of *Burkholderia pseudomallei* Isolates from Melioidosis Cases in Magway Division, Myanmar. Ph.D. Thesis, University of Medicine 1, Yangon, Myanmar, 2012.

23. Chu, C.S.; Winearls, S.; Ling, C.; Torchinsky, M.B.; Phyo, A.P.; Haohankunnathum, W.; Turner, P.; Wuthiekanun, V.; Nosten, F. Two fatal cases of melioidosis on the Thai-Myanmar border. *F1000Research* **2014**, *3*, 4. [CrossRef] [PubMed]

24. Kyi, M.M.; Kyi, T.T.; Thit, S.S.; Aung, N.M. A forgotten disease of Myanmar origin. *Myanmar Med. J.* **2014**, *56*, 55–58.

25. Brummaier, T.; Ling, C.; Chu, C.S.; Wuthiekanun, V.; Haohankhunnatham, W.; McGready, R. Subcutaneous abscess formation in septic melioidosis, devoid of associated risk factors. *IDCases* **2016**, *4*, 23. [CrossRef] [PubMed]

26. Myat, T.O.; Prasad, N.; Thinn, K.K.; Win, K.K.; Htike, W.W.; Zin, K.N.; Murdoch, D.R.; Crump, J.A. Bloodstream infections at a tertiary referral hospital in Yangon, Myanmar. *Transact. R. Soc. Trop. Med. Hyg.* **2014**, *108*, 692–698. [CrossRef] [PubMed]

27. Wuthiekanun, V.; Langa, S.; Swaddiwudhipong, W.; Jedsadapanpong, W.; Kaengnet, Y.; Chierakul, W.; Day, N.P.; Peacock, S.J. Short report: Melioidosis in Myanmar: Forgotten but not gone? *Am. J. Trop. Med. Hyg.* **2006**, *75*, 945–946. [PubMed]

28. Pumpuang, A.; Dunachie, S.J.; Phokrai, P.; Jenjaroen, K.; Sintiprungrat, K.; Boonsilp, S.; Brett, P.J.; Burtnick, M.N.; Chantratita, N. Comparison of o-polysaccharide and hemolysin co-regulated protein as target antigens for serodiagnosis of melioidosis. *PLoS Negl. Trop. Dis.* **2017**, *11*, e0005499. [CrossRef] [PubMed]

29. Lubell, Y.; Mahidol-Oxford Research Unit, Bangkok, Thailand. Unpublished work. 2018.

30. Win, M.M.; Aung, W.W.; Thu, H.M.; Wah, T.T.; Aye, K.M.; Htwe, T.T.; Htay MT and San, K.K. The environmental study on melioidosis in agricultural farms of Thanlyin and Hmawbi Townships. In Proceedings of the 44th Myanmar Health Research Congress, Yangon, Myanmar, 5–9 January 2016.

31. Ministry of Health. *Health in Myanmar 2014*; Ministry of Health: Nay Pyi Taw, Myanmar, 2014.

32. Aye Aye Hlaing. Opium in Myanmar (1885–1948). Ph.D. Thesis, University of Mandalay, Mandalay, Myanmar, 2008.

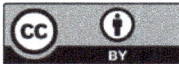

Tropical Medicine and
Infectious Disease

MDPI

Article

Melioidosis in Papua New Guinea and Oceania

Jeffrey M. Warner [1,2,*] and Bart J. Currie [3,4] (ORCID)

1   Australian Institute of Tropical Health and Medicine, James Cook University, Townsville 4811, Australia
2   College of Public Health, Medical and Veterinary Sciences, James Cook University,
    Townsville 4811, Australia
3   Global and Tropical Health Division, Menzies School of Health Research, Charles Darwin University,
    Darwin, NT 0815, Australia; Bart.currie@menzies.edu.au
4   Department of Infectious Diseases, Royal Darwin Hospital, Darwin, NT 0815, Australia
*   Correspondence: jeffrey.warner@jcu.edu.au; Tel.: +61-429474977

Received: 31 January 2018; Accepted: 6 March 2018; Published: 15 March 2018

Abstract: Melioidosis has only been sporadically reported throughout Melanesia and the Pacific region since the first report from Guam in 1946; therefore, its contribution to the disease burden in this region is largely unknown. However, the outcome of a small number of active surveillance programs, serological surveys, and presumptive imported cases identified elsewhere provide an insight into its epidemiology and potential significance throughout the region. Both clinical cases and environmental reservoirs have been described from the rural district of Balimo in the Western Province of Papua New Guinea and from the Northern Province of New Caledonia. In both these locations the incidence of disease is similar to that described in tropical Australia and *Burkholderia pseudomallei* isolates are also phylogenetically linked to Australian isolates. Serological evidence and presumptive imported cases identified elsewhere suggest that melioidosis exists in other countries throughout the Pacific. However, the lack of laboratory facilities and clinical awareness, and the burden of other infections of public health importance such as tuberculosis, contribute to the under-recognition of melioidosis in this region.

Keywords: Papua New Guinea; Oceania; melioidosis

1. History

The Western Pacific is home to the island communities of Oceania, including 15 countries within Melanesia, Micronesia, Polynesia, and Australasia (Figure 1). Each of these countries has diverse geography, demography, and socio-economic status. Melioidosis within Australasia will not be discussed in this review.

The first reported cases of melioidosis in Oceania outside Australasia were from two military personal stationed on Guam during World War II [1]. In Papua New Guinea (PNG), melioidosis seems sporadic. The first reports were from animals kept in a zoo in the urban capital of Port Moresby in 1963 [2–4]. The first human case from PNG was recorded in 1965 from a patient referred to Port Moresby General Hospital from Gemo Island, the then-leprosarium [5]. A case of melioidosis reported from Sydney was reported in a man with a history of World War II service in PNG [6]. Similarly, Kingston, a year later, reported from the same repatriation hospital a case of presumptive reactivation illness from an individual 24 years after World War II military service in Milne Bay, PNG [7]. In New Caledonia, *Burkholderia pseudomallei* was first isolated from soil as part of an animal health program in 1984 [8] and the first human case was reported in 1999 [9].

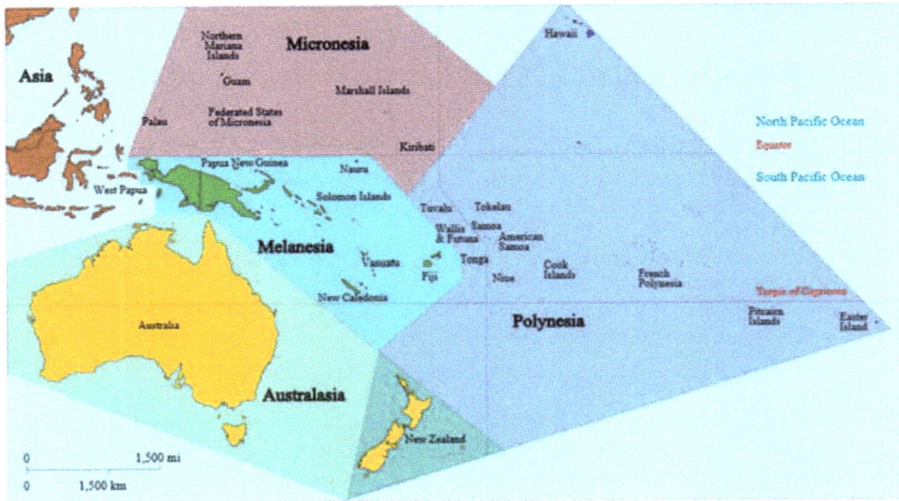

Figure 1. Map of Oceania based on the United Nations geoscheme M49 coding classification, devised by the United Nations Statistics Division.

2. Review of Confirmed Human Melioidosis Cases

2.1. Melioidosis Is Rare in PNG's Urban Capital

Since PNG independence in 1975, seven cases of culture-confirmed melioidosis have been reported from the PNG capital Port Moresby as a result of active case detection [10–13]. De Buse and colleagues reported a five-year-old boy presenting with pyrexia of unknown origin (PUO), who failed to respond to malaria treatment. Two from three blood cultures taken revealed *Staphylococcus aureus*. During exhaustive clinical work-up, *B. pseudomallei* along with *S. aureus* was recovered from a pus-filled nodule excised from the abdominal wall. Subcutaneous abscesses appeared which, upon culture, grew *B. pseudomallei*. Lee and Naraqi undertook a retrospective study in a review of Gram-negative pneumonia presenting in adults at Port Moresby General Hospital between February 1977 and May 1979. Of the 3500 adult in-patients during this time, 550 had been admitted with acute pneumonia. Of the 80 patients with Gram-negative bacteraemia, four were found to have primary pneumonia caused by *B. pseudomallei*. One of the cases was melioidosis pneumonia with left side consolidation and cavitation resembling pulmonary tuberculosis. The patient was a 36-year-old female who presented acutely ill with fever, cough, and pleuritic chest pain. She had a past history of tuberculosis but no other traditional co-morbidity factors were described.

Melioidosis was included in a prospective study of adult atypical pneumonia at Port Moresby General Hospital over a ten-month period, reported in 1991 [14]. Of the 175 adults admitted to the study, none revealed evidence of melioidosis using culture or indirect haemagglutination (IHA) serology. Currie described a report of melioidosis in PNG presenting in a 28-year-old highland man residing in Port Moresby with fulminating pneumonia [12]. The patient had a history of excessive alcohol consumption, smoking, and glucose intolerance; he died a day after admission.

Between 2000 and 2002, laboratory surveillance for *B. pseudomallei* at the Port Moresby General Hospital Pathology Department and at the Central Public Health Laboratory, Port Moresby, was undertaken. From 2285 blood cultures tested from patients at Port Moresby General Hospital, two (0.09%; 95% CI 0.01–0.32%) were positive for *B. pseudomallei*. In an attempt to determine the prevalence of melioidosis in the tuberculosis (TB) patient cohort in Port Moresby, 1309 sputum samples from 529 patients were selectively cultured for *B. pseudomallei*; only 1/1309 was positive for *B. pseudomallei* [13].

These studies confirm that melioidosis does exist in the urban capital but it is rare, despite the large and increasing population and increasing numbers with risk factors such as diabetes and hazardous alcohol use [15].

2.2. Melioidosis Hotspot: The Balimo Region of the Western Province, PNG

In contrast to the rare reports of melioidosis in Port Moresby, a focus of endemicity has been reported and studied in the remote Balimo region of the Western Province. Following an unpublished clinical report of melioidosis in this community in 1983 [16], two periods of active case detection were conducted as part of a broader development of microbiology facilities in the 1990s. Over an 18-month period this resulted in the diagnosis of eight culture-confirmed cases [17]. A feature of the disease in this region is childhood predilection with chronic presentation, which can mimic TB. Sero-epidemiology revealed a seroprevalence in some village communities as high as those in regions in northern Australia. In the environment, particularly sites that children frequent, *B. pseudomallei* was isolated (in 2.6% of 274 soil samples overall) [18]. Of 13 clinical and 26 environmental isolates analysed, only three multi-locus sequence type (MLST)-derived genotypes have been described—the most common being ST267, with the others (ST667 and ST668) differing from ST267 by only one SNP in the *ace* gene [19]. Further phylogenetic analysis shows the origins of these isolates to be in the Australian clade, yet some characteristics of the Asian isolates are also evident. It has therefore been proposed that the ancient land mass that joined Australia and New Guinea 20,000 years ago during the last ice age provided a land bridge, which may have facilitated movement of ancestral stains of *B. pseudomallei* from Australia to Asia via PNG [19].

Since the late 1990s, further cases of suspected melioidosis from Balimo District Hospital have been noted and some have been confirmed with culture of *B. pseudomallei*. However, the majority go unreported due to a downgrading of laboratory and clinical facilities over recent decades in Balimo as in many other rural locations in PNG. This includes no resident medical staff being present in Balimo and only sporadically-available bacteriological culture facilities. In this community the emergence of multidrug-resistant tuberculosis has also complicated the clinical diagnosis of melioidosis. Only when the diagnostic capacity for infectious diseases is improved will the true burden of melioidosis be realised and managed in this community.

2.3. Elsewhere in Oceania

Since the first description in Guam, melioidosis elsewhere in Oceania has been equally sporadic and reports are opportunistic. Several cases in Australia have been attributed to infection acquired in Fiji [20,21]. There is seroprevalence evidence from East Timor [22], but to date, no confirmed culture of *B. pseudomallei*. Only in New Caledonia has melioidosis been more thoroughly studied and reported.

Similar to in PNG, the first melioidosis studies in New Caledonia were conducted and reported by animal health workers [8]. The first human case was reported in 1999 [9]; since then, 19 melioidosis cases have been reported and studied [23–25]. As seems the case in PNG, melioidosis in New Caledonia is mostly restricted to one regional province, although whether there are biogeographic, demographic, or simply healthcare access factors at play can be only determined through a thorough and structured epidemiological and environmental study across the dispersed islands of that nation. As in Australia and other endemic regions, the most common presentation is community-acquired pneumonia, which may mimic TB, yet 32% presented with chronic disease including skin lesions.

As is the case in the Balimo region of PNG, there is evidence in New Caledonia of a persistent, dominant clonal strain as defined by MLST, with ST292 being the most common in the highly-endemic east coast region. All isolates analysed with MLST were shown to cluster—along with the other isolates from Melanesia—within the Australian clade rather than the Asian clade [25].

In recent years there has been a cluster of fatal melioidosis cases on the island of Yap, located in the Federated States of Micronesia (Figure 1) [26,27]. This is currently being investigated by the US Centers for Disease Control.

3. Current Recommendations and Availability of Measures against Melioidosis

The studies of melioidosis from isolated communities within this region highlight the difficulties in diagnosing and treating melioidosis without appropriate laboratory and clinical facilities. It is likely—as it almost certainly remains the case today in Balimo—that the disease carries very high mortality in such circumstances. In many of these communities, the gold-standard parenteral antibiotics meropenem and ceftazidime are not available. In these communities, cotrimoxazole or even chloramphenicol may be the only available antibiotics for therapy of suspected or confirmed melioidosis.

4. Awareness of Melioidosis, and Current and Future Challenges

Melioidosis is not a notifiable disease in any country in Oceania outside Australasia; as a result, the general awareness of the disease in this region is poor. With such limited data and such poor ability to obtain quality data, it is therefore unwise to generalise regarding the significance of melioidosis in Oceania. However, the evidence so far gathered and reported suggests that melioidosis is rare in urban centres, where microbiology facilities are able to detect the organism, but is likely to remain undiagnosed in some rural communities that lack the healthcare systems needed to identify it. With the development of an enhanced rural medical workforce plus laboratory facilities, perhaps including the introduction of non-culture-based detection methods that do not rely on extensive laboratory expertise, this may change. However, the burden of other diseases of public health importance such as multidrug-resistant TB, may yet overwhelm these developing health systems.

The spatial clustering of clinical melioidosis linked to parameters of the environmental reservoir, the diversity of the geography, and the limited ability to diagnose infection in this region, support the need for the establishment of a systematic remote sensing study to predict, identify, and locate regions that may harbour unrevealed melioidosis. Until these studies are conducted, melioidosis will remain an under-recognised, enigmatic condition, with high mortality rates.

Acknowledgments: The work described in this review is supported in part by the BHP Community Trust, James Cook University and the National Health and Medical Research Council (Project Grants 1098337 and 1131932 [the HOT NORTH initiative]).

Author Contributions: J.M.W. and B.J.C. wrote the paper.

Conflicts of Interest: The authors declare no conflict of interest.

References

1. Mirick, G.S.; Zimmerman, H.M.; Maner, G.D. Melioidosis on Guam. *JAMA* **1946**, *130*, 1063–1067. [CrossRef]
2. Egerton, J. Bovine melioidosis. *Aust. Vet. J.* **1963**, *40*, 34–35. [CrossRef]
3. Egerton, J.R. Melioidosis in a tree climbing kangaroo. *Aust. Vet. J.* **1963**, *39*, 243–244. [CrossRef]
4. Rampling, A. Porcine melioidosis in the territory of Papua New Guinea. *Aust. Vet. J.* **1964**, *40*, 241. [CrossRef]
5. Rowlands, J.B.; Curtis, P.G. A case of melioidosis in Papua and New Guinea. *Med. J. Aust.* **1965**, *2*, 494–496. [PubMed]
6. Newland, R.C. Chronic melioidosis: A case in Sydney. *Pathology* **1969**, *1*, 149–152. [CrossRef] [PubMed]
7. Kingston, C.W. Chronic or latent melioidosis. *Med. J. Aust.* **1971**, *2*, 618–621. [PubMed]
8. Domenech, J.; Lucet, P.; Desoutter, D.; Daynès, P.; Fortineau, O.; Colas, F.; Lechapt, M. An animal health survey. *Revue d'Elevage et de Médecine Vétérinaire de Nouvelle-Calédonie* **1984**, *2*, 1–8. (In French)
9. Poirier, N. Melioidosis: A Propos of a Clinical Case Observed in New Caledonia: Epidemiology, Clinical and Therapeutic Aspects. Ph.D. Thesis, Université de Rennes 1, Rennes, France, 2001.
10. De Buse, P.J.; Henderson, A.; White, M. Melioidosis in a child in Papua New Guinea: Successful treatment with kanamycin and trimethoprim-sulphamethoxazole. *Med. J. Aust.* **1975**, *2*, 476–478. [PubMed]
11. Lee, L.; Naraqi, S. Primary Gram-negative pneumonia in adults in Papua New Guinea. *PNG Med. J.* **1980**, *23*, 174–178.
12. Currie, B. Melioidosis in Papua New Guinea: Is it less common than in tropical Australia? *Trans. R. Soc. Trop. Med. Hyg.* **1993**, *87*, 417. [CrossRef]

13. Warner, J.M.; Pelowa, D.B.; Currie, B.J. Melioidosis—An uncommon but also under-recognized cause of pneumonia in Papua New Guinea. *PNG Med. J.* **2010**, *53*, 176–179.
14. Barnes, D.J.; Gottlieb, T.; Naraqi, S.; Benn, R. The role of viruses and atypical organisms in the pathogenesis of adult pneumonia in Papua New Guinea. *PNG Med. J.* **1991**, *34*, 13–16.
15. The National Statistical Office. *Final Figures–Papua New Guinea*; The National Statistical Office: Waigani, Papua New Guinea, November 2013. Available online: http://www.nso.gov.pg/index.php/document-library?view=download&fileId=65 (accessed on 1 March 2018).
16. Reece, A.S. *A Clinical Report: The Experience of the Balimo Health Centre with the Clinical Syndrome of Melioidosis, Including a Suggested Diagnostic, Therapeutic and Epidemiological Program*; Balimo Health Centre: Balimo, Papua New Guinea, 1984.
17. Warner, J.M.; Pelowa, D.B.; Currie, B.J.; Hirst, R.G. Melioidosis in a rural community of Western Province, Papua New Guinea. *Trans. R. Soc. Trop. Med. Hyg.* **2007**, *101*, 809–813. [CrossRef] [PubMed]
18. Warner, J.M.; Pelowa, D.B.; Gal, D.; Rai, G.; Mayo, M.; Currie, B.J.; Govan, B.; Skerratt, L.F.; Hirst, R.G. The epidemiology of melioidosis in the Balimo region of Papua New Guinea. *Epidemiol. Infect.* **2008**, *136*, 965–971. [CrossRef] [PubMed]
19. Baker, A.; Pearson, T.; Price, E.P.; Dale, J.; Keim, P.; Hornstra, H.; Greenhill, A.; Padilla, G.; Warner, J. Molecular phylogeny of *Burkholderia pseudomallei* from a remote region of Papua New Guinea. *PLoS ONE* **2011**, *6*, e18343. [CrossRef] [PubMed]
20. Corkill, M.M.; Cornere, B. Melioidosis: A new disease to New Zealand. *N. Z. Med. J.* **1987**, *100*, 106–107. [PubMed]
21. Currie, B.J. Menzies School of Health Research, Darwin, NT, Australia. Unpublished work. 2015.
22. Armstrong, P.K.; Anstey, N.M.; Kelly, P.M.; Currie, B.J.; Martins, N.; Dasari, P.; Krause, V. Seroprevalence of *Burkholderia pseudomallei* in East Timorese refugees: Implications for healthcare in East Timor. *Asian J. Trop. Med. Public Health* **2005**, *36*, 1496.
23. Le Hello, S.; Currie, B.J.; Godoy, D.; Spratt, B.G.; Mikulski, M.; Lacassin, F.; Garin, B. Melioidosis in New Caledonia. *Emerg. Infect. Dis.* **2005**, *11*, 1607–1609. [CrossRef] [PubMed]
24. Estivals, M.; du Couedic, L.; Lacassin, F.; Mermond, S.; Levenes, H. Septicemia, bilateral community-acquired pneumonia and empyema due to *Burkholderia pseudomallei* (melioidosis) with a favorable outcome following prolonged specific antibiotic therapy. *Rev. Mal. Respir.* **2008**, *25*, 319–322. [CrossRef]
25. Melot, B.; Colot, J.; Lacassin, F.; Tardieu, S.; Lapisardi, E.; Mayo, M.; Price, E.P.; Sarovinch, D.S.; Currie, B.J.; Goarant, C. Melioidosis in New Caledonia: A dominant strain in a transmission hotspot. *Epidemiol. Infect.* **2016**, *144*, 1330–1337. [CrossRef] [PubMed]
26. Melioidosis Disease Found in Yap Lab Test. Available online: http://www.mvariety.com/regional-news/62874-melioidosis-disease-found-in-yap-lab-test (accessed on 1 March 2018).
27. Yap-EpiNet-8 Feb 2014. Available online: https://www.facebook.com/Yap-Epi-Net-388433107955645/?hc_ref=ARRW79jS3cmeVtRnWmOoRhhoJ5PsLRvS5efkHJfMn93WMtYYLz39U7t_99JBAVohElw&fref=nf (accessed on 1 March 2018).

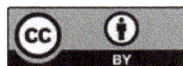

Tropical Medicine and Infectious Disease

MDPI

Article

Melioidosis in the Philippines

Peter Franz M. San Martin [1,*] [ID] , **Joseph C. Chua** [1] , **Ralph Louie P. Bautista** [1] , **Jennifer M. Nailes** [2] ,
Mario M. Panaligan [3] **and David A. B. Dance** [4,5,6] [ID]

[1]   Department of Physiology, College of Medicine, University of the East—Ramon Magsaysay Memorial
     Medical Center Inc., Aurora Boulevard, Quezon City 1113, Philippines; joseph_c_chua@yahoo.com (J.C.C.);
     rlpbautista@gmail.com (R.L.P.B.)
[2]   Department of Preventive and Community Medicine, College of Medicine, University of the
     East—Ramon Magsaysay Memorial Medical Center Inc., Aurora Boulevard, Quezon City 1113, Philippines;
     jmnailes@uerm.edu.ph
[3]   Department of Medicine, College of Medicine, University of the East—Ramon Magsaysay Memorial
     Medical Center Inc., Aurora Boulevard, Quezon City 1113, Philippines; mmpanaligan@gmail.com
[4]   Lao-Oxford-Mahosot Hospital-Wellcome Trust Research Unit, Microbiology Laboratory, Mahosot Hospital,
     Vientiane, Laos; David.d@tropmedres.ac
[5]   Centre for Tropical Medicine and Global Health, Nuffield Department of Clinical Medicine,
     Old Road Campus, University of Oxford, Oxford OX3 7FZ, UK
[6]   Faculty of Infectious and Tropical Diseases, London School of Hygiene and Tropical Medicine,
     London WC1E 7HT, UK
*   Correspondence: petersanmartinmd@gmail.com; Tel.: +63-2-715-0861

Received: 11 August 2018; Accepted: 3 September 2018; Published: 5 September 2018

Abstract: The first documented case of melioidosis in the Philippines occurred in 1948. Since then, there have been sporadic reports in the literature about travelers diagnosed with melioidosis after returning from the Philippines. Indigenous cases, however, have been documented rarely, and under-reporting is highly likely. This review collated all Philippine cases of melioidosis published internationally and locally, as well as unpublished case series and reports from different tertiary hospitals in the Philippines. In total, 25 papers and 41 cases were identified. Among these, 23 were indigenous cases (of which 20 have not been previously reported in the literature). The most common co-morbidity present was diabetes mellitus, and the most common presentations were pulmonary and soft tissue infections. Most of the cases received ceftazidime during the intensive phase, while trimethoprim-sulfamethoxazole was given during the eradication phase. The known mortality rate was 14.6%, while 4.9% of all cases were reported to have had recurrence. The true burden of melioidosis in the country is not well defined. A lack of awareness among clinicians, a dearth of adequate laboratories, and the absence of a surveillance system for the disease are major challenges in determining the magnitude of the problem.

Keywords: melioidosis; Philippines; *Burkholderia pseudomallei*

---

1. Introduction and History of Melioidosis in the Philippines

Melioidosis, or Whitmore's disease, is a potentially lethal infection caused by the Gram-negative bacterium *Burkholderia pseudomallei*. Its clinical presentation is so diverse that the diagnosis relies heavily on laboratory culture.

During the past few decades, melioidosis has emerged as an important public health concern, especially in the South East Asian (SEA) region and northern Australia [1]. The increase in global interest in the disease was a consequence of the rising number of reported cases, both within endemic areas and among travelers, the occurrence of cases in areas not previously known to be endemic; and also, its potential use as an agent of bioterrorism.

After the disease was first described by Alfred Whitmore and C.S. Krishnaswami in 1912 [1–3], initially the majority of cases reported were from the SEA region. Reviews of the global distribution of the disease showed that cases have been found in the tropical and subtropical regions, mainly between 20° north and 20° south of the equator—which includes the Philippines [2,4]. A recent modelling study suggested that there could be as many as 9000 cases and 4500 deaths, due to melioidosis occurring in the Philippines each year [5]. Certainly, nowhere near that number are being diagnosed, so how likely is this to be true?

The first documented case of human melioidosis in the Philippines occurred in 1948 in a 25-year-old American soldier who presented with weight loss and symptoms of pneumonia. Diagnosis was established through guinea pig inoculation of sputum and lymph node pus [6]. This was not long after the disease had first been recognized in countries like Vietnam [7] and Indonesia [8], and before the first indigenous case was described in Thailand [9]. However, in contrast to other SEA countries, there has been little development with regards to defining the epidemiology of the disease in the Philippines. A further case in an American soldier was reported in 1957, although his illness had started many years earlier, while he was stationed in the Philippines [10]. Sporadic cases were reported thereafter in people who had either transited or stayed in the country. Some of these individuals also had a history of travel to other parts of SEA, hence the evidence that the infection was acquired in the Philippines was inconclusive [2]. However, in others, such as the first case diagnosed in Taiwan in 1985, there was strong circumstantial evidence that infection was acquired in the Philippines during a near-drowning incident in a river near Manila [11].

Cases have not been limited to humans: For example, an isolate from a horse from the Philippines was included in a taxonomic study published in 1956, although no further clinical details are available about this case [12]. Then in 1992, a number of primates imported from the Philippines to the United Kingdom were involved in an outbreak of melioidosis [13]. However, there have been no other cases among animals from the Philippines reported in the literature thereafter.

Indigenous cases, meaning those with no apparent travel history to other endemic areas, and who were diagnosed and treated in the Philippines, had never been reported in the literature until 2002, when a 49-year-old farmer from Bulacan in the Philippines presented with pain and swelling of the left shoulder and was found to have melioidosis after *Burkholderia pseudomallei* was isolated from blood [14]. The second indigenous case, and the first case published in an international journal, was reported as recently as 2016 [15]. The patient was a farmer from Isabela with no history of travel outside the country, who was diagnosed and treated in a hospital in Metro Manila.

The preponderance of reports of melioidosis among travelers from the Philippines, and the paucity of indigenous cases, leads us to suspect that the disease is being grossly under-reported in the country. This article describes the evidence for, and distribution of, melioidosis in the Philippines by reviewing reports published in international and local publications and unpublished case reports that were obtained from tertiary hospitals and local subspecialty organizations. These cases were examined to determine common patient profiles, disease presentations, modes of diagnosis, treatment received, and outcomes.

2. Materials and Methods

2.1. Review of Publications

Published reports citing cases of culture-confirmed melioidosis from the Philippines were collected. The melioidosis website (www.melioidosis.info) served as the main starting point for the search, as it already contains a database of published case reports by country. In addition, PubMed and Google Scholar were searched, using various combinations of keywords (and MESH terms, where applicable) such as Philippines, Filipino, Southeast Asia, melioidosis, Whitmore's disease, *Burkholderia pseudomallei*, and *Pseudomonas pseudomallei*. The bibliography of each reference was searched for further cases. Finally, the personal EndNote database of one of us (DABD) was searched for references that had been missed. From each reference, relevant information about each case was extracted, such as age, sex, co-morbidities, risk factors, type of infection, mode of diagnosis, treatment received, outcome, country where diagnosed, and year of diagnosis.

2.2. Collection of Locally Published and Unpublished Cases from the Philippines

Local medical journals and university papers available in the National Library of the Philippines, different universities, and hospitals were searched for any mention of local cases of melioidosis. Inquiries regarding cases of melioidosis were made to the Philippine Society for Microbiology and Infectious Diseases, the Research Institute for Tropical Medicine, and other medical centers. Consent to use the data was obtained from the authors of unpublished case series and reports that were collected.

3. Results and Discussion

A total of 25 articles, either single case reports or case series, describing culture-confirmed melioidosis in the Philippines were collected (Tables 1 and 2). Of these 25 papers, only 11 were listed in the melioidosis.org database—although those not included had either been published or presented at international conferences recently (between 2015 and 2017). This also included four unpublished local reports which were obtained from different tertiary hospitals in Metro Manila. Only one of these reports related to a case of melioidosis in an animal [13].

A total of 41 human cases was included in these articles, with 18 cases involving travelers and 23 indigenous cases. Among the indigenous cases, 20 were from the four previously unpublished reports. Of these four unpublished papers, two were case series derived from a 3- to 5-year chart review of patients that were culture-positive for *B. pseudomallei* from their respective institution, and the other two were single case reports. Diagnosis was established via culture-based technique and VITEK among indigenous cases. No additional molecular confirmatory tests were performed for these specimens.

The patients were between the ages of 21 and 82 years, with a mean of 50.2 years (Table 3). The patients were predominantly (85.4%) male. This is consistent with the epidemiologic data from some other endemic areas [16–18]. Data on risk factors were limited, but only six patients were known to be working in the agricultural sector. Geographical data were available for 20 indigenous cases, where 11 were from areas with moderate to high rice production in the Philippines (Isabela, Pampanga, and Bulacan). Figure 1 shows the geographical distribution of the reported cases in the Philippines, and annual rice production per province. Although the number of cases in Metro Manila is inconsistent with the expected high incidence of melioidosis among rice farmers, the authors suspected that these patients had previous exposure to agricultural areas. In addition, the proximity and access to diagnostic facility could have caused the relatively higher proportion of cases in Manila. All the indigenous cases were diagnosed in tertiary hospitals in Metro Manila, which generally have better-equipped laboratory and diagnostic facilities than most provincial hospitals, and it is likely that many patients are going undiagnosed outside the city.

Table 1. Clinical characteristics of culture confirmed cases of melioidosis in the Philippines from published case reports.

Year Published	Age	Sex	Place Diagnosed	Co-Morbidities/Risk Factors	Melioidosis Type	Method of Diagnosis	Antibiotics	Outcome	Reference
1948	25	M	No data	No data	Pulmonary	Sputum culture (guinea pig inoculation)	No data	No data	Gutner and Fisher [6]
1957	32	M	USA	No data	Cutaneous/soft tissue	Sputum culture (guinea pig inoculation); tissue (rib and femoral mass) culture	PEN, SD, STR, CLI, CHL	Recurrent	Prevatt and Hunt [10]
1975	54	M	USA	Lung carcinoma	Pulmonary	Sputum and bronchial washing cultures	TET, CHL	Died	Mays and Ricketts [19]
1976	21	M	USA	None	Pulmonary	Sputum culture	PEN, KAN, SXT	Improved	John [20]
1978	23	M	USA	None	Pulmonary	Sputum culture	TET, CHL, KAN, SXT	Improved	Fuller et al. [21]
1985	46	F	Taiwan	Drowning	Pulmonary	Blood culture	CEF, AMK	Improved	Lee et al. [11]
1994	40	M	Canada	Diabetes mellitus	Pulmonary	Sputum culture	CAZ	Improved	Turner et al. [22]
2002	49	M	Philippines	Diabetes mellitus	Disseminated (joint, pulmonary)	Blood culture	IPM, AMC, SXT	Improved	Ereno et al. [14]
2008	64	M	USA	Diabetes mellitus, coronary artery disease, hypertension	Pulmonary, osteomyelitis	Paraspinal abscess culture, PCR, isolate sent to CDC for confirmation	MEM, SXT	Improved	Falade et al. [23]
2009	61	M	USA	Metabolic syndrome	Pulmonary	Blood culture and pleural fluid culture, PCR	IMP, TGC, SXT, DOX	Improved	Duplessis and Maguire [24]
2010	45	F	Philippines	Diabetes mellitus	Pulmonary	Blood culture	TZP, CLI, AZM	Died	Velasco et al. [25]
2011	50	M	Brunei	Diabetes mellitus	Liver, spleen, cellulitis	Blood culture	No Data	Improved	Pande et al. [26][1]
2011	41	M	Brunei	Diabetes mellitus	Cellulitis, pulmonary, liver	Blood culture	No Data	Improved	Pande et al. [26][1]
2014	62	M	Canada	Diabetes mellitus, Sjogren syndrome, chronic kidney disease, Stevens-Johnson syndrome secondary to amoxicillin, schistosomiasis, warm autoimmune hemolytic anemia	Musculoskeletal	Blood culture and PCR	LVX, MET, DOX, SXT	Improved	Chagla et al. [27]
2015	60	M	South Korea	None	Pulmonary	Tissue (lung) and sputum culture	No data	Improved	Kim et al. [28]

Table 1. *Cont.*

Year Published	Age	Sex	Place Diagnosed	Co-Morbidities/Risk Factors	Melioidosis Type	Method of Diagnosis	Antibiotics	Outcome	Reference
2015	68	M	USA	Diabetes mellitus, coronary artery disease, hypertension, paroxysmal SVT	Splenic	Splenic abscess culture	CAZ, DOX, SXT	Improved	Guo et al. [29]
2016	44	M	Philippines	Diabetes mellitus	Hepatic	Liver abscess culture	MEM, SXT	Improved	San Martin et al. [15]
2016	67	F	USA	Diabetes mellitus, cardiovascular disease, tuberculosis	Mycotic aneurysm	Blood culture, PCR, isolate sent to CDC for confirmation	MEM, SXT	Died	Hemarajata et al. [30]
2017	60	M	USA	Diabetes mellitus, hypertension, dyslipidemia	Fever, loss of appetite, myalgia, weight loss	Blood culture, isolate sent to CDC for confirmation	CAZ, SXT	Improved	Singh and Mahmood [31]
2017	82	M	USA	Hypertension, hyperlipidemia, osteoarthritis	Mycotic aneurysm	Blood culture	CAZ	Improved	Panginnikod et al. [32]
2018	41	M	Japan	Unknown	Pulmonary, septic arthritis (soft tissue)	Blood culture	DOR	Died	Hadano et al. [33]

AMC = amoxicillin-clavulanic acid; AMK = amikacin; AZM = azithromycin; CAZ = ceftazidime; CEF = cephalothin; CHL = chloramphenicol; CLI = clindamycin; CLR = clarithromycin; CLT = chlortetracycline; DOX = doxycycline; DOR = doripenem; FEP = cefepime; IPM = imipenem; KAN = kanamycin; LVX = levofloxacin; MEM = meropenem; MET = metronidazole; PEN = penicillin; SD = sulfadizine; SXT = trimethoprim-sulfamethoxazole; TGC = tigecycline; TZP = piperacillin-tazobactam; CIP = ciprofloxacin. [1] These were Filipino cases diagnosed in Brunei. The infection could have been either be acquired from the Philippines or during their stay in Brunei.

Table 2. Clinical characteristics of confirmed cases of melioidosis in the Philippines from unpublished case reports and series.

Year Diagnosed	Age	Sex	Co-Morbidities/Risk Factors	Melioidosis Type	Culture Specimen	Antibiotics	Outcome	Reference
2010	54	M	Diabetes mellitus	Pulmonary	Sputum	TZP, CLR	Improved	Masbang [34]
2010	62	M	Diabetes mellitus, cardiovascular disease	Disseminated (cutaneous/soft tissue, pulmonary)	Blood	CAZ, SXT	Improved	Masbang [34]
2010	55	M	Heavy alcohol consumption	Pulmonary, neurologic	Bronchial washing	MEM, CAZ, SXT	Improved	Masbang [34]
2011	66	M	Squamous cell lung carcinoma, hypertension, heavy smoker	Pulmonary	Sputum	MEM, AMC	Improved	Masbang [34]

Table 2. *Cont.*

Year Diagnosed	Age	Sex	Co-Morbidities/Risk Factors	Melioidosis Type	Culture Specimen	Antibiotics	Outcome	Reference
2011	54	F	Diabetes mellitus, hypertension	Pulmonary	Blood	FEP	Improved	Masbang [34]
2012	60	M	Hypertension	Pulmonary	Sputum	MEM, SXT	Improved	Masbang [34]
2013	45	M	Diabetes mellitus	Neurologic	Sputum	MEM, CAZ, DOX	Improved	Masbang [34]
2014	57	F	Lung adenocarcinoma, hypertension	Pulmonary	Blood	CAZ, LVX	Died	Masbang [34]
2014	38	F	Breast cancer	Pulmonary	Endotracheal aspirate	CAZ	Died	Masbang [34]
2014	64	M	Hypertension	Cutaneous/soft tissue	Abscess	CAZ	No data	Masbang [34]
2014	47	M	Cardiovascular disease	Pulmonary	Sputum	CAZ	No data	Masbang [34]
2014	59	M	Pulmonary tuberculosis	Pulmonary, cutaneous/soft tissue	Blood, sputum, and wound swab	FEP, CLI, MEM, SXT, TB antibiotics (Isoniazid, Rifampicin, Ethambutol, Pyrazinamide)	Improved	Ocampo [35]
2013	40	M	Diabetes mellitus, poultry worker	Disseminated (soft tissue, liver, intra-abdominal infection)	Abscess	CAZ, SXT, DOX	Improved	Yap et al. [36]
2009	34	M	Diabetes mellitus	Pulmonary	Blood	CAZ, SXT	Improved	Santos [37]
2008	36	M	Diabetes mellitus	Hepatic	Abscess	CAZ, SXT	Improved	Santos [37]
2012	59	M	Diabetes mellitus	Disseminated (cutaneous, joint, pulmonary)	Synovial fluid, wound swab	CAZ, SXT, DOX	Improved	Santos [37]
2009, 2012	44	M	Diabetes mellitus	Soft tissue (parotid), neurologic (chronic and recurrent)	Abscess	2009: CAZ, CIP; 2012: CAZ DOX, CHL [1]	Recurrent	Santos [37]
2009	50	M	Diabetes mellitus, hypertension, coronary artery disease	Pulmonary	Pleural fluid	CAZ, SXT, DOX	Improved	Santos [37]
2011	43	M	Diabetes mellitus, hypertension	Neurologic	Frontal cortex abscess	CAZ, SXT	Improved	Santos [37]
2009	58	M	Diabetes mellitus, hypertension	Urinary tract, CKD	Urine	CAZ, SXT	Improved	Santos [37]

AMC = amoxicillin-clavulanic acid; AMK = amikacin; AZM = azithromycin; CAZ = ceftazidime; CEF = cephalothin; CHL = chloramphenicol; CLI = clindamycin; CLR = clarithromycin; CLT = chlortetracycline; DOR = doripenem; DOX = doxycycline; FEP = cefepime; IPM = imipenem; KAN = kanamycin; LVX = levofloxacin; MEM = meropenem; MET = metronidazole; PEN = penicillin; SD = sulfadizine; SXT = trimethoprim-sulfamethoxazole; TGC = tigecycline; TZP = piperacillin-tazobactam; CIP = ciprofloxacin. [1] Case readmitted after three years, due to recurrence of melioidosis.

Table 3. Summary of clinical characteristics of culture-confirmed cases of melioidosis in the Philippines.

Clinical Characteristics	Number of Cases
Mean Age	50.2
Sex	
Male	35 (85.4%)
Female	6 (14.6%)
Comorbidities	
Diabetes mellitus	24 (58.5%)
Cardiovascular disease	11 (26.82%)
Cancer	4 (9.76%)
Pulmonary tuberculosis	2 (4.9%)
Chronic kidney disease	1 (2.4%)
Drowning	1 (2.4%)
Heavy alcohol consumption	1 (2.4%)
Hyperlipidemia	1 (2.4%)
Osteoarthritis	1 (2.4%)
Organs involved	
Pulmonary	22 (53.7%)
Soft tissue	12 (29.3%)
Hepatic	5 (12.2%)
Neurologic	4 (9.76%)
Splenic	2 (4.9%)
Mycotic aneurysm	2 (4.9%)
Osteomyelitis	1 (2.4%)
Positive cultures	
Blood	17 (41.5%)
Respiratory (sputum)	16 (39.0%)
Abscess pus	7 (17.1%)
Wound swab/Tissue	3 (7.3%)
Synovial fluid	1 (2.4%)
Outcome	
Improved	22 (53.7%)
Relapsed	2 (4.9%)
Died	6 (14.6%)
No Data	5 (12.2%)

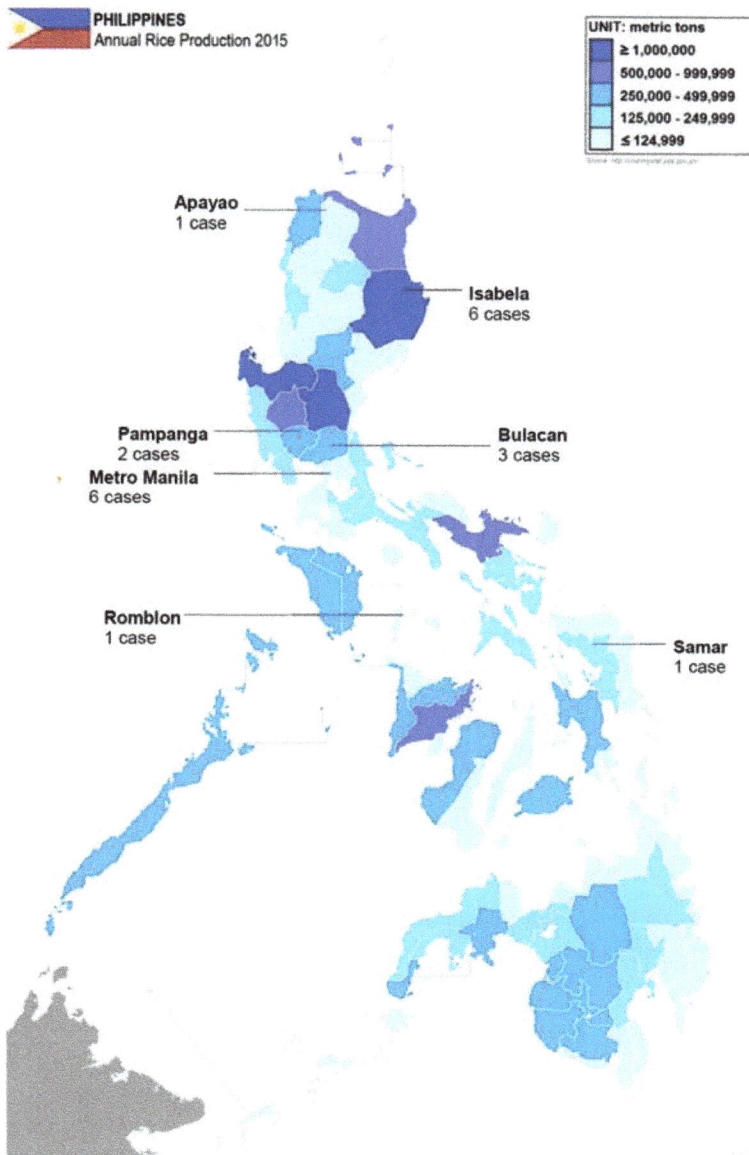

Figure 1. Distribution of indigenous cases of melioidosis in the Philippines (reported from 2002 to 2016) and the amount of rice production per province. Original image imported from: https://commons. wikimedia.org/wiki/File:Philippine_provinces_Annual_Rice_Production_2015.png.

The most common co-morbidity was diabetes mellitus, comprising 58.5% of cases, followed by cardiovascular disease (which includes hypertension and coronary artery disease) at 26.82%. Diabetes mellitus is the most common co-morbidity and risk factor found in the literature [16,38,39].

With the steadily increasing prevalence of type 2 diabetes in the Philippines [40], it is likely that the incidence of melioidosis will increase correspondingly.

Pneumonia and soft tissue infection were present in 53.7% and 29.3% of cases respectively, which again is consistent with the melioidosis literature from elsewhere [17]. Pulmonary diseases, particularly pneumonia, chronic lower respiratory tract diseases, and tuberculosis, are among the top 10 causes of mortality in the Philippines [41]. Since melioidosis may be difficult to differentiate from other respiratory diseases, it is possible that many cases labelled simply as 'pneumonia' or other respiratory infections may actually have melioidosis. A high index of suspicion, and good laboratory support, are necessary to make a specific diagnosis of melioidosis. Furthermore, co-infection with *B. pseudomallei* and *Mycobacterium tuberculosis* was seen in two patients in this review, which presents a further diagnostic and therapeutic challenge to clinicians. Other than pulmonary cases, four neurological cases were reported among indigenous cases. Although, conclusions could not be drawn, due to limited number of cases, this should be subject for further investigation if this type of melioidosis occur more frequently in the country.

All cases were diagnosed by culture studies. Bacteremia was found in 41.5% of cases. The most common antibiotic used were ceftazidime and trimethoprim-sulfamethoxazole for the intensive phase and eradication phase, respectively. Most of the cases received the recommended antibiotic treatment for melioidosis [42] such as ceftazidime (43.59%), meropenem (12.82%), trimethoprim-sulfamethoxazole (53.84%), and amoxicillin-clavulanic acid (5.13%). Those treated with different antibiotics were cases diagnosed earlier than 1990s, and those indigenous cases which followed the result of the antibiotic sensitivity test. The reported recurrence rate among all cases were 4.9%, while the mortality rate was 12.6%. This, however, could be an underestimate due to lack of data and follow-up.

Failure to consider melioidosis, which requires specific treatment, may be contributing to the continued high mortality from pulmonary diseases in the Philippines. Local clinical guidelines do not include ceftazidime and meropenem as empiric treatment unless classified as high-risk community-acquired pneumonia, healthcare-associated pneumonia, or those at risk for multidrug-resistant organisms.

4. Challenges

The greatest challenges for the Philippines are to raise awareness of melioidosis amongst clinicians and laboratory staff, and to improve the availability of facilities capable of making a laboratory diagnosis of the disease. During our enquiries with colleagues and local institutions about case reports, many of those who responded admitted to being unfamiliar with melioidosis. Also, melioidosis is rarely included in the curriculum of medical schools within the Philippines. It is notable that the majority of the earlier cases in this series were diagnosed in travelers to other countries, albeit only 21 cases occurring over 70 years, implying considerable under-diagnosis of indigenous cases. However, there are some encouraging signs, particularly, the fact that four unpublished reports, comprising 20 indigenous cases seen over a relatively short span of seven years, were identified. This suggests an increasing awareness of the disease among physicians, resulting in improved diagnosis and reporting. However, these were all diagnosed in Metro Manila, which is unlikely to be the area of highest incidence in a country where the environment is predicted to be widely suitable for *B. pseudomallei* [5], and the incidence of melioidosis in more rural areas requires further investigation. Areas such as those in Mindanao, which are a highly rural area, post additional challenge since access to health care facilities is another existing issue. However, this will require the strengthening of medical laboratories in these areas, and education of staff in how to detect and identify *B. pseudomallei*.

Although the most common presentation of *B. pseudomallei* infection is pneumonia, the 2016 community-acquired pneumonia (CAP) guidelines in the Philippines do not even mention melioidosis as a differential diagnosis. There is no national surveillance system for melioidosis, nor is the disease included in the list of notifiable disease in the Philippines [43].

5. Conclusions and Recommendations

This report highlights the fact that melioidosis is indeed endemic in the Philippines but is likely to be grossly under-reported. The clinical and epidemiological characteristics of the disease in the Philippines, albeit based on limited data, are consistent with those described in published literature from other countries. Furthermore, the data show that this condition has been successfully diagnosed and treated in the country with increasing frequency over the past few years.

Further studies should be done on the extent and impact of this disease within the country. It is recommended that a program of education of clinicians and laboratory staff about melioidosis should be initiated, ideally starting at medical schools, and especially targeted at rural areas that are likely to have the highest incidence of melioidosis. Furthermore, consideration should be given to making the disease statutorily notifiable. This would provide more accurate information about the clinical characteristics and distribution of the disease within the Philippines. Soil sampling studies should also be undertaken in order to establish the geographic distribution of this microorganism, as well as enable analysis of the population structure. Genotyping of bacterial isolates are in progress in order to determine if indigenous strains were different than those identified elsewhere in Southeast Asia or Australia. Studies should also be undertaken to describe the current knowledge and attitudes of Filipino clinicians regarding melioidosis.

Author Contributions: Conceptualization, P.F.M.S.M. and D.A.B.D.; Data Curation, P.F.M.S.M. and J.C.C.; Methodology, P.F.M.S.M., J.C.C., R.L.P.B.; Investigation, P.F.M.S.M., J.C.C., R.L.P.B.; Resources, J.M.N. and M.M.P.; Supervision: D.A.B.D. and M.M.P.; Visualization: J.C.C., R.L.P.B.; Project administration, P.F.M.S.M. and J.M.N.; Writing original draft, P.F.M.S.M., J.C.C., R.L.P.B.; Writing review and editing, P.F.M.S.M., D.A.B.D., M.M.P.

Funding: This research received no external funding.

Acknowledgments: Authors would like to extend their sincerest gratitude to Armin Masbang, Lisette Ocampo, Suzanne Santos, and Emily Yap for sharing their unpublished case reports and case series.

Conflicts of Interest: The authors declare no conflict of interest.

References

1. Cheng, A.C.; Currie, B.J. Melioidosis: Epidemiology, pathophysiology, and management. *Clin. Microbiol. Rev.* **2005**, *18*, 383–416. [CrossRef] [PubMed]
2. Dance, D.A. Melioidosis: The tip of the iceberg? *Clin. Microbiol. Rev.* **1991**, *4*, 52–60. [CrossRef] [PubMed]
3. Whitmore, A. An account of a glanders-like disease occurring in Rangoon. *J. Hyg.* **1913**, *13*, 1–34. [CrossRef] [PubMed]
4. Smith, C.J.; Allen, J.C.; Embi, M.N.; Othman, O.; Razak, N.; Ismail, G. Human melioidosis: An emerging medical problem. *MIRCEN J.* **1987**, *3*. [CrossRef]
5. Limmathurotsakul, D.; Golding, N.; Dance, D.A.B.; Messina, J.P.; Pigott, D.M.; Moyes, C.L.; Rolim, D.B.; Bertherat, E.; Day, N.P.; Peacock, S.J.; et al. Predicted global distribution of *Burkholderi pseudomallei* and burden of melioidosis. *Nat. Microbiol.* **2016**, *1*. [CrossRef] [PubMed]
6. Gutner, L.B.; Fisher, M.W. Chronic melioidosis: Discussion, case report, and special studies. *Ann. Intern. Med.* **1948**, *28*, 1157–1169. [CrossRef]
7. Pons, R.; Advier, M. Melioidosis in Cochin China. *J. Hyg.* **1927**, *26*, 28–30. [CrossRef] [PubMed]
8. De Moor, C.E.; Soekarnen Walle, N. Melioidosis op Java. *Mededeeling uit het Geneeskundig Laboratorium te Weltevreden* **1932**, *72*, 1618–1635.
9. Chittivej, C.; Buspavanich, S.; Chaovanasai, A. Melioidosis with case report in a Thai. *R. Thai Army Med. J.* **1955**, *68*, 11–17.
10. Prevatt, A.L.; Hunt, J.S. Chronic systemic melioidosis. *Am. J. Med. Sci.* **1957**, *23*, 810–823. [CrossRef]
11. Lee, N.; Wu, J.L.; Lee, C.H.; Tsai, W.C. *Pseudomonas pseudomallei* infection from drowning: The first reported case in Taiwan. *J. Clin. Microbiol.* **1985**, *22*, 352–354. [PubMed]
12. Wetmore, P.W.; Gochenour, W.S. Comparative studies of the genus *Malleomyces* and selected *Pseudomonas* species. *J. Bacteriol.* **1956**, *72*, 79–89. [PubMed]

13. Dance, D.A.; King, C.; Aucken, H.; Knott, C.D.; West, P.G.; Pitt, T.L. An outbreak of melioidosis in imported primates in Britain. *Vet. Rec.* **1992**, *130*, 525–529. [CrossRef] [PubMed]

14. Ereno, I.L.; Mariano, N.; Reyes, J.; Amando, C. Melioidosis: A case report. *Philipp. J. Microbiol. Infect. Dis.* **2002**, *31*, 125–133.

15. Martin, P.F.M.S.; Teh, C.S.C.; Casupang, M.A.J. Melioidosis: A rare cause of liver abscess. *Case Rep. Hepatol.* **2016**, *2016*. [CrossRef] [PubMed]

16. Kingsley, P.V.; Leader, M.; Nagodawithana, N.S.; Tipre, M.; Sathiakumar, N. Melioidosis in Malaysia: A review of case reports. *PLoS Negl. Trop. Dis.* **2016**, *10*, e0005182. [CrossRef] [PubMed]

17. Meumann, E.M.; Cheng, A.C.; Ward, L.; Currie, B.J. Clinical features and epidemiology of melioidosis pneumonia: Results from a 21-year study and review of the literature. *Clin. Infect. Dis.* **2012**, *54*, 362–369. [CrossRef] [PubMed]

18. Churuangsuk, C.; Chusri, S.; Hortiwakul, T.; Charernmak, B.; Silpapojakul, K. Characteristics, clinical outcomes and factors influencing mortality of patients with melioidosis in southern Thailand: A 10-year retrospective study. *Asian Pac. J. Trop. Med.* **2016**, *9*, 256–260. [CrossRef] [PubMed]

19. Mays, E.E.; Ricketts, E.A. Melioidosis: Recrudescence associated with bronchogenic carcinoma twenty-six years following initial geographic exposure. *Chest* **1975**, *68*, 261–263. [CrossRef] [PubMed]

20. John, J.F., Jr. Trimethoprim-sulfamethoxazole therapy of pulmonary melioidosis. *Am. Rev. Respir. Dis.* **1976**, *114*, 1021–1025. [CrossRef] [PubMed]

21. Fuller, P.B.; Fisk, D.E.; Byrd, R.B.; Griggs, G.A.; Smith, M.R. Treatment of pulmonary melioidosis with combination of trimethoprim and sulfamethoxazole. *Chest* **1978**, *74*, 222–224. [CrossRef] [PubMed]

22. Turner, M.O.; Lee, V.T.; FitzGerald, J.M. Melioidosis in a diabetic sailor. *Chest* **1994**, *106*, 952–954. [CrossRef] [PubMed]

23. Falade, O.O.; Antonarakis, E.S.; Kaul, D.R.; Saint, S.; Murphy, P.A. Clinical problem-solving. Beware of first impressions. *N. Engl. J. Med.* **2008**, *359*, 628–634. [CrossRef] [PubMed]

24. Duplessis, C.; Maguire, J.D. Melioidosis masquerading as community-acquired pneumonia: A case report demonstrating efficacy of intrapleural fibrinolytic therapy. *J. Travel. Med.* **2009**, *16*, 74–77. [CrossRef] [PubMed]

25. Velasco, A.B.; Untalan, C.A.; Visperas, J.C. Melioiodisis presenting as severe community acquired pneumonia. *Am. J. Respir. Crit. Care* **2010**, *181*. [CrossRef]

26. Pande, K.C.; Kadir, K.A. Melioidosis of the extremities in Brunei Darussalam. *Singap. Med. J.* **2011**, *52*, 346–350.

27. Chagla, Z.; Aleksova, N.; Quirt, J.; Emery, J.; Kraeker, C.; Haider, S. Melioidosis in a returned traveller. *Can. J. Infect. Dis. Med. Microbiol.* **2014**, *25*, 225–226. [CrossRef] [PubMed]

28. Kim, S.W.; Kwon, G.-Y.; Kim, B.; Kwon, D.; Shin, J.; Bae, G.-R. Imported melioidosis in South Korea: A case series with a literature review. *Osong Public Health Res. Perspect.* **2015**, *6*, 363–368. [CrossRef] [PubMed]

29. Guo, R.F.; Wong, F.L.; Perez, M.L. Splenic abscesses in a returning traveler. *Infect. Dis. Rep.* **2015**, *7*. [CrossRef] [PubMed]

30. Hemarajata, P.; Baghdadi, J.D.; Hoffman, R.; Humphries, R.M. *Burkholderia pseudomallei*: Challenges for the clinical microbiology laboratory. *J. Clin. Microbiol.* **2016**, *54*, 2866–2873. [CrossRef] [PubMed]

31. Singh, M.; Mahmood, M. Melioidosis: The great mimicker. *J. Community Hosp. Intern. Med. Perspect.* **2017**, *7*, 245–247. [CrossRef] [PubMed]

32. Panginikkod, S.; Ramachandran, A.; Bollimunta, P.; Habibi, R.; Kumar Arjal, R.; Gopalakrishnan, V. *Burkholderia* aortic aneurysm: A case report and review of the literature. *Case Rep. Infect. Dis.* **2017**. [CrossRef] [PubMed]

33. Hadano, Y. Imported melioidosis in Japan: A review of cases. *Infect. Drug Resist.* **2018**, *11*, 163–168. [CrossRef] [PubMed]

34. Masbang, A.N. *Melioidosis in the Philippines—Its Emergence from Obscurity: A Case Series*; St. Luke's Hospital: Quezon City, Philippines, 2015; unpublished work.

35. Ocampo, L.D.M. *Septicemic Melioidosis and Pulmonary Tuberculosis Co-Infection: A Case Report*; Chinese General Hospital: Metro Manila, Philippines, 2014; unpublished work.

36. Yap, E.M.; Rosario, M.; Inductivo-Yu, I. Liver abscess harbors melioidosis: A rare finding in a potentially endemic community. In Proceedings of the APASL Single Topic Conference, Kaohsiung, Taiwan, 10–12 June 2016; National Kidney and Transplant Institute: Metro Manila, Philippines, 2016, unpublished work.

37. Santos, S.V.; Coronel, R.F.; Bergantin, M.R.G.; Delgado, J.S. *Demographic Characteristics and Clinical Profile of Adult Patients with Burkholderia pseudomallei Infection at the University of Santo Tomas Hospital: A Case Series*; University of Santo Thomas: Metro Manila, Philippines, 2014; unpublished.

38. Hassan, M.R.; Pani, S.P.; Peng, N.P.; Voralu, K.; Vijayalakshmi, N.; Mehanderkar, R.; Aziz, N.A.; Michael, E. Incidence, risk factors and clinical epidemiology of melioidosis: A complex socio-ecological emerging infectious disease in the Alor Setar region of Kedah, Malaysia. *BMC Infect. Dis.* **2010**, *10*, 302. [CrossRef] [PubMed]

39. Simpson, A.J.; Newton, P.N.; Chierakul, W.; Chaowagul, W.; White, N.J. Diabetes mellitus, insulin, and melioidosis in Thailand. *Clin. Infect. Dis.* **2003**, *36*. [CrossRef] [PubMed]

40. Jimeno, C.A.; Kho, S.A.; Matawaran, B.J.; Duante, C.A.; Jasul, G.V. Prevalence of diabetes mellitus and pre-diabetes in the Philippines: A sub-study of the 7th National Nutrition and Health Survey (2008). *Philipp. J. Intern. Med.* **2015**, *53*, 1–8.

41. World Health Organization. Philippines: WHO Statistical Profile. Country Statistics and Global Health Estimates by WHO and UN Partners. Available online: http://www.who.int/gho/countries/phl.pdf?ua=1 (accessed on 1 July 2018).

42. Dance, D. Treatment and prophylaxis of melioidosis. *Int. J. Antimicrob. Agents* **2014**, *43*, 310–318. [CrossRef] [PubMed]

43. World Health Organization. Surveillance System in the Philippines—World Health Organization. Available online: www.wpro.who.int/philippines/mediacentre/features/surveillanceresponseevd.pdf (accessed on 1 July 2018).

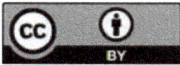

Tropical Medicine and
Infectious Disease

MDPI

Review

Melioidosis in Singapore: Clinical, Veterinary, and Environmental Perspectives

Siew Hoon Sim [1,†], Catherine Ee Ling Ong [1,†], Yunn Hwen Gan [2], Dongling Wang [1],
Victor Wee Hong Koh [1], Yian Kim Tan [1], Michelle Su Yen Wong [1], Janet Seok Wei Chew [1],
Sian Foong Ling [1], Brian Zi Yan Tan [3], Agnes Zhengyu Ye [3], Patrick Chuan Kiat Bay [4],
Wai Kwan Wong [3], Charlene Judith Fernandez [3], Shangzhe Xie [5], Praveena Jayarajah [5],
Tasha Tahar [5], Pei Yee Oh [5], Sonja Luz [5], Jaime Mei Fong Chien [6], Thuan Tong Tan [6],
Louis Yi Ann Chai [7,8,9], Dale Fisher [7,8], Yichun Liu [1], Jimmy Jin Phang Loh [1] and
Gladys Gek Yen Tan [1,*]

[1] Defence Medical and Environmental Research Institute, DSO National Laboratories, Singapore 117510,
    Singapore; ssiewhoo@dso.org.sg (S.H.S.); catong@dso.org.sg (C.E.L.O.); dongling@dso.org.sg (D.W.);
    kweehong@dso.org.sg (V.W.H.K.); tyiankim@dso.org.sg (Y.K.T.); wsuyen@dso.org.sg (M.S.Y.W.);
    cseokwei@dso.org.sg (J.S.W.C.); lsianfoo@dso.org.sg (S.F.L.); lyichun@dso.org.sg (Y.L.);
    jimmyloh@dso.org.sg (J.J.P.L.)
[2] Department of Biochemistry, Yong Loo Lin School of Medicine, National University of Singapore, Singapore
    117597, Singapore; bchganyh@nus.edu.sg
[3] Laboratories Group, Agri-Food & Veterinary Authority of Singapore, Singapore 718827, Singapore;
    Brian_TAN@ava.gov.sg (B.Z.Y.T.); agnes_ye@ava.gov.sg (A.Z.Y.); Wong_Wai_Kwan@ava.gov.sg (W.K.W.);
    Charlene_FERNANDEZ@ava.gov.sg (C.J.F.)
[4] Food Establishment Regulation Group, Agri-Food & Veterinary Authority of Singapore, Singapore 608550,
    Singapore; chuan_kiat@ava.gov.sg
[5] Conservation, Research and Veterinary Services, Wildlife Reserves Singapore, Singapore 729826, Singapore;
    shangzhe.xie@wrs.com.sg (S.X.); praveenajayarajah@yahoo.com (P.J.); tasha.tahar@wrs.com.sg (T.T.);
    peiyee.oh@wrs.com.sg (P.Y.O.); sonja.luz@wrs.com.sg (S.L.)
[6] Department of Infectious Diseases, Singapore General Hospital, Singapore 169608, Singapore;
    Jaime.chien.m.f@singhealth.com.sg (J.M.F.C.); tan.thuan.tong@sgh.com.sg (T.T.T.)
[7] Division of Infectious Diseases, Department of Medicine, National University Health System, Singapore
    119228, Singapore; louis_chai@nuhs.edu.sg (L.Y.A.C.); mdcfda@nus.edu.sg (D.F.)
[8] Department of Medicine, Yong Loo Lin School of Medicine, National University of Singapore, Singapore
    117597, Singapore
[9] National University Cancer Institute, Singapore 119074, Singapore
* Correspondence: tgekyen@dso.org.sg; Tel.: +65-6485-7205
† These authors contributed equally to this report.

Received: 7 February 2018; Accepted: 7 March 2018; Published: 12 March 2018

Abstract: Melioidosis is a notifiable infectious disease registered with the Ministry of Health (MOH) and Agri-Food & Veterinary Authority (AVA), Singapore. From a clinical perspective, increased awareness of the disease has led to early detection and treatment initiation, thus resulting in decreasing mortality rates in recent years. However, the disease still poses a threat to local pet, zoo and farm animals, where early diagnosis is a challenge. The lack of routine environmental surveillance studies also makes prevention of the disease in animals difficult. To date, there have been no reports that provide a complete picture of how the disease impacts the local human and animal populations in Singapore. Information on the distribution of *Burkholderia pseudomallei* in the environment is also lacking. The aim of this review is to provide a comprehensive overview of both published and unpublished clinical, veterinary and environmental studies on melioidosis in Singapore to achieve better awareness and management of the disease.

Trop. Med. Infect. Dis. **2018**, *3*, 31

Keywords: melioidosis; *B. pseudomallei*; Singapore; clinical; veterinary; environmental

1. Introduction

Melioidosis is an infectious disease associated with high mortality and morbidity in endemic regions of Southeast Asia and northern Australia [1]. The etiological agent, *Burkholderia pseudomallei*, can be found in the soil and water in these endemic regions. Infection generally occurs through inhalation, ingestion or contact of skin wounds with contaminated soil, dust particles or water [2]. Melioidosis, also known as the great mimicker, can result in highly diverse disease manifestations, often complicating diagnosis and delaying treatment [3–6]. Other than humans, *B. pseudomallei* can also infect a wide range of animals including goats, sheep, camels, birds, crocodiles, kangaroos, etc. [7,8]. The zoonotic potential of *B. pseudomallei* (Bp) has also been reported [7,9]. Due to the hardy nature of the bacterium, it is able to survive in the most nutrient-limiting environments, such as distilled water [10,11].

The first case of melioidosis in Singapore was reported in 1920 [12]. Since the 1980s, rapid urbanization has occurred within the country, and today it is mainly dominated by high-rise buildings and well-developed infrastructure. However, despite its urbanized setting, melioidosis still exists in Singapore, with an overall annual incidence of 0.6–2.4 per 100,000 of the population between the years 2000 and 2015, as reported by MOH [13]. Furthermore, animal cases of melioidosis were reported as early as in the 1980s by AVA (formerly called Primary Production Department). In this review article, we describe the clinical, veterinary and environmental aspects of melioidosis in Singapore.

2. Clinical Aspects

2.1. Disease Epidemiology

Prior to 1989, there were only two published reports on the epidemiology of the disease in the country. Tan et al. (1990) [14] reported a sudden increase in the number of cases from 5 cases in 1987 to 36 and 24 cases in the years 1988 and 1989, respectively, and attributed the increase to the generation of infective aerosols as a result of soil excavation activities conducted around the island. The disease was also a concern among healthy military personnel due to involvement with soil-related training programs during these early years. Between 1987 and 1994, 23 cases (including 4 fatal cases) were reported [15].

Three separate studies addressing the epidemiology of melioidosis were conducted, from 1989 to 1996, 1998 to 2007, and 2003 to 2014 [16–18]. The mean annual number of melioidosis cases reported during these three study periods were 46, 70, and 44, respectively. The higher mean annual number observed during the period from 1998 to 2007 was related to a melioidosis outbreak in 2004, which was associated with higher-than-average rainfall [17]. A molecular typing study confirmed that this 2004 outbreak was caused by highly heterogeneous *B. pseudomallei* isolates, rather than a single virulent strain [19]. In the last-mentioned epidemiological study, spanning 2003–2014, a progressive 10% reduction in the incidence of melioidosis cases was noted. However, the last 2 years (2015–2016) have seen a rise in the number of melioidosis cases diagnosed (Figure 1). The early case-fatality rate, as exemplified by the 98 cases that occurred during the 2004 surge, was 52.6% [17]. The mortality rate has since fallen to 18.4%, possibly as a result of increased disease awareness and earlier recognition by clinicians, and prompt institution of definitive antimicrobial treatment.

In Singapore, the recent overall annual melioidosis incidence rate was 1.1 per 100,000 population. The incidence rate was higher in those of Malay and Indian ethnicity (2.4 and 2.1 per 100,000 respectively) [18]. Males were predominantly affected, which can possibly be attributed to their involvement in outdoor occupational or recreational activities [16–18]. Systemic melioidosis primarily affects older individuals with underlying medical conditions, with the highest disease incidence rate being reported in the population cohort ≥45 years of age. Diabetes mellitus is the key co-morbidity, reported in 47.9% to 56.7% of the diagnosed cases [16–18]. Patients with renal impairment were also at higher risk of infection.

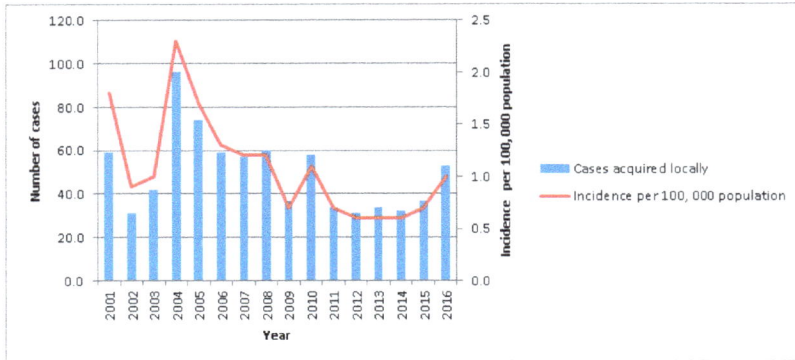

Figure 1. Annual number of human melioidosis cases from 2003 to 2016 in Singapore.

2.2. Clinical Features of Melioidosis Patients

In Singapore, the major systemic presentations of melioidosis are bacteraemia (60.3%), deep organ abscesses (40.7%) and pneumonia (33.1%) [18]. In contrast to *B. pseudomallei* bacteraemia cases, the incidence of cases presenting as pneumonia is on the decline. Conventionally, antimicrobial regimens containing *B. pseudomallei*-active agents (e.g., ceftazidime or a carbapenem) have been utilized for treatment of severe community-acquired pneumonia in Singaporean intensive care units. For deep abscesses, the primary organs involved are liver, prostate and spleen, and these are often seen in patients with poorly-controlled diabetes. The incidence of deep organ abscesses appears to be on the rise [18,20,21]. Localized soft tissue infections have been seen, and some of these cases may be linked to local trauma or inoculation. These patients often do not have diabetes or compromised immunity, in contrast to the patients with bacteraemia or deep abscesses.

Singapore has also seen its share of melioidosis cases with uncommon clinical presentations. For example, in 2006, there was a case of melioidosis osteomyelitis reported in a 32-year-old diabetic man, who also had infection in the spleen and liver [22]. In another case, a 37-year-old Italian man possibly acquired melioidosis through inhalation of dust generated by helicopter rotor blades during business travel to Singapore. He developed bacteraemia, pneumonia, splenic abscess and osteomyelitis of the head of humerus [23].

Involvement of the cardiovascular system, a rare occurrence associated with high morbidity and relapse rates, has also been observed in melioidosis cases in Singapore [24]. Rao et al. (2009) [25] reported two cases presenting with abdominal aortic pseudo-aneurysms requiring both medical and surgical intervention, with only one surviving. A relapsing case of meningitis caused by *B. pseudomallei* following inadequate treatment of the primary episode of melioidosis mycotic aneurysm was also reported by Chlebicki et al. (2008) [26]. Between 1997 and 2000, five cases presenting with brain abscess were also reported [27]. Successful treatment was achieved with drainage coupled with antibiotics, although two of the cases failed to achieve complete neurological recovery [28].

2.3. Diagnosis

In Singapore, the reference standard for the diagnosis of melioidosis is based on the culture of *B. pseudomallei* from clinical specimens [3,29], along with relevant clinical presentations. Biochemical tests including API 20NE (bioMerieux, Lyon, France) and Vitek 2 GN card (bioMerieux, Lyon, France) are also conducted to confirm the biochemical properties of the isolated *B. pseudomallei*. Since the occurrence of 4 deaths in 23 melioidosis cases among apparently young and healthy military personnel between 1987 and 1994, melioidosis has been a priority consideration for Singapore's clinicians [15,30]. Risk factors including activities entailing soil and water contact, as well as underlying co-morbidities such as diabetes and renal disease, will also raise diagnostic concerns among the clinicians [31].

A disadvantage of culture-based diagnosis is the delay of some days. Molecular methods such as Bp-specific polymerase chain reactions (PCR) targeting bacterial DNA fragments provide rapid diagnosis for melioidosis, but are not routinely used in local clinical laboratories and the sensitivity of PCR can be low, especially with blood specimens [32,33]. While a serological test alone cannot offer a definitive diagnosis of melioidosis, especially in endemic areas [34], seropositivity is an indicator of exposure to *B. pseudomallei*. The most commonly used serological test for a melioidosis diagnosis is indirect hemagglutination assay (IHA), which has been well evaluated and accepted since it is cost-effective and has a short turnaround time, although in other countries it has been reported to lack both sensitivity and specificity [3].

In Singapore, the IHA with a cut-off ratio of ≥1:16 for seropositivity was first established by Yap et al. (1991) [35]. The DSO Clinical Diagnostic Services Laboratory (CDSL) has been ISO15189 accredited for performing the IHA test to facilitate melioidosis diagnosis for local samples. The laboratory has conducted IRB-approved studies (Singhealth Centralized Institutional Review Board, DSO IRB committee) and performed IHA tests on serum samples collected from culture-confirmed melioidosis cases, clinically unconfirmed cases, and healthy volunteers from 2004 to 2016. Based on unpublished data (Table 1), it has been observed that all of the culture-confirmed melioidosis cases were also positive by IHA, 54.8% with very high (≥1:512) and 38.7% with high (1:128 to 1:256) titers. In contrast, the two large cohorts (992 and 1027 cases) with suspected melioidosis or clinically unconfirmed infection were mostly negative in the IHA test (89.4% and 86.5%, respectively). Furthermore, of 109 healthy volunteers, 23 (21.1%) had low positive results (1:16 to 1:64) and one subject (0.9%) was highly positive with an IHA titer of 1:128, suggesting previous exposure to *B. pseudomallei*, possibly due to engagement in prior outdoor activities. The IHA is thus considered more useful in Singapore than elsewhere, and those with high or very high IHA titers are considered likely either to be melioidosis cases with active Bp infection or individuals who have had prior exposure to *B. pseudomallei*.

Table 1. IHA results on serum samples collected from culture-confirmed melioidosis patients, suspected melioidosis cases presenting to local hospitals and healthy volunteers from 2004 to 2016 [36].

Study Groups	Subject Information/Year of Blood Collection	Number (%) of Subjects with Different Levels of IHA Titer			
		Very High Positive ≥1:512	High Positive 1:128 to 1:256	Low Positive 1:16 to 1:64	Negative ≤1:8
Culture-confirmed melioidosis (*n* = 31)	Acute, relapsed and recovered cases with a mean age of 52.5 years old/2004–2013	17 (54.8%)	12 (38.7%)	2 (6.5%)	0 (0%)
Clinically unconfirmed infection (*n* = 992)	Patients with an active infection/2006	31 (3.1%)	21 (2.1%)	54 (5.4%)	886 (89.4%)
Clinically unconfirmed infection (*n* = 1027)	Patients with an active infection/2016	18 (1.8%)	20 (1.9%)	101 (9.8%)	888 (86.5%)
Healthy volunteers (*n* = 109)	Age range: 18–60 mean age: 33.1 years old/2004–2013	0 (0%)	1 (0.9%)	23 (21.1%)	85 (78.0%)

2.4. Treatment

Clinicians in Singapore, particularly physicians, intensivists and emergency department specialists, have melioidosis in mind early when a suspicious clinical pattern presents. Empiric antibiotics are generally started pending culture results. Hence, ceftazidime or a carbapenem are featured in local empiric antibiotic guidelines for severe community-acquired pneumonia for this reason. The treatment for melioidosis in Singapore is conducted in accordance with international guidelines, consisting of an initial intensive phase followed by an extended eradication phase [37]. As initial empiric therapy for suspected melioidosis or for intensive phase treatment for confirmed melioidosis, either ceftazidime or meropenem is administered intravenously. The duration of treatment for the intensive phase is at least 2 weeks. Some clinicians may extend treatment duration to 4 weeks or beyond, in circumstances such as multiple large deep organ abscesses or extensive multi-lobar pneumonia. In addition, while not in the standard guidelines, some physicians also add oral trimethoprim-sulfamethoxazole during the intensive phase for the perceived benefit of good penetration into deep organs and lungs as well as the anecdotal emergence of ceftazidime resistance, despite the fact that such a practice has not been proven to be more efficacious [38]. The eradication phase is long, lasting at least 3 months, and consists of oral trimethoprim-sulfamethoxazole as the backbone of therapy. Locally, some physicians may opt to add in a second agent, either amoxicillin-clavulanate or doxycycline, in addition to trimethoprim-sulfamethoxazole. Drug tolerance is always a concern during the extended treatment periods, and so close follow-up is advised. In addition, due to the high prevalence of glucose-6-phosphate dehydrogenase (G6PD)-deficiency in this region, G6PD screening is advised before commencement of trimethoprim-sulfamethoxazole. For patients who are intolerant or who have known sulfonamide allergy, the combination of amoxicillin-clavulanate plus doxycycline is used, although this regimen is perceived to be less efficacious than one containing trimethoprim-sulfamethoxazole. Eradication therapy is considered adequate and ceases when follow-up clinical, radiological and biochemical (e.g., inflammatory markers such as C-reactive protein) assessments document complete resolution. Otherwise, the eradication phase treatment may be extended beyond 3 months. In some circumstances (e.g., disease complexity or drug allergy), treatment may deviate from the standard antibiotic regimens [31]. In Singapore, antibiotic susceptibility testing is routinely performed on *B. pseudomallei*, with alternative antibiotics used when resistance to the standard antibiotics is detected. In 2010, Kung et al. [39] reported a patient with mediastinal lymphadenitis, who developed resistance to ceftazidime during the course of treatment. One of us has managed another patient with melioidosis, whose isolate developed ceftazidime resistance on treatment, in 2008 [40]. The patient relapsed with overwhelming bacteraemia and rapidly demised, prompting some clinicians to favor initial antibiotic therapy with a combination of two active antibiotics.

The management of deep organ abscesses is challenging. There is a need to ensure adequate drug penetration into the abscess cavity for adequate treatment, often necessitating an extended duration of treatment. To reduce the microbial burden, some local clinicians advocate radiologically-guided drainage of abscesses, where possible, especially in the liver and prostate. The rationale for such an invasive procedure is multi-fold: (i) for diagnostic microbiological confirmation of the disease, (ii) for *B. pseudomallei* susceptibility testing, (iii) to reduce the microbial burden, and (iv) to shorten treatment duration.

For severe septic melioidosis cases, in addition to antibiotic therapy, treatment in an intensive care unit (ICU) with strict glycemic control [41] is also employed to improve the outcome [31]. Careful use of anti-diabetic therapy in diabetic patients with septic melioidosis is recommended, and a recent study by Liu et al. (2014) [42] highlighted the occurrence of more severe complications in diabetic patients receiving sulphonylurea due to the suppression of the host inflammatory response by the drug.

3. Veterinary Aspects

3.1. Prevalence and Surveillance of Animal Melioidosis

Singapore has a diverse population of animals. For livestock animals, there are a total of 5 poultry layer farms, 4 dairy (3 cattle and 1 goat) farms, 220 fish farms (food and ornamental) and 11 horse establishments (racing and equestrian) [43]. As of 2016, the pet population, comprising dogs, cats, birds, fish, and small mammals, is estimated to be 780,100 [44]. In addition, there is a zoological collection of 16,134 animals, consisting of 949 different species of Pisces, Amphibia, Reptilia, Aves and Mammalia in Wildlife Reserves Singapore (WRS).

In Singapore, animal melioidosis cases are notifiable to AVA. To date, AVA has documented 454 confirmed melioidosis cases between 1983 and 2016, comprising isolates from wild animals (including the zoo animals at WRS), pet animals from local veterinary clinics, farm animals, and the environment, such as outdoor multipurpose fields and ponds. At WRS, 37 sporadic cases in 26 animal species were documented between 1983 and 2017 (Table 2). Notably, gorillas appeared to be highly susceptible to melioidosis. In 1984, a total of 4 imported gorillas (2 from Monaco and 2 from Bristol zoo, imported between 1982 and 1983) succumbed to melioidosis. Additionally, of another 2 gorillas imported from Dublin zoo in 1992, one succumbed to melioidosis six months after importation. The other was subsequently returned to Dublin zoo in 1993. *B. pseudomallei* was cultured from various organs of these five deceased gorillas (Table 2). It was postulated that various factors, including social dynamics, diet and housing, had resulted in increased susceptibility of these gorillas to *B. pseudomallei* infection.

Clinical signs can differ within each animal species, depending on the site of infection [45]. Based on past observations, the first clinical signs in infected animals were non-specific and consisted of inappetence, lethargy and diarrhea. In some cases, infected animals can even succumb to infection within one or two days without showing visible signs of disease. As previously reported, one key feature of animal melioidosis was the formation of abscesses in one or multiple organs [7,46]. At WRS, the most common sites of lesions in infected animals were the liver (Figure 2) and lungs (Figure 3). Lung lesions were more commonly seen in primates [47], whereas liver lesions were more common among the avian cases (78%). It is also interesting to note that lung lesions have never been seen in the avian cases.

With the increase in global trade of animals for food, zoological exhibitions and as pets, importation and movement of subclinically-infected animals poses a significant risk to local animal populations due to the propensity of *B. pseudomallei* for long latency periods. These animals can shed *B. pseudomallei* in their faeces or through ruptured abscesses during the stressful transport process and change in environment, which might serve as a source of infection or environmental contamination when they are in close contact with naïve animals [48,49].

There is no formal active surveillance program for melioidosis in local pet, zoo or farm animals. In Singapore, farm animals are mainly reared for dairy products and eggs, and are not slaughtered for meat. In addition, only pasteurized milk is allowed to be sold for consumption. To date, there has only been a single instance in which *B. pseudomallei* was isolated from the spleen of a clinically healthy dairy goat from a local farm in 2014. However, subsequent sampling of the goats in the farm did not yield any positive cases. As part of Singapore's food safety program, AVA conducts post-mortem inspection on imported livestock, i.e., pigs and accompanying viscera (spleen, liver, kidneys) at the local pig abattoir. The inspection involves visual checks, palpation and, where necessary, incision to check for abnormalities, including abscesses. Carcasses and viscera with multiple abscesses/pyemia will not enter the food chain, as they will be condemned and subsequently incinerated if the examination findings are consistent between AVA inspectors and Supervising Inspectors (SI). In addition, AVA conducts regular microbiological surveillance on the condemned carcasses and viscera (liver, lymph node, lung, spleen and kidney), which includes *B. pseudomallei* culture, to monitor the health status of imported livestock. From January 2008 to December 2016, a total of 1696 samples were collected, of which 341 (20%) were positive for *B. pseudomallei*. Thus, the risk of transmission from infected animals to humans through the consumption of meat and animal products would be deemed negligible.

Ongoing work is being done to analyze the strains isolated from animals. The local farms also have good animal husbandry practices in place and are required to report any abnormal clinical signs observed. Furthermore, the health status of farm animals is also inspected regularly by AVA. These additional measures provide some forms of surveillance for any first signs of disease in farm animals.

Trop. Med. Infect. Dis. **2018**, 3, 31

Table 2. Summary of animal melioidosis cases in WRS parks from 1983 to 2017 [50].

	Species	Number	Year of Diagnosis	Organ from Which *B. pseudomallei* Was Isolated						
				Blood	Lung	Liver	Kidney	Spleen	Gonad	Skin
Primates	Gorilla (*Gorilla gorilla*)	5	1983/1992	x	x	x	x			
	Southern pig-tailed macaque (*Macaca nemestrina*)	1	1992		x					
	Chimpanzee (*Pan troglodytes*)	2	1985/1990		x		x			
	Müller's Bornean gibbon (*Hylobates muelleri*)	2	1989/1992		x			x		
	Mandrill (*Mandrillus sphinx*)	1	1990					x		
	Golden lion tamarin (*Leontopithecus rosalia*)	2	1995/1996		x	x				
	Siamang (*Symphalangus syndactylus*)	1	2005			x				
	Lesser spot-nosed guenon (*Cercopithecus petaurista*)	1	1996		x					
	Debrazza's monkey (*Cercopithecus neglectus*)	1	1998		x					
	Douc langur (*Simia nemaeus*)	1	1992		x					
Herbivores	Eastern grey kangaroo (*Macropus giganteus*)	2	1986/1989		x		x			
	Indochinese hog deer (*Hyelaphus annamiticus*)	1	2013		x					
	Camel (*Camelus dromedaries*)	1	1994		x					
	Llama (*Lama glama*)	1	1994		x					
	Nile hippopotamus (*Hippopotamus amphibious*)	1	1996			x				
	Red lechwe (*Kobus leche*)	2	1998/2007			x		x		
	Indian sambar (*Rusa unicolor*)	1	2003			x				
	Chinese goral (*Naemorhedus griseus*)	1	2008							x
Carnivores	Cape hunting dog (*Lycaon pictus pictus*)	1	1990	x						
Birds	Southern cassowary (*Casuarius casuarius*)	1	1985					x		
	Southern crowned pigeon (*Goura scheepmakeri*)	1	1987						x	
	Moustached parakeet (*Psittacula alexandri*)	1	1998			x				
	Palm cockatoo (*Probosciger terrimus*)	2	1991/1996			x				
	Salmon-crested cockatoo (*Cacatua moluccensis*)	2	1998/2014			x				
	Humboldt penguin (*Spheniscus humboldti*)	1	1987			x				
	Bird of paradise (exact species unknown)	1	1986			x				

x: organ of animal species where *B. pseudomallei* was isolated.

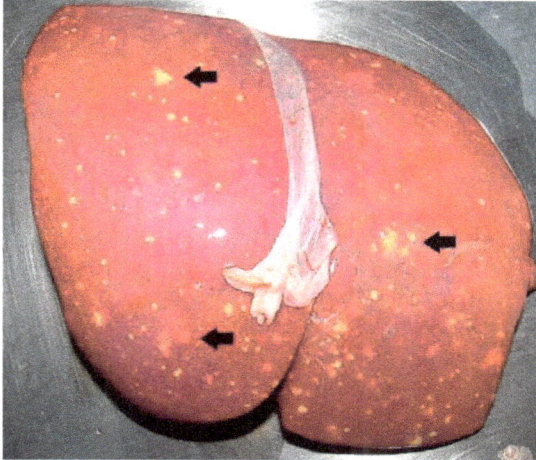

Figure 2. Multifocal abscess (black arrows) in the liver of a Douc langur with melioidosis.

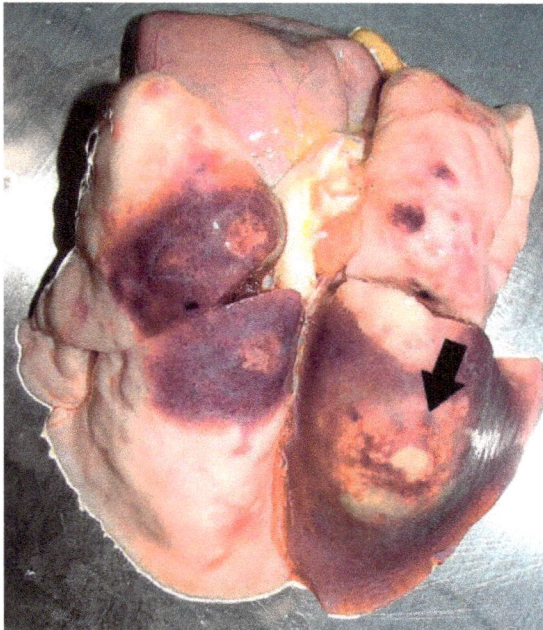

Figure 3. Large abscess in the left caudal lung lobe (black arrow) of a Douc langur with melioidosis.

3.2. Laboratory Diagnosis for Animal Melioidosis

The diagnosis of melioidosis in animals requires the isolation and identification of *B. pseudomallei*, usually from swabs or abscesses from affected organs. Diagnosis of the reported animal cases is usually obtained through post-mortem examination, unless the presenting clinical sign is a lesion on the skin, as observed in a Chinese goral (*Naemorhedus griseus*) in 2008. Upon detection of the disease, environmental sampling from the surrounding soil and water where the animals reside is conducted as part of the investigation procedure for source attribution.

In all cases, the standard Ashdown media or modified Ashdown broth containing colistin and crystal violet [51] are used for the isolation of *B. pseudomallei*. Further confirmation is achieved through phenotypic characterization using biochemical tests, including the API 20NE kit or Vitek GN card, and genotypic characterization using *B. pseudomallei*-specific real-time PCR [52].

3.3. Treatment and Prevention of Melioidosis in Zoo Animals

In Singapore, animals suspected of having melioidosis are generally given supportive treatment, which may include fluid therapy, anti-inflammatories and antibiotics. In the four parks managed by WRS, as a preventive measure against melioidosis, proper water hygiene and environmental surveillance are conducted to identify for the presence of *B. pseudomallei* in the exhibit areas. Quarterly environmental sampling is conducted before introducing susceptible species into the parks. For instance, between February 2016–2017, a total of 450 soil samples and 54 water samples were collected from four sites, namely the Butterfly Park, Kidzworld, Chimpanzee Exhibit and Polar Bear Exhibit. All samples were negative for *B. pseudomallei* by both culture and real-time PCR. The Chimpanzee Exhibit was positive for *B. multivorans* in May 2016, but subsequent soil and water samples collected from the same site were negative for the bacterium.

4. Environmental Melioidosis

4.1. Prevalence and Environmental Surveillance of B. pseudomallei

For a country long known to be endemic for melioidosis, Singapore has surprisingly few publications on the isolation, distribution, prevalence and spread of the pathogen in the local environment. After the first case of melioidosis in 1920 [12], the next report on environmental isolation of *B. pseudomallei* was in 1971 [53]. In this study, 8 of the 136 surface water samples collected within the city of Singapore were positive for *B. pseudomallei* (isolation rate of 5.9%) (Table 3). In 1995, Yap et al. [54] documented the recovery of 3 isolates from water samples collected from a moat within an animal enclosure in Singapore Zoological Gardens (now known as WRS), where the gorillas had earlier succumbed to melioidosis. Additionally, two soil isolates were obtained from an island off mainland Singapore where two fatal human cases of melioidosis had been reported, and one isolate from a residential compound where a pet German shepherd dog had died (Table 3) [54]. To date, the most extensive environmental surveillance of *B. pseudomallei* in Singapore involved the collection of 395 soil samples during the period 1992 to 1996 for epidemiological investigation of the disease [16]. Seven of the soil samples obtained from 3 different sites were positive for the pathogen (Table 3) [16].

Between 2000 and 2013, DSO National Laboratories executed a number of projects on environmental surveillance of *B. pseudomallei* (unpublished) (Table 4). One of these environmental surveillance studies was conducted in the island off mainland Singapore where Yap et al. (1995) [54] had previously reported the isolation of *B. pseudomallei*. Among the 188 soil samples collected from fields, plantations and reclaimed lands (*n* = 98, 62 and 28, respectively), and 16 water samples from streams or puddles, 3 soil samples from plantations (4.8%) and 2 water samples (12.5%) were positive for *B. pseudomallei*. In 2001, through collaborative efforts with WRS and Prof Paul Ananth Tambyah from the National University Hospital (NUH), 43 soil samples and 3 water samples were collected from 3 animal enclosures. No *B. pseudomallei* was isolated.

Table 3. Literature review of environmental surveillance for *B. pseudomallei* in Singapore.

Type of Environmental Sample	Terrain/Location	Isolation Protocol	No. Collected	No. Positive	Percentage (%)	Interesting Correlations *	Reference
Surface water	Forest around buildings, roadside drains, sports fields	Hamster inoculation method [55]; colony identification on MacConkey agar.	21 44 43 28	1 0 2 5	4.8 0.0 4.6 18.0	- - Rainfall Rainfall; low lying field	[53]
	Different localities where melioidosis patients had sustained injuries or had direct contact prior to their onset of illness	TSB with crystal violet (5 mg/L) and colistin (20 mg/L); colony identification on Ashdown agar.	46	0	0.0	-	[16]
Water	Moat within animal enclosure in Singapore Zoological Gardens (WRS)	Hamster inoculation method [55]; colony identification on MacConkey's agar.	Unknown	3	N.D.	4 gorillas succumbed to melioidosis; both animal and water isolates belonged to same RE II type.	[54]
Soil	Island off Singapore	Hamster inoculation method [55]; colony identification on MacConkey agar.	Unknown	2	N.D.	2 patients staying on the island died of melioidosis (see Table 5). Pet German shepherd succumbed to melioidosis; both animal and soil isolates belonged to same RE II type.	[54]
	Residential compound		4	1	25.0		
	Different localities where melioidosis patients had sustained injuries or had direct contact prior to their onset of illness	TSB with crystal violet (5 mg/L) and colistin (20 mg/L) enrichment; colony identification on Ashdown agar.	395	7	1.8	Genotype (by REA-PFGE) of Bp isolated from 4 samples in 1 locality similar to that isolated from elbow abscess of adult who had sustained injury at same locality.	[16]

* Correlations observed or hypothesized by the authors.

Table 4. Environmental surveillance of *B. pseudomallei* in Singapore between 2000 and 2013 [56].

Sample Source	Terrain/Location	Year	No. Collected	No. Positive	Percentage Positive (%)	Type of Study	Interesting Correlations *
	Fields, island	2000/01	98	0	0	Repeated Sampling at sites reported by Yap et al. [54]	
	Plantations, island	2000/01	62	3	3.1	Repeated Sampling at sites reported by Yap et al. [54]	
	Reclaimed land, island	2000/01	28	0	0	Repeated Sampling at sites reported by Yap et al. [54]	
	Animal enclosure 1	2001	18	0	0	Collaboration with SZG.	
	Animal enclosure 2	2001	13	0	0	Collaboration with SZG.	
	Animal enclosure 3	2001	8	0	0	Collaboration with Dr. Paul A. Tambyah, NUH	
	Animal enclosure 4	2001	4	0	0	Collaboration with Dr. Paul A. Tambyah, NUH	
	Park A	2005	15	0	0	Environmental Surveillance at 9 locations	
Soil	Park B	2005	5	0	0	Environmental Surveillance at 9 locations	Refer to Table 5
	Park C	2005	90	3	3.3	Environmental Surveillance at 9 locations	
	Park D	2005	100	1	1.0	Environmental Surveillance at 9 locations	
	Nature Reserve A	2005	79	0	0	Environmental Surveillance at 9 locations	
	Nature Reserve B	2005	30	0	0	Environmental Surveillance at 9 locations	
	Nature Reserve C	2005	90	0	0	Environmental Surveillance at 9 locations	
	Disturbed soil area A	2005	259	0	0	Environmental Surveillance at 9 locations	
	Disturbed soil area B	2005	63	0	0	Environmental Surveillance at 9 locations	
	Forested hill, southern island	2013	55	1	1.8	Environmental Surveillance project in 2013	
	Water from streams/puddles, island	2000/01	16	2	12.5	Repeated sampling at sites reported by Yap et al. [54]	
Water	Moat within animal enclosure 2	2001	3	0	0	Collaboration with SZG.	Refer to Table 5
	Water behind animal enclosure 3	2001	1	0	0	Collaboration with Dr Paul A. Tambyah, NUH	
	Run-off from forested hill, southern island	2013	1	0	0	Environmental surveillance project in 2013	
Rainwater	Forested hill, southern island	2013	9	0	0	Environmental Surveillance project in 2013	

SZG-Singapore Zoological Gardens; * Correlations observed or hypothesized by the authors.

Between 2003 and 2005, environmental surveillance of *B. pseudomallei* was carried out at 9 locations on mainland Singapore and 731 soil samples were collected. Two of these locations (Park C and Park D) tested positive for *B. pseudomallei*, with isolation rates of 1.0% and 3.3%, respectively (Table 4). Data from a subsequent surveillance project carried out from January to April 2013 showed that the isolation rate of *B. pseudomallei* from soil samples collected from a forested hill in a southern island off Singapore was 1.8%. However, rainwater and water samples collected from run-off from the forested hill were negative for *B. pseudomallei* (Table 4).

It is worth noting that environmental surveillance studies to identify the source of infection are confounded by the small area of Singapore, and the movement of the general population all over the island. In addition, technical and funding issues, and the difficulty in getting approval from regulatory bodies and private institutions have also hindered these environmental surveillance studies.

4.2. Detection of B. pseudomallei in Environmental Samples

Optimizing protocols for sample collection and laboratory processing for the isolation and identification of *B. pseudomallei* is one of the many technical challenges faced in environmental surveillance studies. Due to the diverse range of colony morphotypes of *B. pseudomallei* when cultured on Ashdown agar, considerable expertise is required for visual identification of the bacterial colonies [57]. The hamster inoculation method used by Thin et al. (1971) [53] is a long and tedious process, making it challenging to sample extensive areas and collect large numbers of samples. Similarly, Yap et al. (1995) [54] adopted a 'small and sampling-biased' approach in their study, thus limiting the extent of sampling area.

Following the dissemination of an internationally-recognized SOP for environmental sampling of *B. pseudomallei* by the Detection of Environmental *Burkholderia pseudomallei* Working Party (DEBWorP) in 2012, samples could be collected systematically and processed more efficiently [58]. Using this SOP, DSO embarked on an extensive island-wide environmental surveillance project for comprehensive understanding of the distribution, prevalence, spread, and characterization of environmental *B. pseudomallei* in the Singapore environment (manuscript in preparation). Moreover, with the recent success of the air sampling methodology reported by Currie et al. (2015) [59], we will be reassessing our air sampling protocols to increase our chances of isolating the pathogen from the air in Singapore.

4.3. Correlation between Environmental Isolates and Animal/Clinical Isolates

There have so far been few successes in directly correlating clinical isolates with environmental isolates in the Singapore context. Using restriction endonuclease (RE) analysis with pulsed-field gel electrophoresis (REA-PFGE), Heng et al. (1989) [16] reported that the genotype of *B. pseudomallei* isolated from 4 soil samples in a locality was similar to that isolated from an elbow abscess of an adult who sustained an injury at the location. However, Yap et al. (1995) [54] reported that the genotypes of clinical isolates from 2 patients who died of melioidosis whilst staying in an island off Singapore did not match those recovered from the soil. Instead, the study had more successes with animal isolates—restriction endonuclease profiles of *B. pseudomallei* isolates obtained from infected gorillas in Singapore Zoological Gardens matched the isolates obtained from the surrounding moat of the animal enclosure. In addition, a soil isolate obtained from a residential compound matched the genotype of an isolate from a pet German shepherd dog that succumbed to the disease [54] (Table 3). It is likely that the relatively smaller and well-defined boundaries of the animal enclosure and residential compound increased the chances of locating the environmental source.

Advanced technologies, such as microarrays and multi-locus sequence typing (MLST) have allowed more detailed study of the clinical, animal and environmental *B. pseudomallei* isolates in Singapore. Sim et al. (2008 [47] performed high-resolution comparative genomic analysis to determine the relatedness of 94 *B. pseudomallei* isolates from Southeast Asian origins, and demonstrated a core genome and an accessory genome comprising of 86% and 14% of the genes (respectively) in the Bp K96243 genome. Of these isolates, 68 were isolated from clinical (n = 35), animal (n = 17) and environmental (*n* = 16) sources from Singapore. Bp 22, isolated from a fatal melioidosis case in a young and healthy individual in the 1980s, was amongst the clinical isolates studied. Seven environmental *B. pseudomallei* isolates, including Bp DB and Bp DC [54], Bp 12-40, Bp 15-10, Bp 15-40, Bp SW1 and Bp SW 9 isolated by DSO National Laboratories (herein referred as DSO isolates for easy reference), were obtained in the vicinity of the origin of Bp 22. Unsupervised clustering of the accessory genomes showed that Bp 22 and the DSO isolates belonged to a broad 'Environmental' cluster [47]. Interestingly, Bp DB and Bp DC did not cluster together with the 'Environmental' isolates, but belonged to a broad 'Animal' cluster, instead [47] (Table 5). The results achieved with MLST analysis of these isolates was in alignment with the genome clustering data, with Bp 22 and the DSO isolates belonging to ST423, and Bp DB and Bp DC belonging to ST51 (Table 5) [60].

Table 5. Correlation of clinical and environmental *B. pseudomallei* isolates from an island off Singapore [61].

Isolate	Source	Isolated by	Accessory Genome Clade [47]	Sequence Type (MLST) [60]	Genomic Clade (WGS) [60]
22	Human, clinical	Yap et al. (1995) [54]	Environmental clade	ST423	N.D.
DB	Soil, environmental	Yap et al. (1995) [54]	Animal clade	ST51	A
DC	Soil, environmental	Yap et al. (1995) [54]	Animal clade	ST51	A
15-10	Soil, environmental	DSO 2000/01	Environmental clade	ST423	B
15-40	Soil, environmental	DSO 2000/01	Environmental clade	ST423	B
12-40	Soil, environmental	DSO 2000/01	Environmental clade	ST423	B
SW1	Water, environmental	DSO 2000/01	Environmental clade	ST423	B
SW9	Water, environmental	DSO 2000/01	Environmental clade	ST423	B

Furthermore, using whole genome sequencing (WGS), which provides a higher resolution of isolate matching, the seven environmental isolates were resolved into 2 clades: Clade A, which comprised Bp DB and Bp DC; and Clade B, which was made up of DSO isolates [60]. Unfortunately, the clinical isolate, Bp 22, was not included in this study. To examine the relatedness of Bp 22 with DSO isolates, the genome sequence of Bp 22 was obtained from a DSO in-house sequencing project and compared with the genome sequences of the seven environmental isolates. Using Phylogenetic Tree Building Service by PATRIC v3.5.7 (https://www.patricbrc.org/app/PhylogeneticTree), we determined that Bp 22 was indeed closely related to the 5 DSO isolates and was distinctly different from Bp DB and Bp DC (Figure 4).

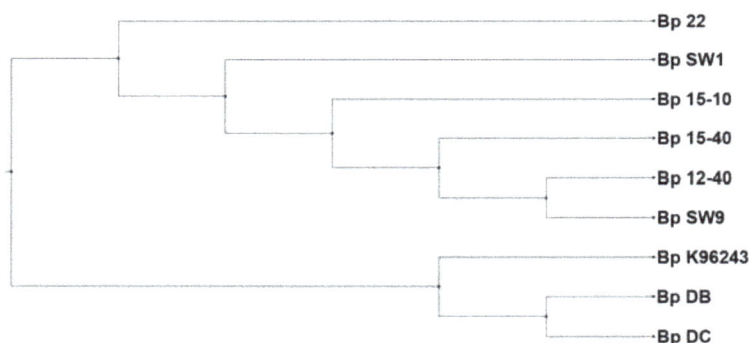

Figure 4. Whole genome phylogeny tree of clinical and environmental isolates from same locale in Singapore. Phylogenetic tree generated using Phylogenetic Tree Building Service by PATRIC v3.5.7 (https://www.patricbrc.org/app/PhylogeneticTree), depicting the relationships of the clinical isolate Bp22 and environmental isolates obtained from an island off Singapore. Bp K96243 was included as a reference isolate.

4.4. Characterization of Environmental B. pseudomallei Isolates from Singapore

While much attention has been paid to characterization of clinical isolates, the environmental isolates from Singapore have been largely neglected in most studies. The antibiograms of clinical isolates from Singapore have been investigated in detail in various studies, reporting consistent susceptibility to ceftazidime, imipenem, amoxicillin-clavulanate, chloramphenicol and tetracycline [14,62,63]. Unfortunately, similar studies of environmental *B. pseudomallei* isolates has not been conducted. Currently, there are only a few studies of the virulence and pathogenesis of environmental isolates. Lee et al. (2010) [64] reported the successful infection of tomato plants by two local soil isolates (Bp 77/96 and Bp 109/96). However, these *B. pseudomallei* isolates did not infect rice plants.

In terms of genome characterization of environmental isolates, the most extensive study was reported by Nandi et al. (2015) [60] involving WGS of more than 100 *B. pseudomallei* genomes, including 13 local environmental isolates. These 13 isolates were collected from various sites in Singapore and belonged to only three sequence types (STs), namely ST51, ST300 and ST423 (*n* = 7, 1 and 5 respectively), hence implying a much lower diversity than in Thailand, where nine STs could be identified from a single sampling site [65].

5. Conclusions

In recent decades, in the clinical setting in Singapore, melioidosis has gained considerable notoriety, with early disease consideration and improved management practices resulting in low mortality rates from the disease. However, it still poses a high threat to animal populations, as early detection and treatment in animals is hindered by variability in clinical course of the disease and the lack of a vaccine for disease prevention. Moving forward, AVA and WRS will be using molecular characterization and typing of the existing isolates to better understand the relationship between the *B. pseudomallei* strains present in the environment and those infecting the different animal populations in Singapore.

Environmental sampling remains a challenge, as isolation of *B. pseudomallei* can be affected by many parameters. Continued efforts in improving protocols and greater support from regulatory authorities for conducting environmental surveillance studies would help identify endemic areas, following which control measures could be applied to reduce disease incidence, particularly in the animal population.

Acknowledgments: The authors would like to thank the following funding sources from the Ministry of Defence, Singapore, and Wildlife Reserves Singapore, WRS, to conduct the studies mentioned in this review. We would also like to thank Placido Ronald Palapal for his contribution on AVA's meat inspection program.

Author Contributions: S.H.S., C.E.L.O., D.W., V.W.H.K., Y.K.T., M.S.Y.W., J.S.W.C. and S.F.L. conducted the experiments. S.H.S., C.E.L.O., Y.H.G., D.W., B.Z.Y.T., A.Z.Y.Y., P.C.K.B., W.K.W., C.J.F., S.X., P.J., T.T., P.Y.O., S.L., J.M.F.C., T.T.T., L.Y.A.C., D.F. and J.J.P.L. contributed to drafting this manuscript. S.H.S., Y.L. and G.G.Y.T. contributed to the organization of the manuscript. S.H.S., C.E.L.O., Y.L., J.J.P.L. and G.G.Y.T. wrote the manuscript.

Conflicts of Interest: The authors declare no conflict of interest.

References

1. Dance, D.A. Melioidosis: The tip of the iceberg? *Clin. Microbiol. Rev.* **1991**, *4*, 52–60. [CrossRef] [PubMed]
2. Thomas, A.D.; Spinks, G.A.; D'Arcy, T.L.; Norton, J.H.; Trueman, K.F. Evaluation of four serological tests for the diagnosis of caprine melioidosis. *Aust. Vet. J.* **1988**, *65*, 261–264. [CrossRef] [PubMed]
3. Cheng, A.C.; Currie, B.J. Melioidosis: Epidemiology, pathophysiology, and management. *Clin. Microbiol. Rev.* **2005**, *18*, 383–416. [CrossRef] [PubMed]
4. White, N.J. Melioidosis. *Lancet* **2003**, *361*, 1715–1722. [CrossRef]
5. Chan, H.P.; Yip, H.S. Mediastinal lymphadenopathy: Melioidosis mimicking tuberculosis. *Trop. Med. Health* **2015**, *43*, 93–94. [CrossRef] [PubMed]

6. Wijekoon, S.; Prasath, T.; Corea, E.M.; Elwitigala, J.P. Melioidosis presenting as lymphadenitis: A case report. *BMC Res. Notes* **2014**, *7*, 364. [CrossRef] [PubMed]

7. Choy, J.L.; Mayo, M.; Janmaat, A.; Currie, B.J. Animal melioidosis in Australia. *Acta. Trop.* **2000**, *74*, 153–158. [CrossRef]

8. Dance, D.A. Melioidosis as an emerging global problem. *Acta. Trop.* **2000**, *74*, 115–119. [CrossRef]

9. Elschner, M.C.; Hnizdo, J.; Stamm, I.; El-Adawy, H.; Mertens, K.; Melzer, F. Isolation of the highly pathogenic and zoonotic agent *Burkholderia pseudomallei* from a pet green iguana in Prague, Czech Republic. *BMC Vet. Res.* **2014**, *10*, 283. [CrossRef] [PubMed]

10. Moore, R.A.; Tuanyok, A.; Woods, D.E. Survival of *Burkholderia pseudomallei* in water. *BMC Res. Notes* **2008**, *1*, 11. [CrossRef] [PubMed]

11. Pumpuang, A.; Chantratita, N.; Wikraiphat, C.; Saiprom, N.; Day, N.P.; Peacock, S.J.; Wuthiekanun, V. Survival of *Burkholderia pseudomallei* in distilled water for 16 years. *Trans. R. Soc. Trop. Med. Hyg.* **2011**, *105*, 598–600. [CrossRef] [PubMed]

12. Stanton, A.T.; Fletcher, W. Melioidosis. Studies from the institute of medical research, Federated Malay States. *Bull* **1932**, *21*, 8–9.

13. Limmathurotsakul, D.; Golding, N.; Dance, D.A.; Messina, J.P.; Pigott, D.M.; Moyes, C.L.; Rolim, D.B.; Bertherat, E.; Day, N.P.; Peacock, S.J.; et al. Predicted global distribution of *Burkholderia pseudomallei* and burden of melioidosis. *Nat. Microbiol.* **2016**, *1*, 15008. [CrossRef] [PubMed]

14. Tan, A.L.; Ang, B.S.; Ong, Y.Y. Melioidosis: Epidemiology and antibiogram of cases in Singapore. *Singap. Med. J.* **1990**, *31*, 335–337.

15. Lim, M.K.; Tan, E.H.; Soh, C.S.; Chang, T.L. *Burkholderia pseudomallei* infection in the Singapore Armed Forces from 1987 to 1994 - an epidemiological review. *Ann. Acad. Med. Singap.* **1997**, *26*, 13–17. [PubMed]

16. Heng, B.H.; Goh, K.T.; Yap, E.H.; Loh, H.; Yeo, M. Epidemiological surveillance of melioidosis in Singapore. *Ann. Acad Med. Singap.* **1998**, *27*, 478–484. [PubMed]

17. Lo, T.J.; Ang, L.W.; James, L.; Goh, K.T. Melioidosis in a tropical city state, Singapore. *Emerg. Infect. Dis.* **2009**, *15*, 1645–1647. [CrossRef] [PubMed]

18. Pang, L.; Harris, P.N.A.; Seiler, R.L.; Ooi, P.L.; Cutter, J.; Goh, K.T.; Cook, A.R.; Fisher, D.; Chai, L.Y.A. Melioidosis, Singapore, 2003–2014. *Emerg. Infect. Dis.* **2018**, *24*. [CrossRef] [PubMed]

19. Liu, Y.; Loh, J.P.; Aw, L.T.; Yap, E.P.; Lee, M.A.; Ooi, E.E. Rapid molecular typing of *Burkholderia pseudomallei*, isolated in an outbreak of melioidosis in Singapore in 2004, based on variable-number tandem repeats. *Trans. R. Soc. Trop. Med. Hyg.* **2006**, *100*, 687–692. [CrossRef] [PubMed]

20. Yip, S.K.; Ang, B.S.; Tan, J. Clinics in diagnostic imaging (57). *Singap. Med. J.* **2001**, *42*, 41–43.

21. Tan, A.P.; Pui, M.H.; Tan, L.K. Imaging patterns in melioidosis. *Australas. Radiol.* **1995**, *39*, 260–264. [CrossRef] [PubMed]

22. Ng, W.M.; Kwan, M.K.; Merican, A.M. Melioidotic osteomyelitis treated with antibiotic-calcium hydroxyapatite composite: Case report with four-year follow-up. *Singap. Med. J.* **2006**, *47*, 71–74.

23. Amadasi, S.; Dal Zoppo, S.; Bonomini, A.; Bussi, A.; Pedroni, P.; Balestrieri, G.; Signorini, L.; Castelli, F. A case of melioidosis probably acquired by inhalation of dusts during a helicopter flight in a healthy traveler returning from Singapore. *J. Travel. Med.* **2015**, *22*, 57–60. [CrossRef] [PubMed]

24. Li, P.H.; Chau, C.H.; Wong, P.C. Melioidosis mycotic aneurysm: An uncommon complication of an uncommon disease. *Respir. Med. Case Rep.* **2015**, *14*, 43–46. [CrossRef] [PubMed]

25. Rao, J.; Kaushal, A.S.; Hoong, C.K. Abdominal aortic pseudoaneurysm secondary to melioidosis. *Asian J. Surg.* **2009**, *32*, 64–69. [CrossRef]

26. Chlebicki, M.P.; Kurup, A.; Sin, Y.K. *Burkholderia pseudomallei* meningitis following inadequate treatment of melioidotic mycotic aneurysm. *Singap. Med. J.* **2008**, *49*, e219–221.

27. Lath, R.; Rajshekhar, V.; George, V. Brain abscess as the presenting feature of melioidosis. *Br. J. Neurosurg.* **1998**, *12*, 170–172. [CrossRef] [PubMed]

28. Chadwick, D.R.; Ang, B.; Sitoh, Y.Y.; Lee, C.C. Cerebral melioidosis in Singapore: A review of five cases. *Trans. R. Soc. Trop. Med. Hyg.* **2002**, *96*, 72–76. [CrossRef]

29. Limmathurotsakul, D.; Peacock, S.J. Melioidosis: A clinical overview. *Br. Med. Bull.* **2011**, *99*, 125–139. [CrossRef] [PubMed]

30. Chong, W.S. Dermatology in the military field: What physicians should know? *World J. Clin. Cases* **2013**, *1*, 208–211. [CrossRef] [PubMed]

31. Foong, Y.W.; Tan, N.W.; Chong, C.Y.; Thoon, K.C.; Tee, N.W.; Koh, M.J. Melioidosis in children: A retrospective study. *Int. J. Dermatol.* **2015**, *54*, 929–938. [CrossRef] [PubMed]

32. Meumann, E.M.; Novak, R.T.; Gal, D.; Kaestli, M.E.; Mayo, M.; Hanson, J.P.; Spencer, E.; Glass, M.B.; Gee, J.E.; Wilkins, P.P.; et al. Clinical evaluation of a type III secretion system real-time PCR assay for diagnosing melioidosis. *J. Clin. Microbiol.* **2006**, *44*, 3028–3030. [CrossRef] [PubMed]

33. Chantratita, N.; Wuthiekanun, V.; Limmathurotsakul, D.; Thanwisai, A.; Chantratita, W.; Day, N.P.; Peacock, S.J. Prospective clinical evaluation of the accuracy of 16s rRNA real-time PCR assay for the diagnosis of melioidosis. *Am. J. Trop. Med. Hyg.* **2007**, *77*, 814–817. [PubMed]

34. Wuthiekanun, V.; Chierakul, W.; Langa, S.; Chaowagul, W.; Panpitpat, C.; Saipan, P.; Thoujaikong, T.; Day, N.P.; Peacock, S.J. Development of antibodies to *Burkholderia pseudomallei* during childhood in melioidosis-endemic northeast Thailand. *Am. J. Trop. Med. Hyg.* **2006**, *74*, 1074–1075. [PubMed]

35. Yap, E.H.; Chan, Y.C.; Ti, T.Y.; Thong, T.W.; Tan, A.L.; Yeo, M.; Ho, L.C.; Singh, M. Serodiagnosis of melioidosis in Singapore by the indirect haemagglutination test. *Singap. Med. J.* **1991**, *32*, 211–213.

36. Liu, Y.; Sim, S.H.; Wang, D. IHA results on serum samples collected from culture-confirmed melioidosis patients, suspected melioidosis cases presenting to local hospitals and healthy volunteers from 2004 to 2016. Defence Medical and Environmental Research Institute, DSO National Laboratories: Singapore, Unpublished work. 2018.

37. Wiersinga, W.J.; Currie, B.J.; Peacock, S.J. Melioidosis. *N. Engl. J. Med.* **2012**, *367*, 1035–1044. [CrossRef] [PubMed]

38. Chierakul, W.; Anunnatsiri, S.; Short, J.M.; Maharjan, B.; Mootsikapun, P.; Simpson, A.J.; Limmathurotsakul, D.; Cheng, A.C.; Stepniewska, K.; Newton, P.N.; et al. Two randomized controlled trials of ceftazidime alone versus ceftazidime in combination with trimethoprim-sulfamethoxazole for the treatment of severe melioidosis. *Clin. Infect. Dis.* **2005**, *41*, 1105–1113. [CrossRef] [PubMed]

39. Kung, C.T.; Lee, C.H.; Li, C.J.; Lu, H.I.; Ko, S.F.; Liu, J.W. Development of ceftazidime resistance in *Burkholderia pseudomallei* in a patient experiencing melioidosis with mediastinal lymphadenitis. *Ann. Acad. Med. Singap.* **2010**, *39*, 945-3. [PubMed]

40. Fisher, D. Division of infectious diseases, Department of Medicine, National University Health System, Singapore. Unpublished work. 2008.

41. Suputtamongkol, Y.; Chaowagul, W.; Chetchotisakd, P.; Lertpatanasuwun, N.; Intaranongpai, S.; Ruchutrakool, T.; Budhsarawong, D.; Mootsikapun, P.; Wuthiekanun, V.; Teerawatasook, N.; et al. Risk factors for melioidosis and bacteremic melioidosis. *Clin. Infect. Dis.* **1999**, *29*, 408–413. [CrossRef] [PubMed]

42. Liu, X.; Foo, G.; Lim, W.P.; Ravikumar, S.; Sim, S.H.; Win, M.S.; Goh, J.G.; Lim, J.H.; Ng, Y.H.; Fisher, D.; et al. Sulphonylurea usage in melioidosis is associated with severe disease and suppressed immune response. *PLoS Negl. Trop. Dis.* **2014**, *8*, e2795. [CrossRef] [PubMed]

43. *Annual Report 2016/17: Handled with Care*; Agri-Food & Veterinary Authority of Singapore: Singapore, 2017.

44. *Pet Care in Singapore, Industry Overview*; Euromonitor International: Singapore, 2016; pp. 1–55.

45. Sprague, L.D.; Neubauer, H. Melioidosis in animals: A review on epizootiology, diagnosis and clinical presentation. *J. Vet. Med. B. Infect. Dis. Vet. Public Health* **2004**, *51*, 305–320. [CrossRef] [PubMed]

46. Tonpitak, W.; Sornklien, C.; Chawanit, M.; Pavasutthipaisit, S.; Wuthiekanun, V.; Hantrakun, V.; Amornchai, P.; Thaipadungpanit, J.; Day, N.P.; Yingst, S.; et al. Fatal melioidosis in goats in Bangkok, Thailand. *Am. J. Trop. Med. Hyg.* **2014**, *91*, 287–290. [CrossRef] [PubMed]

47. Sim, S.H.; Yu, Y.; Lin, C.H.; Karuturi, R.K.; Wuthiekanun, V.; Tuanyok, A.; Chua, H.H.; Ong, C.; Paramalingam, S.S.; Tan, G.; et al. The core and accessory genomes of *Burkholderia pseudomallei*: Implications for human melioidosis. *PLoS Pathog.* **2008**, *4*, e1000178. [CrossRef] [PubMed]

48. Currie, B.J.; Fisher, D.A.; Howard, D.M.; Burrow, J.N.; Selvanayagam, S.; Snelling, P.L.; Anstey, N.M.; Mayo, M.J. The epidemiology of melioidosis in Australia and Papua New Guinea. *Acta Trop.* **2000**, *74*, 121–127. [CrossRef]

49. Ketterer, P.J.; Webster, W.R.; Shield, J.; Arthur, R.J.; Blackall, P.J.; Thomas, A.D. Melioidosis in intensive piggeries in south eastern Queensland. *Aust. Vet. J.* **1986**, *63*, 146–149. [CrossRef] [PubMed]

50. Xie, S. Conservation, Research and Veterinary Services, Wildlife Reserves Singapore, Singapore. Unpublished work. 2018.

51. Walsh, A.L.; Wuthiekanun, V.; Smith, M.D.; Suputtamongkol, Y.; White, N.J. Selective broths for the isolation of *Pseudomonas pseudomallei* from clinical samples. *Trans. R. Soc. Trop. Med. Hyg.* **1995**, *89*, 124. [CrossRef]

52. Supaprom, C.; Wang, D.; Leelayuwat, C.; Thaewpia, W.; Susaengrat, W.; Koh, V.; Ooi, E.E.; Lertmemongkolchai, G.; Liu, Y. Development of real-time PCR assays and evaluation of their potential use for rapid detection of *Burkholderia pseudomallei* in clinical blood specimens. *J. Clin. Microbiol.* **2007**, *45*, 2894–2901. [CrossRef] [PubMed]

53. Thin, R.N.; Groves, M.; Rapmund, G.; Mariappan, M. *Pseudomonas pseudomallei* in the surface water of Singapore. *Singap. Med. J.* **1971**, *12*, 181–182.

54. Yap, E.H.; Thong, T.W.; Tan, A.L.; Yeo, M.; Tan, H.C.; Loh, H.; Teo, T.P.; Thong, K.T.; Singh, M.; Chan, Y.C. Comparison of *Pseudomonas pseudomallei* from humans, animals, soil and water by restriction endonuclease analysis. *Singap. Med. J.* **1995**, *36*, 60–62.

55. Strauss, J.M.; Groves, M.G.; Mariappan, M.; Ellison, D.W. Melioidosis in Malaysia. Ii. Distribution of *Pseudomonas pseudomallei* in soil and surface water. *Am. J. Trop. Med. Hyg.* **1969**, *18*, 698–702. [CrossRef] [PubMed]

56. Ong, C.E.L.; Koh, V.W.H.; Tan, Y.K.; Wong, M.S.Y.; Chew, J.S.W. Environmental surveillance of B. pseudomallei in Singapore between 2000 and 2013. Defence Medical and Environmental Research Institute, DSO National Laboratories: Singapore, Unpublished work. 2018.

57. Chantratita, N.; Wuthiekanun, V.; Boonbumrung, K.; Tiyawisutsri, R.; Vesaratchavest, M.; Limmathurotsakul, D.; Chierakul, W.; Wongratanacheewin, S.; Pukritiyakamee, S.; White, N.J.; et al. Biological relevance of colony morphology and phenotypic switching by *Burkholderia pseudomallei*. *J. Bacteriol.* **2007**, *189*, 807–817. [CrossRef] [PubMed]

58. Limmathurotsakul, D.; Wuthiekanun, V.; Amornchai, P.; Wongsuwan, G.; Day, N.P.; Peacock, S.J. Effectiveness of a simplified method for isolation of *Burkholderia pseudomallei* from soil. *Appl. Environ. Microbiol.* **2012**, *78*, 876–877. [CrossRef] [PubMed]

59. Currie, B.J.; Price, E.P.; Mayo, M.; Kaestli, M.; Theobald, V.; Harrington, I.; Harrington, G.; Sarovich, D.S. Use of whole-genome sequencing to link *Burkholderia pseudomallei* from air sampling to mediastinal melioidosis, Australia. *Emerg. Infect. Dis.* **2015**, *21*, 2052–2054. [CrossRef] [PubMed]

60. Nandi, T.; Holden, M.T.; Didelot, X.; Mehershahi, K.; Boddey, J.A.; Beacham, I.; Peak, I.; Harting, J.; Baybayan, P.; Guo, Y.; et al. Burkholderia pseudomallei sequencing identifies genomic clades with distinct recombination, accessory, and epigenetic profiles. *Genome Res.* **2015**, *25*, 129–141. [CrossRef] [PubMed]

61. Ong, C.E.L. Correlation of clinical and environmental B. pseudomallei isolates from an island off Singapore. Defence Medical and Environmental Research Institute, DSO National Laboratories: Singapore, Unpublished work. 2018.

62. Sivalingam, S.P.; Sim, S.H.; Aw, L.T.; Ooi, E.E. Antibiotic susceptibility of 50 clinical isolates of *Burkholderia pseudomallei* from Singapore. *J. Antimicrob. Chemother.* **2006**, *58*, 1102–1103. [CrossRef] [PubMed]

63. Tan, A.L.; Tan, M.L. Melioidosis: Antibiogram of cases in Singapore 1987–2007. *Trans. R. Soc. Trop. Med. Hyg.* **2008**, *102* (Suppl. 1), S101–S102. [CrossRef]

64. Lee, Y.H.; Chen, Y.; Ouyang, X.; Gan, Y.H. Identification of tomato plant as a novel host model for *Burkholderia pseudomallei*. *BMC Microbiol.* **2010**, *10*, 28. [CrossRef] [PubMed]

65. Chantratita, N.; Wuthiekanun, V.; Limmathurotsakul, D.; Vesaratchavest, M.; Thanwisai, A.; Amornchai, P.; Tumapa, S.; Feil, E.J.; Day, N.P.; Peacock, S.J. Genetic diversity and microevolution of *Burkholderia pseudomallei* in the environment. *PLoS Negl. Trop. Dis.* **2008**, *2*, e182. [CrossRef] [PubMed]

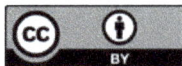

Tropical Medicine and
Infectious Disease

MDPI

Review

Melioidosis in South America

Dionne B. Rolim [1,2,*], **Rachel Ximenes R. Lima** [1], **Ana Karoline C. Ribeiro** [1], **Rafael M. Colares** [1], **Leoniti D. Q. Lima** [1], **Alfonso J. Rodríguez-Morales** [3], **Franco E. Montúfar** [4,5,6] and **David A. B. Dance** [7,8,9]

[1] Post-Graduation Program in Medical Sciences, University of Fortaleza (UNIFOR),
    Fortaleza CE 60811-905, Brazil; quel0505@gmail.com (R.X.R.L.); anakarolfreire@gmail.com (A.K.C.R.);
    rafaelmcolares@gmail.com (R.M.C.); leadanquei@gmail.com (L.D.Q.L.)
[2] Medicine School, Ceara State University (UECE), Fortaleza CE 60714-903, Brazil
[3] Public Health and Infection Research Group, Faculty of Health Sciences, Universidad Tecnologica de Pereira,
    Pereira 660003, Risaralda, Colombia; ajrodriguezmmd@gmail.com
[4] Infectious Diseases Section, Pablo Tobón Uribe Hospital, Medellín 05001000, Colombia;
    frmontufar@yahoo.com
[5] Pulmonology Unit, León XIII Clinic of Antioquia University, Medellín 05001000, Colombia
[6] Research Group in Respiratory and Infectious Diseases (GIERI), Medellín 05001000, Colombia
[7] Lao-Oxford-Mahosot Hospital-Wellcome Trust Research Unit, Microbiology Laboratory, Mahosot Hospital,
    Vientiane, Laos; david.d@tropmedres.ac
[8] Centre for Tropical Medicine & Global Health, University of Oxford, Oxford OX3 7FZ, UK
[9] London School of Hygiene and Tropical Medicine, London WC1E 7HT, UK
*   Correspondence: dionnerolim@unifor.br; Tel.: +55-859-9994-1263

Received: 12 March 2018; Accepted: 31 May 2018; Published: 5 June 2018

Abstract: Melioidosis is an emerging disease in the Americas. This paper reviews confirmed cases, the presence of *Burkholderia pseudomallei* and the organization of national surveillance policies for melioidosis in South America. Confirmed cases in humans have been reported from Ecuador, Venezuela, Colombia, Brazil, and Peru. The bacterium has been isolated from the environment in Brazil and Peru. The state of Ceará, northeastern region of Brazil, is the only place where specific public strategies and policies for melioidosis have been developed. We also discuss the urgent need for health authorities in South America to pay greater attention to this disease, which has the potential to have a high impact on public health, and the importance of developing coordinated strategies amongst countries in this region.

Keywords: melioidosis; *Burkholderia pseudomallei*; South America

1. Introduction

Melioidosis is an infectious disease caused by *Burkholderia pseudomallei*, an environmental bacterium that is being detected with increasing frequency across the world but that has only attracted attention in the Americas in the past few years. Limmathurotsakul et al., in a recent review, estimated that some 165,000 cases of the disease occurred each year in tropical areas of the globe, accounting for approximately 89,000 deaths [1]. In this study, a substantial part of South America, including northern, north-eastern and mid-western regions of Brazil, northeastern Colombia and south-western Venezuela, and parts of Peru, Guyana, Suriname, Paraguay, Bolivia and Argentina, was considered to represent a suitable environment for the bacterium [1].

Melioidosis is known to occur in the American continent; however, the true distribution of the disease is undetermined. In South America, northeastern Brazil is known to be a definite endemic area [1] and, by 2015, it had accounted for 32 of the 48 (67%) published cases from the whole continent (Table 1) [2]. This study broadens the perspective on melioidosis in South America by reviewing reported cases and exploring the organisation of public policies. Despite the relative paucity of published cases, melioidosis undoubtedly deserves to be included in the lists of infectious diseases of potential epidemiologic importance in the region.

Table 1. Published Cases of Melioidosis in South America.

Case	Age	Gender	Year of Diagnosis	Country of Diagnosis	Country Where Infection Was Most Likely Acquired	Outcome	References
1	30	M	1962	Ecuador	Ecuador	Died	[3]
2	50	M	1995	Venezuela	Venezuela	Survived	[4]
3	60	M	1998	Colombia	Colombia	Survived	[5]
4	65	M	1998	Colombia	Colombia	Survived	[5]
5	50	M	2000	Venezuela	Venezuela	Survived	[4]
6	66	M	2003	Portugal	Venezuela	Survived	[6]
7	10	F	2003	Colombia	Colombia	Died	[5]
8	40	M	2003	Colombia	Colombia	Died	[5]
9	15	M	2003	Brazil	Brazil	Died	[7–10]
10	14	F	2003	Brazil	Brazil	Died	[7–10]
11	10	M	2003	Brazil	Brazil	Died	[7–10]
12	12	F	2003	Brazil	Brazil	Survived	[7–10]
13	50	M	2003	Netherlands	Brazil	Died	[11]
14	46	F	2004	Colombia	Colombia	Survived	[5]
15	28	M	2005	Spain	Colombia	Survived	[5]
16	52	M	2005	Colombia	Colombia	Survived	[5]
17	17	F	2005	Brazil	Brazil	Survived	[12]
18	30	M	2005	Brazil	Brazil	Died	[2,13]
19	22	M	2008	Colombia	Colombia	Survived	[14]
20	17	M	2008	Brazil	Brazil	Died	[15]
21	69	M	2008	Brazil	Brazil	Died	[16,17]
22	48	M	2009	Brazil	Brazil	Survived	[17]
23	47	M	2010	Brazil	Brazil	Survived	[17]
24	28	M	2010	Brazil	Brazil	Died	[18]
25	29	M	2010	Brazil	Brazil	Died	[2]
26	56	M	2010	Brazil	Brazil	Survived	[2]
27	53	M	2011	Brazil	Brazil	Survived	[2]
28	3	M	2011	Brazil	Brazil	Died	[2]
29	56	M	2011	Brazil	Brazil	Died	[2]
30	7	M	2011	Brazil	Brazil	Survived	[2]
31	29	M	2011	Brazil	Brazil	Survived	[2]
32	21	M	2012	Brazil	Brazil	Died	[2]
33	82	F	2012	Brazil	Brazil	Died	[2]
34	31	M	2012	Colombia	Colombia	Survived	[5]
35	36	M	2013	Colombia	Colombia	Survived	[19,20]
36	19	F	2016	Peru	Peru	Died	[21]
37	68	M	2013	Brazil	Brazil	Died	[2]
38	57	M	2014	Brazil	Brazil	Died	[2]
39	42	M	2014	Brazil	Brazil	Survived	[2]
40	57	M	2014	Brazil	Brazil	Survived	[2]
41	50	M	2014	Brazil	Brazil	Died	[2]
41	72	M	2014?	Colombia	Colombia	Survived	[22]
42	42	M	2015	Brazil	Brazil	Survived	[2]
43	13	F	2015	Brazil	Brazil	Died	[23]
44	64	M	2016	Brazil	Brazil	Survived	[23]
45	58	M	2016	Brazil	Brazil	Died	[23]
46	54	M	2016	Brazil	Brazil	Survived	[23]
47	100	M	2017	Brazil	Brazil	Died	[23]
48	4	F	2017	Brazil	Brazil	Survived	[23]

2. Review of Published Melioidosis Cases and the Presence of *B. pseudomallei*

In 1962, in Ecuador, Biegeleisen reported the first case of melioidosis in South America [3]. Fifteen years later, French researchers reported the isolation of *B. pseudomallei* from Brazilian and Peruvian soil [24,25]. Since these early descriptions, only sporadic human cases of melioidosis had been reported in four countries by the 1990s: Venezuela, Colombia, Brazil and Peru (in order of first reporting)

(Figure 1) [2,13,21]. A genetic study, which included isolates from Ecuador, Venezuela and Brazil, suggested that isolates of *B. pseudomallei* from Central and South America probably had an African origin and were most likely imported between 1650 and 1850, as a result of colonization and the slave trade [26].

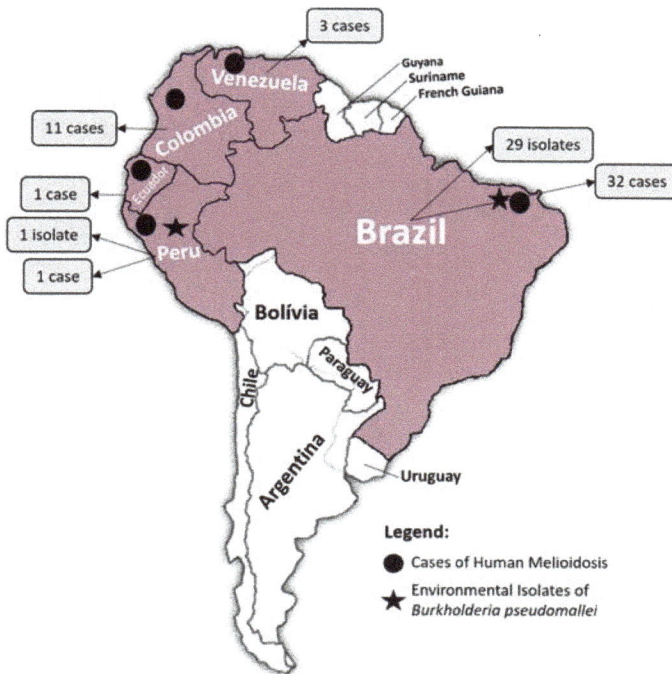

Figure 1. Melioidosis in South America.

2.1. Venezuela, Colombia and Peru

Three cases of human melioidosis have been described in Venezuela from 1995 to 2003 [4,6]. In Colombia, after the first report in 1998 [27], a total of 11 further cases have been described up to 2015 (Table 1) [1–6,13,14,19–22,24–29]. Initially, the reports were clustered in the region of Antioquia, where there is a university referral hospital, although two cases were reported from other regions. In Peru, despite the initial report of environmental isolation, it was not until 2016 that the first human case was reported [21].

2.2. Brazil

The first documented cases of melioidosis in Brazil occurred in 2003 in the state of Ceará, located in the Northeastern region. Four siblings acquired acute infection after recreational exposure at the town dam and three of them died within a week [7–10]. By 2017, 30 cases had been diagnosed in Ceará [2,11,15–18,23]. Characterisation of clinical and environmental *B. pseudomallei* from Ceará showed that considerable genetic diversity is present [30]. Apart from this, there are only two other states with confirmed cases in Brazil: a case reported in 2007 in the state of Mato Grosso, located in the Midwestern region [12] and the other in Alagoas, also located in Northeastern region (Figure 2) [2].

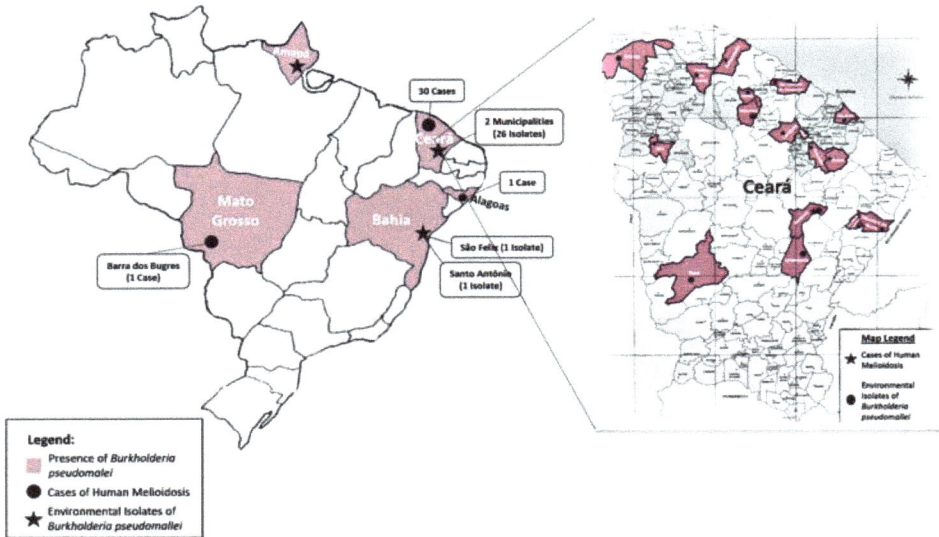

Figure 2. Melioidosis in Brazil.

2.3. Environmental Isolation

Besides the environmental isolation of *B. pseudomallei* reported in Peru and Brazil in 1977 [25], it has also been isolated in the Brazilian states of Ceará [31] and Amapá [32], located in the Northern region. The first attempts at environmental isolation in Brazil were made in 1973 in rice plantations in rural São Paulo, but these were unsuccessful [33].

2.4. Animal Melioidosis

There have been no reports of melioidosis in animals anywhere in South America.

3. Surveillance and Public Policies in South America

Limmathurotsakul et al. estimated the respective annual incidence and mortality of melioidosis in South American countries to be as follows: Brazil, 872 and 339; Colombia, 157 and 64; Venezuela, 103 and 40; Peru, 39 and 16; Argentina, 18 and 7; Paraguay, 13 and 5; and Bolivia, 13 and 7. [1]. These numbers are relatively small in comparison to the estimated number of cases in Asia. Nonetheless, if accurate this means that more than 1200 cases and nearly 500 deaths could be occurring annually in South America, the majority of which are going undetected and untreated. So whilst it is clearly not the top priority for public health authorities in the region, melioidosis still warrants some attention. What, then, is the position in South America as far as public health policies are concerned?

Fifteen years have passed since melioidosis was first diagnosed and documented in Brazil. There is not, however, any national recognition of it as a public health problem. Undoubtedly there are many reasons why melioidosis has not been prioritized. Other well-known and high-impact infectious diseases, such as chikungunya and Zika virus infection, have competed for attention and resources. Ceará is the only state that has developed specific policies and undertaken research into the disease. The first plan was established in 2004 following the family cluster described above, with the proposal of epidemiologic surveillance for the Secretaria de Saúde do Ceará (SESA), a government organization [34]. This document led to the publication of decree 1786/2005 establishing melioidosis as compulsorily notifiable in the state. Although there is an official national list of notifiable diseases, each federal unit has the autonomy to make its own list according to local needs. Since then, measures to enhance surveillance and management of melioidosis in Ceará have been established gradually, such as the development of a complete protocol in Brazilian Portuguese covering issues such as: definition of a suspect case, notification and environmental investigations; procedures for diagnosis and treatment, workflows for the submission of laboratory samples, and recommendations for prevention. Other activities were developed: professional training materials, dissemination of information about melioidosis at local, regional and national scientific events, research and development, the use of new media and educational technology (for example, the establishment of a web site: https://www.melioidose.com.br), trials of developing prospective surveillance in health services, and raising laboratory diagnostic capacity. However, it would be fair to say that the success of these initiatives has been limited. Professional awareness remains restricted to small groups of physicians in Fortaleza, the state capital of Ceará. In addition, the general population does not know about the disease, with rare exceptions such as in the locations where cases have been confirmed.

The scarcity and limited capabilities of microbiology laboratories in most regions of Brazil is also important in this respect. Preliminary studies in Ceará have demonstrated that few laboratories are able to identify *B. pseudomallei*. In this state, most cases have occurred in small communities and the diagnosis was only made when patients were transferred to larger reference centres located in Fortaleza or the northern and southern regions of the state.

As far as the rest of South America is concerned, there are no policies relating to melioidosis and no formal surveillance for the disease. Even in Colombia, where the greatest number of cases outside Brazil have been detected, there are currently no specific or general public policies relating to melioidosis.Currently, in Colombia the National Institute of Health conducts indirect surveillance through the surveillance of antimicrobial resistance, but melioidosis is not statutorily notifiable and is thus likely to be under-recognised. However, a pilot study to identify cases of melioidosis in Colombia has recently been initiated. This collaborative study involving the US CDC, Tephinet, the National Institute of Health and some of the larger referral hospitals in Antioquia, will develop an epidemiological surveillance protocol and attempt to identify new cases of melioidosis, which will be confirmed using techniques such as MALDI-TOF and molecular methods.Once the collaborative project is completed, the newly identified cases and a more formal melioidosis surveillance program for Colombia will be announced. Concern over the emergence of melioidosis recently led to the first meeting focused on 'Melioidosis in the Americas' in Bogota in April 2018, which was attended by representatives from Brazil, Colombia, Dominican Republic, Ecuador, Haiti, Panama, Paraguay, Peru, Puerto Rico, Trinidad and Tobago, and the USA. A pamphlet on melioidosis in Spanish was developed, which could used by public health stakeholders to improve recognition of the disease in Latin America. It is hoped that this meeting will be the basis for further collaborations and perhaps even a regional network to share information to improve melioidosis surveillance.

4. Current Challenges and Perspective

The biggest challengesrelating to melioidosis in South America are:

1.   To raise professional and government awareness that this disease is present.
2.   To alert clinicians to the fact that its early detection is critical if lives are to be saved.

In Ceará, new approaches have been designed such as the inclusion of melioidosis in the curriculum of professional physicians, and the development of capacity amongst laboratory staff. The Brazilian health system is organized according to the Sistema Único de Saúde (SUS), geared to address the priorities for the local population. A recent pilot study involved the provision of information about melioidosis to community health agents in cities and towns in rural areas. These agents are part of the Family Health Strategy, a pillar of the development of primary care. Historically, these professionals have played a major role in reducing the mortality from infectious diseases in infants, such as diarrhoea, pneumonia, and measles [35]. Considering the environmental, social and geographic context of melioidosis, it is possible that using this network might help to raise the awareness of melioidosis in the wider community. Lessons learned in Brazil might then be extended to the rest of the continent. In addition, efforts should be made to integrate melioidosis into the infectious diseases agenda of pan-American meetings and organisations such as the Pan-American Health Organisation, in order to raise the profile of the disease and to initiate discussions with national public health organisations, universities and academic communities across the continent. Consideration should be given to making the disease notifiable in countries where it is predicted to be present.

An additional problem for South America is the relative under-development of the diagnostic microbiology sector. This is not something that warrants specific attention as far as melioidosis is concerned, but as laboratory capacity across the continent improves, it will be important to ensure that technicians are trained in the isolation and identification of *B. pseudomallei*. It is hoped that developments in Brazil and Colombia, and the recent meeting in Bogota, will help to catalyse the development of an integrated laboratory network among South American countries.

Although melioidosis is a relatively new disease to South America and the numbers of confirmed cases are as yet small, it is likely that it is being substantially under-diagnosed. It is only by sharing experiences about organizing and planning surveillance activities in different places, taking into consideration the individuality of each set of circumstances, that we may begin to understand the size and extent of the problem. Shared dialogue, discussion and co-ordinated actions in both Portuguese and Spanish may be the first step to reach the goal. We believe that it is essential that health authorities (national, state and municipal) should pay attention to this emerging problem. Investment in strategies already initiated must continue if the lack of knowledge about melioidosis in the continent is to be addressed.

Acknowledgments: Thanks go to the Fundação Cearense de Apoio ao Desenvolvimento Cientifico e Tecnológico (FUNCAP-Programa de Pesquisa para SUS(PPSUS)-13695866-4) for financial support.

Conflicts of Interest: The authors declare no conflict of interest.

References

1. Limmathurotsakul, D.; Golding, N.; Dance, D.A.B.; Messina, J.P.; Pigott, D.M.; Moyes, C.L.; Rolim, D.B.; Bertherat, E.; Day, N.P.J.; Peacock, S.J.; et al. Predicted global distribution of *Burkholderia pseudomallei* and burden of melioidosis. *Nat. Microbiol.* **2016**, *1*, 15008. [CrossRef] [PubMed]

2. Benoit, T.; Blaney, D.D.; Doker, T.J.; Gee, J.E.; Mindy, G.; Elrod, M.; Rolim, D.B.; Inglis, T.J.J.; Hoffmaster, A.R.; Bower, A.W.; et al. Review article: A review of melioidosis cases in the Americas. *Am. J. Trop. Med. Hyg.* **2015**, *93*, 1134–1139. [CrossRef] [PubMed]

3. Biegeleisen, J.Z., Jr.; Mosquera, R.; Cherry, W.B. A case of human melioidosis: Clinical, epidemiological and laboratory findings. *Am. J. Trop. Med. Hyg.* **1964**, *13*, 89–99. [CrossRef] [PubMed]

4. Redondo, M.C.; Gómez, M.; Landaeta, M.E.; Ríos, H.; Khalil, R.; Guevara, R.N.; Palavecino, S.; Figuera, M.; Caldera, J.; Rivera, R.; et al. Melioidosis presenting as sepsis syndrome: A case report. *Int. J. Infect. Dis.* **2011**, *15*, E217–E218. [CrossRef] [PubMed]

5. Montufar, F.E.; Ochoa, J.E.; Ortega, H.; Franco, L.; Montufar, M.C.; Monsalve, A.; Jaramillo, C.; Zapata, M. Melioidosis in Antioquia, Colombia: An emerging or endemic disease? A cases series. *Int. J. Infect. Dis.* **2015**, *37*, 50–57. [CrossRef] [PubMed]

6. Magalhaes, S.; Paiva, A.; Henrique, R.; Koch, A. Melioidose; diagnostico diferencial de tumor renal. *Acta Urol.* **2003**, *2*, 31.

7. Miralles, I.S.; do Carmo Alves Maciel, M.; Angelo, M.R.F.; Gondini, M.M.; Frota, L.H.F.; dos Reis, C.M.F.; Hofer, E. *Burkholderia pseudomallei*: A case report of a human infection in Ceara, Brazil. *Rev. Inst. Med. Trop. São Paulo* **2004**, *46*, 51–54. [CrossRef] [PubMed]

8. Rolim, D.B.; Vilar, D.C.; Sousa, A.Q.; Miralles, I.S.; de Oliveira, D.; Harnett, G.; O'Reilly, L.; Howard, K.; Sampson, I.; Inglis, T.J.J. Melioidosis, northeastern Brazil. *Emerg. Infect. Dis.* **2005**, *11*, 1458–1460. [CrossRef] [PubMed]

9. Braga, M.D.; Almeida, P.R. First description of an autopsied case of melioidosis in Ceara State. *Rev. Soc. Bras. Med. Trop.* **2005**, *38*, 58–60. [CrossRef] [PubMed]

10. Virginio, C.G.; Teixeira, M.F.; Frota, C.C.; Café, V.S.; Rocha, M.F.; Sidrim, J.J. Phenotypic characterization of three clinical isolates of *Burkholderia pseudomallei* in Ceara, Brazil. *Mem. Inst. Oswaldo Cruz* **2006**, *101*, 95–97. [CrossRef] [PubMed]

11. Aardema, H.; Luijnenburg, E.M.; Salm, E.F.; Bijlmer, H.A.; Visser, C.E.; Van'tWout, J.W. Changing epidemiology of melioidosis? A case of acute pulmonary melioidosis with fatal outcome imported from Brazil. *Epidemiol. Infect.* **2005**, *133*, 871–875. [CrossRef] [PubMed]

12. Barth, A.L.; Silva, F.A.; Hoffmann, A.; Vieira, M.I.; Zavascki, A.P.; Ferreira, A.; da Cunha, L.G., Jr.; Albano, R.M.; de Andrade Marques, E. Cystic fibrosis patient with *Burkholderia pseudomallei* infection acquired in Brazil. *J. Clin. Microbiol.* **2007**, *45*, 4077–4080. [CrossRef] [PubMed]

13. Inglis, T.J.; Rolim, D.B.; Sousa, AQ. Melioidosis in the Americas. *Am. J. Trop. Med. Hyg.* **2006**, *75*, 947–954. [PubMed]

14. Gonzalez, G.; Mantilla, W.A.; Rada, R. Neumonía y osteomielitis por *Burkholderia pseudomallei*, reporte de un casoclínico. *Rev. Med.* **2009**, *17*, 146–149.

15. Couto, M.S.; de AguiarCordeiro, R.; Rocha, M.F.; Grangeiro, T.B.; Leitao Junior, N.P.; de Jesus Pinheiro Gomes Bandeira, T.; Sidrim, J.J.C.; Brilhante, R.S.N. A diagnosis of *Burkholderia pseudomallei* directly in a bronchoalveolar lavage by polymerase chain reaction. *Diagn. Microbiol. Infect. Dis.* **2009**, *65*, 73–75. [CrossRef] [PubMed]

16. Sidrim, J.J.; Rocha, M.F.; Bandeira, T.J.; Cordeiro, R.A.; Carvalho, B.M.; Grangeiro, T.B.; Holanda, M.A.; Valente, L.G.; Costa, A.K.; Brilhante, R.S. Mycotic aneurysm caused by *Burkholderia pseudomallei*: Report of a Brazilian strain genetically related to Thai strains. *Clin. Microbiol. Infect.* **2011**, *17*, 719–721. [CrossRef] [PubMed]

17. Brilhante, R.S.; Bandeira, T.J.; Cordeiro, R.A.; Grangeiro, T.B.; Lima, R.A.; Ribeiro, J.F.; Castelo-Branco, D.S.; Rodrigues, J.; Coelho, I.C.; Magalhães, F.G.; et al. Clinical-epidemiological features of 13 cases of melioidosis in Brazil. *J. Clin. Microbiol.* **2012**, *50*, 3349–3352. [CrossRef] [PubMed]

18. Macedo, R.N.; Rocha, F.A.; Rolim, D.B.; Vilar, D.C.; Araújo, F.M.; Vieira, N.N.; Teixeira, J.R.; Carvalho, M.C.; Oliveira, F.G.; Cavalcanti, L.P. Severe coinfection of melioidosis and dengue fever in northeastern Brazil: First case report. *Rev. Soc. Bras. Med. Trop.* **2012**, *45*, 132–133. [CrossRef] [PubMed]

19. Arellano, C.H.R.; Gómez, G.; Sanjuán, O.I.G. Cough and dyspnea during six years in a young adult with chronic pulmonary melioidosis: Case report. *Med. Lab.* **2013**, *19*, 1–8.

20. Nasner-Posso, K.M.; Cruz-Calderon, S.; Rodriguez-Morales, A.J.; Montufar-Andrade, F.E. Melioidosis: A sporadic or an emerging disease in Colombia? *Enferm. Infecc. Microbiol. Clin.* **2015**, *33*, 206–207. [CrossRef] [PubMed]

21. ProMEDmail. Melioidosis—Peru. 2016. Available online: http://www.promedmail.org/post/4624371 (accessed on 15 February 2018).

22. Carmona, H.E.O.; Duran, L.F. Melioidosis: A case report in the department of Huila—Colombia. *RFS Rev. Fac. Salud Univ. Surcolomb.* **2014**, *6*, 56–59. [CrossRef]

23. Rolim, D.B.; Rodrigues, J.L.N.; Vilar, D.C.F.L.; Ribeiro, A.K.C.; Castelo-Branco, D.S.; Bandeira, T.J.; Cordeiro, R.A.; Brilhante, R.S.; Gonçalves, A.L.M.; Cavalcanti, V.; et al. The epidemiology and clinical spectrum of melioidosis in Brazil: A fifteen-year review. (manuscript in preparation).

24. Galimand, M.; Dodin, A. Le point sur la mélioïdose dans le monde. *Bull. Soc. Path.* **1982**, *75*, 375–383.

25. Dance, D.A. Melioidosis: The tip of the iceberg? *Clin. Microbiol. Rev.* **1991**, *4*, 52–60. [CrossRef] [PubMed]

26. Chewapreecha, C.; Holden, M.T.; Vehkala, M.; Valimaki, N.; Yang, Z.; Harris, S.R.; Mather, A.E.; Tuanyok, A.; De Smet, B.; Le Hello, S.; et al. Global and regional dissemination and evolution of *Burkholderia pseudomallei*. *Nat. Microbiol.* **2017**, *2*, 16263. [CrossRef] [PubMed]

27. Severiche, D. *Pseudomonas pseudomallei* community acquired pneumonia. *Rev. Colomb. Neumol.* **1998**, *10*, 188–192.

28. Montufar, F.E.; Acosta, J.O.; Ortega, H.; Franco, L. Melioidosis in Colombia. An emerging disease. *Chest* **2011**, *140*, 753A. [CrossRef]

29. Guzman-Gomez, L.; Agudo Bilbao, M.; Peiro-Callizo, E.; Salas, C. Melioidosis imported from Colombia to Spain. *Enferm. Infecc. Microbiol. Clin.* **2015**, *33*, 214–216. [CrossRef] [PubMed]

30. Bandeira, T.D.J.P.G.; Castelo-Branco, D.D.S.C.M.; Rocha, M.F.G.; Cordeiro, R.D.A.; Ocadaque, C.J.; Paiva, M.D.A.N.; Brilhante, R.S.N.; Sidrim, J.J.C. Clinical and environmental isolates of *Burkholderia pseudomallei* from Brazil: Genotyping and detection of virulence gene. *Asian Pac. J. Trop. Med.* **2017**, *10*, 945–951. [CrossRef] [PubMed]

31. Rolim, D.B.; Rocha, M.F.G.; Brilhante, R.S.N.; Cordeiro, R.A.; Leitão-Junior, N.P.; Inglis, T.J.J.; Sidrim, J.J.C. Environmental Isolates of *Burkholderia pseudomallei* in Ceará State, Northeastern Brazil. *Appl. Environ. Microbiol.* **2009**, *75*, 215–1218. [CrossRef] [PubMed]

32. Sousa, V.Y.K.; Segovia, J.F.O.; Martins Junior, P.O.; Bezerra, R.S.; Gonçalves, M.C.A.; Pereira, S.W.M.; Vallim, D.C.; Carvalho-Assef, A.P.D.; Hofer, E.; Kanzaki, L.I.B. Molecular studies of the first report of *Burkholderia pseudomallei* isolation from soil collected in the Amapá State, in Northern Brazil. *Int. J. Biol.* **2016**, *8*, 1. [CrossRef]

33. De Castro, A.F.; Campedelli Filho, O.; Giorgi, W.; Rosa, C.A. Melioidosis and its causative agent: *Pseudomonas pseudomallei*. *Rev. Inst. Med. Trop. São Paulo* **1973**, *15*, 43–49. [PubMed]

34. Rolim, D.B. Epidemiological study of first melioidosis outbreak in Brazil. Master's Thesis, Universidade Federal do Ceará, Fortaleza, Brazil, 2004.

35. Mendas, E.V. 25 anos do Sistema Único de Saúde: Resultados e desafios. *Estud. Avançados* **2013**, *27*, 27–34. [CrossRef]

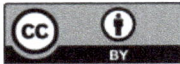

Tropical Medicine and Infectious Disease

MDPI

Article

Melioidosis in Sri Lanka

Enoka M. Corea [1,*] [iD], **Aruna Dharshan de Silva** [2] [iD] and **Vasanthi Thevanesam** [3]

1   Faculty of Medicine, University of Colombo, Colombo 00800, Sri Lanka
2   Faculty of Medicine, Kotelawala Defence University, Ratmalana 10390, Sri Lanka; dslv90@yahoo.com
3   Faculty of Medicine, University of Peradeniya, Peradeniya 2000, Sri Lanka; vasanthithevanesam@yahoo.com
*   Correspondence: enokac@micro.cmb.ac.lk or enokacorea@hotmail.com; Tel.: +94-777-808-439

Received: 31 January 2018; Accepted: 16 February 2018; Published: 21 February 2018

Abstract: Until recently, Sri Lanka was not considered a country with endemic melioidosis. However, an increasing number of cases is being reported. National surveillance for melioidosis was instituted after 2008. A total of 250 culture-positive cases was recorded between 2006 and May 2017. Males predominated (71.6%). The age range was wide (2–92 years) reflecting a ubiquity of exposure. The majority (201/250, 80%) lived in rural areas. All provinces were affected. Case load increased during the two monsoonal periods (67%). There was representation of every population group including farmers (n = 44), housewives (n = 24), school children (n = 10), professionals (n = 5), businesspersons (n = 6), white-collar workers (n = 10) and blue-collar workers (n = 8). Diabetes was the predominant risk factor (n = 163, 65.2%). Clinical presentations included community-acquired sepsis and pneumonia, superficial and deep abscesses, and septic arthritis. Mortality was 20.4% (51/250). A majority (n = 212) of isolates belonged to the YLF (Yersinia-like fimbrial) clade but 38 were BTFC (*B. thailandensis*-like flagellum and chemotaxis). A total of 108 isolates was genotyped and 46 sequence types (STs) were identified, 40 being novel. It is clear that melioidosis is endemic in Sri Lanka with a wide geographic and demographic distribution. There is an urgent need to extend surveillance of melioidosis to under-resourced parts of the country and to populations at high risk.

Keywords: melioidosis; Sri Lanka; epidemiology; *Burkholderia pseudomallei*

1. Introduction and History of Melioidosis in the Country

Sri Lanka lies in the tropics, between 5–10° N of the equator, and within the melioidosis belt. Rice and rice flour comprise the staple diet. Paddy lands are scattered throughout the island where the predominant form of agriculture is rice farming in smallholdings, using traditional farming methods.

Sri Lanka (then Ceylon) (1927), followed British Malaya (now Malaysia and Singapore) (1921) and Cochin China (now Vietnam) (1925/6) as one of the first countries to report melioidosis, after its initial description in Rangoon, Burma (now Myanmar) in 1912 [1]. This report of fatal melioidosis in a European tea broker resident in Sri Lanka was the first from the Indian subcontinent [2] and led to the country being identified as an endemic area [3]. However, this early account was not followed by any further cases. A limited sero-epidemiological survey in hospital-associated populations in 1972 concluded that the disease was unlikely to be of major public health importance in Sri Lanka [4].

Reviews on the global epidemiology of melioidosis and maps depicting the known endemicity of melioidosis included Ceylon/Sri Lanka as an endemic area, based on this single case. Redfearn et al. [5] included Ceylon (Sri Lanka) in their classic map (later reproduced in a much-quoted review by Howe et al. [6]) as an area from which bacteriologically diagnosed cases of melioidosis had been reported. Leelarasamee [7] and Leelarasamee and Bovornkitti [8] listed Sri Lanka as an area where active cases of melioidosis had been seen. Dance, in 1991 [9], comprehensively reviewed the situation in Sri Lanka, identifying it as an area with sporadic isolates but, later, did not specifically refer to it in an update in 2000, probably due to a lack of subsequent cases [10]. Cheng and Currie [11] classified

Sri Lanka, in their review of 2005, as belonging to an 'area with sporadic case reports'. However, a few years later, in spite of the lack of further cases, Currie et al. [12] mapped Sri Lanka (along with the whole Indian subcontinent) as an area endemic for melioidosis and this was echoed by Wiersinga et al. in 2012 [13].

Seven decades after the first case of melioidosis was reported from Sri Lanka, sporadic reports began to surface of infection acquired in Sri Lanka. This included a report of brain and lung abscesses in a Belgian tourist, who had visited the country shortly before his illness [14], infection of a leg wound sustained in the 2004 Indian Ocean tsunami in an Australian man holidaying in Sri Lanka [15], and fatal septicaemia in a Sri Lankan male reported in 2006 [16]. This raised the possibility that melioidosis might be emerging in parts of Sri Lanka. As a result of a World Health Organization-supported laboratory-twinning project, additional cases were confirmed in the Central and Western Provinces in 2006 and 2008 [17,18] and surveillance for melioidosis was commenced. Recently, further cases from Sri Lanka, diagnosed locally and overseas, have been published [19–35].

2. Review of Melioidosis Cases and Presence of *B. pseudomallei* in the Country

A national network of clinical microbiology laboratories in the state and private sector was established. A case definition for surveillance and a laboratory work-up procedure for the routine culture of specimens and preliminary identification of suspected isolates was drawn up. Reference laboratory facilities for confirmation of isolates by polymerase chain reaction (PCR) for the *LPxO* gene [36] and serological testing for antibodies by the indirect haemagglutination assay (IHA) [37] were set up. A standard questionnaire for the collection of demographic, geographic and clinical data was designed. Ethics approval for the study was obtained from the Ethics Review Committee, Faculty of Medicine, University of Colombo.

Primary isolation relied on conventional culture techniques for blood and other sterile fluids, pus, and occasional soft-tissue specimens on routine culture media such as blood and MacConkey agar. Selective agar was not used for specimens from sites with normal flora so it is possible that some cases may have been missed. Suspected *B. pseudomallei* isolates were referred to the reference laboratory for confirmation by PCR. Awareness was raised, chiefly among clinical microbiologists, through lectures, presentations and publications, e-mails and personal communication.

Between 2006 and March 2017, 250 culture-positive cases of melioidosis were identified by the surveillance programme. More than a hundred additional cases were diagnosed and treated as melioidosis on the basis of high antibody titres in the IHA test. However, this article will describe only the culture-confirmed cases.

The number of culture-positive cases increased from year to year (Figure 1).

Melioidosis was prevalent throughout the island with all 9 provinces affected, the highest number being from the Western (*n* = 88), North-Western (*n* = 54) and Eastern (*n* = 33) provinces (Figure 2a). There were no cases at higher elevations (Figure 2b) and only a few cases in the Northern Province, where microbiology services are limited.

The age range of patients was wide (2–92 years), reflecting the ubiquity of soil exposure in the Sri Lankan population (Figure 3).

The majority of patients were men (71.6%), as seen in other settings, probably reflecting occupational soil exposure in a predominantly agricultural society. Unsurprisingly, rural populations were chiefly affected (201/250, 80%). However, only 44 patients were farmers and there was representation of every population group including housewives (*n* = 24), school children (*n* = 10), professionals (including physicians and school principals) (*n* = 5), businesspersons (*n* = 6), white-collar workers including irrigation officers, technicians and clerks (*n* = 10) and blue-collar workers (*n* = 8, including labourers and construction workers). Nine patients (7%) belonged to the defence forces (army, police or civil defence) and 15 (12%) were drivers. Many gave a history of involvement in cultivation. Therefore, melioidosis in Sri Lanka seems not to be a disease limited to rice farmers but an infection related to the outdoor, agricultural, barefoot lifestyle still practised by the majority of the population. The large number of drivers, especially three-wheeler drivers and motorcyclists, in this series is intriguing and a possible explanation is exposure to dust containing *B. pseudomallei*.

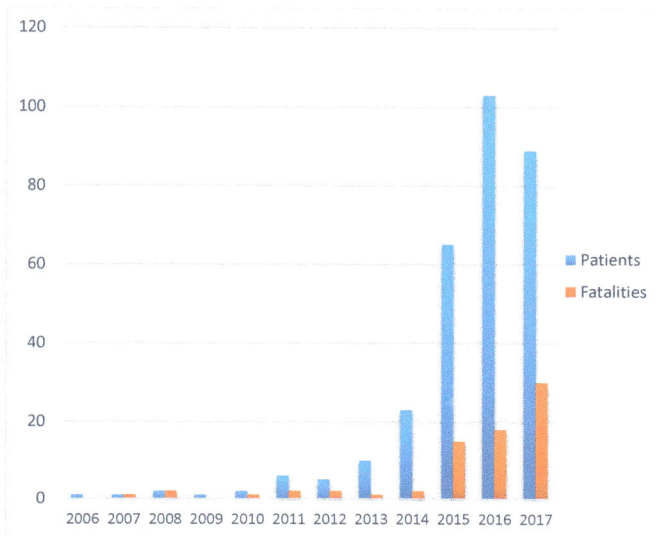

Figure 1. Annual incidence of cases and fatalities (2017 data only up to March).

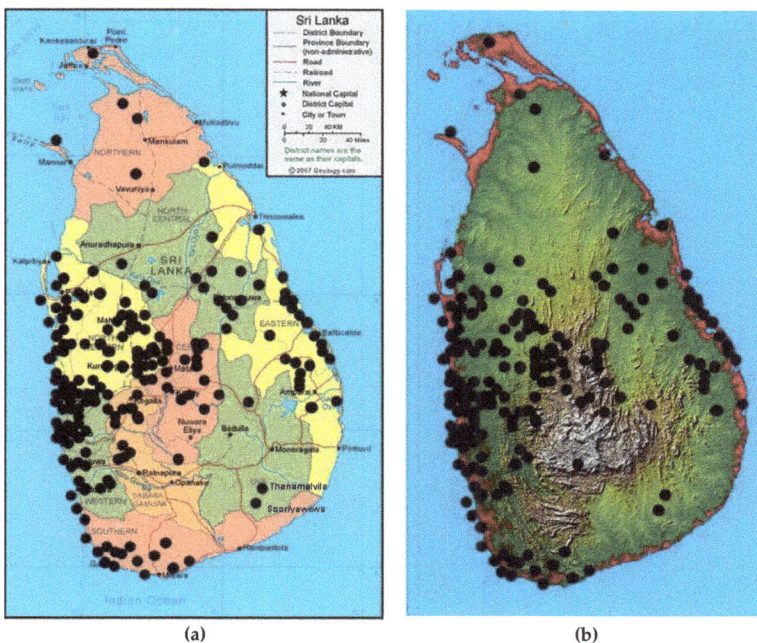

Figure 2. Geographical distribution of melioidosis cases in Sri Lanka. (**a**) By province. (**b**) By topography.

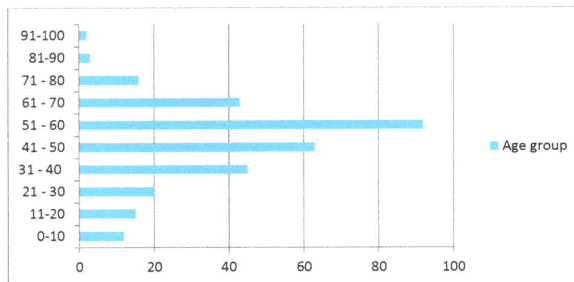

Figure 3. Age distribution of patients with melioidosis in Sri Lanka.

While diabetes was the predominant risk factor, found in 163 cases (65.2%), other organ disease and alcoholism were seen, and thalassemia was a significant risk in children, seen in 3 of our 10 children. Other, more unusual, predisposing causes included IgA nephropathy, dengue haemorrhagic fever, systemic lupus erythematosus (SLE) on prednisolone therapy, and lepromatous leprosy. However, melioidosis was also seen in healthy adults and children with no obvious risk factors (n = 30, 13.2%).

As expected, clinical presentations were varied, ranging from acute sepsis to chronic abscess formation, reflecting the protean nature of this infection and manifesting in the full gamut of its clinical features (Figure 4). As in other series, lung infections predominated followed by musculoskeletal infections including septic arthritis, muscle abscesses and osteomyelitis and abdominal involvement, chiefly abscesses of the liver, spleen or psoas muscle. Skin and soft-tissue abscesses followed. While more than half the patients were blood culture-positive and septic, a few presented with septicaemia only without any obvious focus. Central nervous system infection was seen in the form of meningitis, subdural empyema, cerebral abscess, brain-stem encephalitis, transverse myelitis, Guillain Barré syndrome and status epilepticus. Genitourinary involvement was seen presenting as urinary tract infection or prostatitis. The lymph nodes and salivary glands were the site of infection in many patients. The cardiovascular system was also affected, with one patient presenting with pericardial effusion and one with endocarditis, an extremely rare presentation reported only twice previously in the literature [38,39]. Most patients had involvement of more than one organ or system.

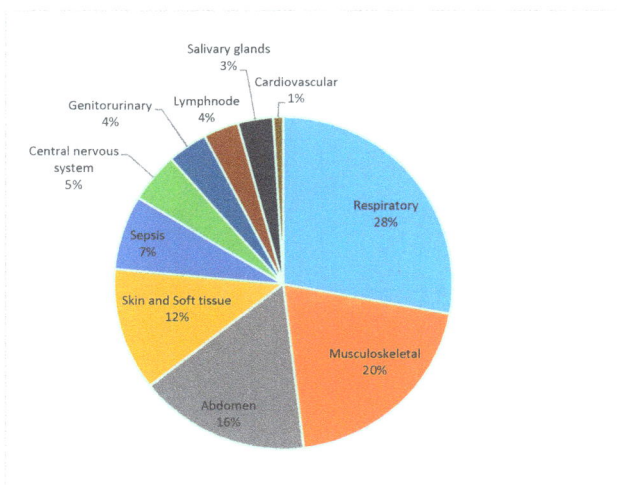

Figure 4. Systems affected by melioidosis in Sri Lankan patients.

It is of note that many patients showed involvement of the lower limbs such as septic arthritis, psoas muscle abscess and cellulitis. Septic arthritis was the primary presentation or complicated the clinical course of many patients. This may reflect bacterial entry by inoculation into the lower limbs consistent with a barefoot lifestyle.

The overall mortality was 20.4% (51/250). This compares favourably with the mortality of melioidosis in northern Australia (14%), as opposed to the mortality in Thailand (49%). However, it is far higher than the 9% mortality recorded in the latter stages of the 20-year study in Darwin [40]. Eight patients had recurrence during this period, including two who had recrudescent disease within two months of discharge whilst on eradication therapy, and four who had recurrences 6 months to 3 years after recovery (the time to recurrence was unknown in two). It is likely that some recurrences were due to non-compliance with the lengthy oral treatment required in the 'eradication phase'.

Looking more closely at the geographical distribution of this infection, melioidosis was present in the wet, intermediate, dry and even arid zones of Sri Lanka. When charting seasonal trends based on rainfall, particularly the south-western and north-eastern monsoons, it was seen that cases occur throughout the year with a trend of two peaks during the monsoons (67% of cases) (Figure 5). This is consistent with studies in many other countries that have shown increased numbers of cases during the rainy season [11]. Flooding has been associated with an increase in the incidence of melioidosis and a sharp peak was seen after torrential rainfall and flooding in May/June 2016.

While most of the cases were sporadic and unrelated to each other, there were some interesting epidemiological clusters. One was melioidosis affecting two thalassaemic siblings from Maha Oya in the Uva Province that occurred six months apart. They had probably been infected during the construction of a new house. The other was a cluster of 10 cases (with 4 deaths) that occurred in Batticaloa in the Eastern Province in October/November 2015 following heavy rains. The deaths included three female patients with severe community-acquired bronchopneumonia, suggesting acquisition via inhalation.

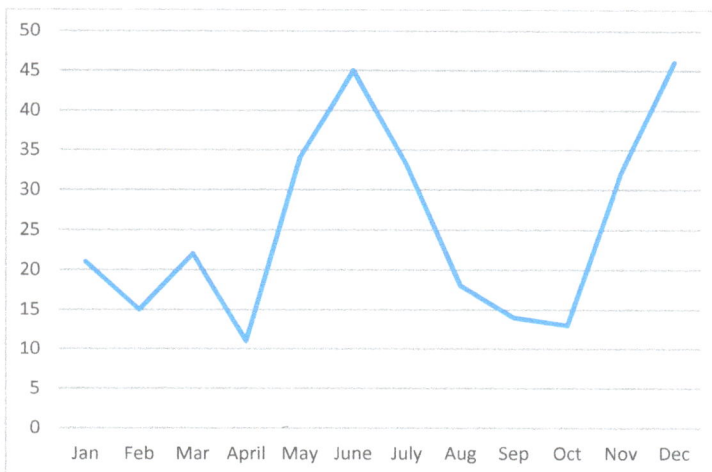

Figure 5. Monthly incidence of melioidosis (combined data for 2006–March 2017).

When the geographic data were plotted on topography and land-use maps of Sri Lanka, an infection-free area, comprising the highlands above 500 m, was noticed (Figure 2B). It seemed that while the distribution of melioidosis predictably coincided with rice-growing areas it appeared to be absent from rubber- and tea-growing regions. It is intriguing to speculate on the reason for this distribution. Is it due to the low temperatures in the hill country or different soil conditions or do the agricultural practices used in tea and rubber cultivation result in a lower risk of exposure? Further research, including soil sampling for *B. pseudomallei* in these areas, is needed to elucidate this question.

A sero-epidemiological study was conducted in 32 blood banks distributed throughout the country on 675 blood donors using the indirect haemagglutination assay between 2011 and 2013. Antibodies to *B. pseudomallei* were quantified and the cut-off for seropositivity was set at an antibody titre of ≥40. The sero-prevalence of antibodies against *B. pseudomallei* in the study population was 7.4% (50/675). To determine demographic, geographic and other risk factors associated with positivity, binary univariate logistic regression analysis was used to generate odds ratios (OR) with 95% confidence intervals (CI). Significance was determined using a p value of <0.05. When the association between province and positivity was explored, donors from the North-Western Province were more likely to be positive than donors from the rest of the country, but the association did not reach statistical significance. Positivity increased progressively with age but this did not reach statistical significance. There was a significantly larger proportion of females who were antibody-positive, 17/139 (12.2%) versus 33/529 (6.2%) of males ($p = 0.019$). A significant association was noted between agriculture/gardening and positivity ($p = 0.032$) and rural location and positivity ($p = 0.022$).

The majority of isolates ($n = 212$) belonged to the YLF (*Yersinia*-like fimbrial) gene cluster which is characteristic of South-East Asian strains. However, 38 of the bacterial strains were of the BTFC (*B. thailandensis*-like flagellum and chemotaxis) gene cluster, which is typically found in northern Australia [41]. Variation in the *bimA* gene was explored in the initial 32 isolates. While the majority of strains ($n = 27$) were *bimA*$_{Bp}$, the variant *bimA*$_{Bm}$, which is rarely found outside Australia, was present in 5 strains [42]. It is interesting to note that two of these patients presented with neurological melioidosis (brain-stem encephalitis and transverse myelitis, respectively), which is known to be associated with the *bimA*$_{Bm}$ gene [43].

Multilocus sequence typing (MLST) [44] of 108 *B. pseudomallei* strains revealed a high diversity, with 46 different sequence types (STs) represented in the collection (Table 1). Of these, 40 were novel sequence types. This molecular epidemiology is more compatible with a bacterium that has been endemic in the country over a long period of time, even millennia, than of one that had been recently introduced. Strains from Sri Lanka cluster separately from strains from South-East Asia and Australia, suggesting separation far back in geological time [45]. Currently Sri Lanka has the largest representation (number of strains submitted) on the public MLST database of all the countries in South Asia (https://pubmlst.org/bpseudomallei/).

Table 1. Sequence types (ST) of *B. pseudomallei* strains from Sri Lanka.

ST	No	ST	No	ST	No	ST	No	ST	No	ST	No
13	2	590		944		1139	3	1147	3	1435	2
132		594	5	1132	8	1140	5	1148		1436	
194		598		1133		1141		1152	2	1437	
202		615		1134		1142	2	1179		1438	
293		655		1135	9	1143	2	1314		1439	
308		733		1136	8	1144		1364		1442	
338		867		1137	18	1145		1413			
474		912	2	1138		1146		1434	6		

In a study summarizing global evidence for the environmental presence of *B. pseudomallei* [46], where 'definite' presence of the bacterium was defined as the detection of *B. pseudomallei* from the environment using culture or a specific PCR, Sri Lanka was classified as a country definitely harbouring the bacterium, based on a report by Inglis et al. [17]. A preliminary study to determine the presence of *B. pseudomallei* in the soil of selected regions in Sri Lanka was undertaken in 2016. Four sites throughout the east–west axis of the island, in close proximity to locations of diagnosed cases of melioidosis, namely Nikaweratiya in the Kurunegala District of the North-Western Province, Hasalaka in the Kandy District of the Central Province and Maha Oya and Kaluwanchikudy in the Ampara and Batticaloa Districts of the Eastern Province, respectively, were studied. Soil samples were taken from rice fields and domestic gardens and subjected to molecular screening, using a quantitative real-time PCR approach with multiple *B. pseudomallei*-specific targets. *B. pseudomallei* was present in all four sites and more than 70% of all samples were *B. pseudomallei*-positive [abstract presented at World Melioidosis Congress (WMC), 2016].

Only one case of animal melioidosis has been reported from Sri Lanka, that of a splenic abscess in a cow that later succumbed to the infection [47].

3. Current Recommendations and Availability of Measures Against Melioidosis

An island-wide, laboratory-based, case-finding system centered on clinical microbiologists is the main surveillance system for melioidosis in Sri Lanka. Clinical microbiologists have expertise in the identification of *B. pseudomallei* in clinical specimens by routine culture. Selective media are not used. Suspected clinical isolates are referred to the reference laboratory for confirmation and a standard datasheet is completed for each culture-confirmed patient. However, it is likely that this method will fail to detect cases in areas not served by clinical microbiologists, such as large areas of the Northern Province, unless the patients are referred to other centres.

Elucidation of the true epidemiology of melioidosis in Sri Lanka requires that it be made a notifiable disease. Steps have been taken to inform the public health authorities of the presence and extent of the infection in the country with a view to adding melioidosis to the list of notifiable diseases in Sri Lanka.

Culture-confirmed cases are treated according to standard published guidelines [48]. Government hospitals, which are well distributed throughout the country, provide treatment free of charge. Intravenous antibiotics for the acute phase and oral antibiotics for the eradication phase are available in all hospitals and there is no out-of-pocket expenditure by the patients. Intensive-care facilities are available in the larger hospitals. The moderately high case fatality rate appears to be related to late diagnosis, rather than to limitations in the availability of effective treatment.

4. Awareness of Melioidosis

Awareness of melioidosis among health care personnel is still inadequate and has probably contributed to the high case fatality rate. Although articles on melioidosis have appeared in the popular press, public awareness of the infection is very low, including among high-risk groups such as rice farmers and other cultivators. Island-wide awareness programmes to alert clinicians and public health authorities to the presence and presentation of melioidosis are needed.

5. Major Achievements

Although sporadic cases of melioidosis have been described previously in Sri Lanka, this study establishes, conclusively, that melioidosis is endemic in Sri Lanka, with a wide geographic and demographic distribution. The absence of melioidosis in the high hills (>500 m above sea level) is noted. This may be due to the low temperatures seen in these areas or the different agricultural practices used in these regions, where tea is the main crop, as opposed to rice as in most other areas of the country. The seasonal nature of the incidence of melioidosis, with an increase during the monsoons, is demonstrated.

The demographic profile of melioidosis in Sri Lanka is described for the first time and is broadly similar to countries with similar climate and agriculture. However, the wide distribution of cases in all strata of society and all grades of occupation is noted. The proposition that the rural, outdoor, agricultural, barefoot lifestyle of the majority of the population poses a general risk of acquisition of melioidosis is postulated. Individuals in the defence forces and construction workers have been confirmed to be at risk, as shown previously, and new risk groups such as housewives and drivers have been identified.

The high rates of co-morbidity in patients in Sri Lanka, compared to other endemic areas such as Thailand and Vietnam, is likely to reflect lower exposure to *B. pseudomallei*, probably due to lower bacterial loads in the environment, so that clinical disease develops mainly in highly susceptible populations.

A higher rate of bacteraemic cases and a lower rate of localized cases were seen in this series and may be an artefact of blood culture-positive patients being investigated more thoroughly. The case profile resembled that described previously in other case series. Neurological melioidosis, which has previously been described mainly in northern Australia, was seen. Musculoskeletal melioidosis was more common and may be the consequence of a barefoot lifestyle.

Genotyping of bacterial strains revealed a high diversity of sequence types, widely distributed throughout the island, confirming that the bacterium is endemic to the country. Strains from Sri Lanka clustered together and separately from the south-east Asian and Australian strains, showing regional specificity.

6. Current and Future Challenges

Increased construction and building activities in Sri Lanka may place construction workers, engineers and the general public at risk. Small-scale farming, gardening and horticulture have become popular for income generation and may increase exposure to this soil bacterium. Climate change has led to an increase in natural disasters, such as storms, landslides and flooding, that expose even healthy persons to high doses and unusual routes of transmission.

Exposure-mitigating practices, such as use of mechanical agriculture and protective clothing when coming into contact with mud and water, may reduce infection with *B. pseudomallei*. However, this may not be feasible due to their lack of acceptability and adverse socioeconomic impact. The use of doxycycline in farmers for leptospirosis prophylaxis may also protect against the acquisition of melioidosis. The evidence base for such strategies needs to be studied. Other 'at risk' occupations such as manual labourers, irrigation, water supply, construction, mining and road repair workers may also need to adopt similar preventive measures, when required. Preventive strategies should include more effective community-based diabetes prevention, detection and control that will reduce the risk of clinical disease. Recrudescent melioidosis should be included in the agenda of migrant health issues, including that of the diaspora that left Sri Lanka following civil disturbances over the past few decades.

Sero-surveillance at the community level may serve to obtain a true reflection of the extent of exposure to *B. pseudomallei* in the community. Targeted sero-surveillance in high-risk groups such as rice farmers, defence personnel and diabetics may help to quantify the risk of clinical disease in these individuals. Studies of the development of antibodies to *B. pseudomallei* during childhood and estimation of the intensity of exposure and incidence of melioidosis in children by IHA testing of a large cohort of children, with each year equally represented, would also add to knowledge of the extent and timing of bacterial exposure.

Soil sampling to detect and quantify the presence of *B. pseudomallei* in soil in Sri Lanka and mapping of the distribution of environmental *B. pseudomallei* will enable identification of high-risk geographic regions where heightened case detection can be implemented. The intriguing lack of infection in the high hills should be explored by soil sampling at different altitudes and from different agricultural settings.

Genotyping of further strains of *B. pseudomallei* will be useful to confirm the diversity of sequence types in Sri Lanka and to explore any associations of genotype with geographical distribution, clinical presentation or virulence and any genetic difference between environmental and clinical strains. The presence of the BTFC and $BimA_{Bm}$ variants in significant numbers in Sri Lanka will have implications for the geographical origins and evolution of the bacterium in geological time. Whole-genome sequencing will allow further discrimination of south-Asian strains from those in Oceania and south-east Asia and help deduce evolutionary relatedness between isolates from these regions.

The One Health concept is founded on the premise that the health of the environment, of animals and humans are inextricably linked. Melioidosis, caused by a soil saprophyte and infecting both animals and humans through soil and water exposure is the ideal candidate infection for the One Health approach to disease mitigation and health promotion. Integrating local, national and global workers in multidisciplinary teams to research this infection with a view to reducing its impact on human and animal populations is essential to this endeavour. Convening such a platform for the south-Asian region, which probably bears the highest burden of melioidosis but where the disease is currently grossly under-diagnosed, is an urgent imperative.

Acknowledgments: The authors acknowledge the contribution of Tim Inglis and Adam Merrit of PathWest, Western Australia, Shivankari Sivam and Harindra Sathkumara of the Genetech Research Institute, Mohan Natesan and Robert Ulrich of USAMRIID, Ivo Steinmetz of the University of Greifswald, Germany, the Laboratory Staff of the Faculty of Medicine, University of Colombo and Genetech Research Institute, and clinical microbiologists of state and private hospitals, contributing clinicians and patients. The research work in Sri Lanka was funded by U.S. Army Medical Research Acquisition Activity (contracts W81XWH-14-C-0071 and W81XWH-16-C-0223).

Author Contributions: E.M.C. drafted the first version. A.D.d.S. and V.T. reviewed and approved the final version.

Conflicts of Interest: The authors declare no conflict of interest.

References

1. Thin, R.N.T.; Brown, M.; Stewart, J.B.; Garrett, C.J. Melioidosis: A report of 10 cases. *Q. J. Med.* **1970**, *39*, 115–127. [PubMed]
2. Denny, C.R.; Nicholls, L. Melioidosis in a European. *Ceylon J. Sci.* **1927**, *2*, 37–40.
3. Manson-Bahr, P.E.C.; Bell, D.R. *Manson's Tropical Diseases*, 19th ed.; Baillière Tindall: London, UK, 1987.
4. Van P, P.F.; See, R.; Soysa, P.E.; Irving, G.S. Seroepidemiological survey of hospital-associated populations in Colombo, Sri Lanka. *Southeast Asian J. Trop. Med. Public Health.* **1976**, *1*, 16–20.
5. Redfearn, M.S.; Palleroni, N.J.; Stanier, R.Y. A comparative study of *Pseudomonas pseudomallei* and *Bacillus mallei*. *J. Gen. Microbiol.* **1966**, *43*, 293–313. [CrossRef] [PubMed]
6. Howe, C.; Sampath, A.; Spotnitz, M. The Pseudomallei group: A review. *J. Infect. Dis.* **1971**, *124*, 598–606. [CrossRef] [PubMed]
7. Leelarasamee, A. Epidemiology of melioidosis. *J. Infect. Dis. Antimicrob. Agents* **1986**, *3*, 84–93.
8. Leelarasamee, A.; Bovornkitti, S. Melioidosis: Review and update. *Rev. Infect. Dis.* **1989**, *11*, 413–425. [CrossRef] [PubMed]
9. Dance, D.A.B. Melioidosis: The tip of the iceberg? *Clin. Microbiol. Rev.* **1991**, *4*, 52–60. [CrossRef] [PubMed]
10. Dance, D.A.B. Melioidosis as an emerging global problem. *Acta Trop.* **2000**, *74*, 115–119. [CrossRef]
11. Cheng, A.C.; Currie, B.J. Melioidosis: Epidemiology, pathophysiology, and management. *Clin. Microbiol. Rev.* **2005**, *18*, 383–416. [CrossRef] [PubMed]
12. Currie, B.J.; Dance, D.A.B.; Cheng, A.C. The global distribution of *Burkholderia pseudomallei* and melioidosis: An update. *Trans. R. Soc. Trop. Med. Hyg.* **2008**, *102*, S1–S4. [CrossRef]
13. Wiersinga, W.J.; Currie, B.J.; Peacock, S.J. Medical progress: Melioidosis. *N. Engl. J. Med.* **2012**, *367*, 1035–1044. [CrossRef] [PubMed]
14. Peetermans, W.E.; Van Wijngaerden, E.; Van Eldere, J.; Verhaegen, J. Melioidosis brain and lung abscess after travel to Sri Lanka. *Clin. Infect. Dis.* **1999**, *28*, 921–922. [CrossRef] [PubMed]
15. ProMED-Mail. Meliodosis, Tsunami-Related (02): Thailand, Request for Information. Available online: http://www.promedmail.org (accessed on 2 February 2005).
16. Jayasekara, K.; Perera, S.; Wijesundere, A. Fatal *Burkholderia pseudomallei* septicaemia. *Ceylon Med. J.* **2006**, *51*, 69–70. [CrossRef] [PubMed]
17. Inglis, T.J.J.; Meritt, A.; Montgomery, J.; Jayasinghe, I.; Thevanesam, V.; McInnes, R. Deployable laboratory response to emergence of melioidosis in central Sri Lanka. *J. Clin. Microbiol.* **2008**, *46*, 3479–3481. [CrossRef] [PubMed]

18. Corea, E.; Thevanasam, V.; Perera, S.; Jayasinghe, I.; Ekanayake, A.; Masakorala, J.; Inglis, T.J.J. Melioidosis in Sri Lanka: An emerging infection. *Sri Lankan J. Infect. Dis.* **2012**, 2, 2–8. [CrossRef]

19. Hesstvedt, L.; Wilhelmsen, M.; Mengshoel, A.T.; Dyrhol-Riise, A.M. Two Norwegian patients with melioidosis presenting with bacteraemia and splenic and prostatic abscesses. *J. Travel Med.* **2011**, 18, 418–421. [CrossRef] [PubMed]

20. Nandasiri, S.; Wimalaratna, H.; Manjula, M.; Corea, E. Transverse myelitis secondary to melioidosis; a case report. *BMC Infect. Dis.* **2012**, 12, 232–236. [CrossRef] [PubMed]

21. Madegedara, D.; Wirasinghe, C. Melioidosis mimicking tuberculosis–Are we missing the diagnosis? *Respire* **2012**, 4, 9–11.

22. Caldera, A.S.; Kumanan, T.; Corea, E. A rare cause of septic arthritis: Melioidosis. *Trop. Doct.* **2013**, 43, 164–166. [CrossRef] [PubMed]

23. Rodrigo, K.M.D.J.; Premaratne, R.; de Silva, H.J.; Corea, E. Melioidosis as a cause of femoral osteomyelitis and multifocal intramuscular abscess around the hip join in a farmer: A case report. *Sri Lankan J. Infect. Dis.* **2013**, 3, 50–54. [CrossRef]

24. Kannangara, L.S.; Samarasekara, G.B.L.; Kularatne, W.N.S.; Corea, E.; Elvitigala, J.; Masakorala, J. Cavitating left upper lobe pneumonia: A case of melioidosis. *Galle Med. J.* **2014**, 19, 23–26. [CrossRef]

25. Wijekoon, S.; Prasath, T.; Corea, E.M.; Elwitigala, J.P. Melioidosis presenting as lymphadenitis: A case report. *BMC Res. Notes* **2014**, 7, 364. [CrossRef] [PubMed]

26. Mathurageethan, M.; Kahathuduwa, C.N.; Badanasinghe, N.; Corea, E.; Fernando, R. Melioidosis associated with chronic osteomyelitis and visceral organ abscesses. *Sri Lanka J. Surg.* **2014**, 32, 41–42. [CrossRef]

27. Arif, M.A.; Abid, M.H.; Renganathan, R.; Siddiqui, K.A. Central and peripheral nervous system involvement in neuromelioidosis. *BMJ Case Rep.* **2015**. [CrossRef] [PubMed]

28. Fernando, M.A.M.; Dassanayake, M.; Corea, E.M.; Herath, H.M.A.D.; Sureka, M. Melioidosis. *Sri Lanka J. Child Health* **2015**, 44, 234–235. [CrossRef]

29. Pathirathne, S.H.; Athukorala, G.P.; Hussain, H.; Nishantha, P.L.B.; Senevirathne, H.M.P.K.; Corea, E.; Siribaddana, A.D. Melioidosis mimicking pulmonary tuberculosis. *Sri Lanka J. Med.* **2015**, 24, 30–32. [CrossRef]

30. Wijekoon, P.W.M.C.S.B.; Bandara, K.A.S.; Kailainathan, A.; Chandrasiri, N.S.; Hapuarachchi, C.T. Guillan-Barre syndrome; A rare complication of melioidosis. A case report. *BMC Infect. Dis.* **2016**, 16, 388. [CrossRef] [PubMed]

31. Dayasiri, M.B.K.C.; Mudiyanse, R.M.; Kudagammana, H.D.W.S.; Rifaya, M.I.; Dissanayaka, P.; Jeyaratnasingham, C.; Nawaratna, U. Melioidosis manifesting as severe emaciation and clinically indolent liver abscesses, in a child with beta thalassemia major. *Sri Lanka J. Child Health* **2016**, 45, 130–133. [CrossRef]

32. Pirasath, S.; Selvaratnam, G.; Kumanan, T.; Pradeepan, J.; Mubarak, F.N. Melioidosis: Emerging infection in northern Sri Lanka. *Int. J. Med. Microbiol. Trop. Dis.* **2016**, 2, 112–114. [CrossRef]

33. Kahandawaarachchi, I.C.I.; Premawansa, G.S.; Warnasuriya, W.; Dassanayake, M.; Corea, E. A case report of co-infection of melioidosis and cutaneous leishmaniasis. *BMC Infect. Dis.* **2017**, 17, 533. [CrossRef] [PubMed]

34. Premaratne, K.K.M.K.; Karunaratne, G.K.D.; Dias, R.; Lamahewage, A.K.; Samarasinghe, M.; Corea, E.; Gunawardena, R.M.T.M. Melioidosis presenting as parotid abscess in children: Two consecutive cases. *Sri Lankan J. Infect. Dis.* **2017**, 7, 116–122. [CrossRef]

35. Weerasinghe, N.P.; Herath, H.M.M.; Liyanage, T.M.U. Isolated septic arthritis of hip joint: A rare presentation of melioidosis. A case report. *BMC Res. Notes* **2018**, 11, 50. [CrossRef] [PubMed]

36. Merritt, A.; Inglis, T.J.J.; Chidlow, G.; Harnett, G. PCR-based identification of *Burkholderia pseudomallei*. *Rev. Inst. Med. Trop. São Paulo* **2006**, 48, 239–244. [CrossRef] [PubMed]

37. Alexander, A.D.; Huxsoll, D.L.; Warner, A.R.; Shepler, V.; Dorsey, A. Serological diagnosis of human melioidosis with indirect haemagglutination and complement fixation tests. *Appl. Microbiol.* **1970**, 20, 825–833. [PubMed]

38. Punyagupta, S. Melioidosis. In *Review of 686 Cases and Presentation of a New Clinical Classification*; Punyagupta, S., Sirisanthana, T., Stapatayavong, B., Eds.; Bangkok Medical Publisher: Bangkok, Thailand, 1989; pp. 217–229.

39. Mansoor, C.A.; Jemshad, A. Meliodosis with endocarditis and massive cerebral infarct. *Ital. J. Med.* **2016**, 10, 55–57.

40. Currie, B.J.; Ward, L.; Cheng, A.C. The epidemiology and clinical spectrum of melioidosis: 540 cases from the 20 year Darwin prospective study. *PLoS Negl. Trop. Dis.* **2010**, 4, e900. [CrossRef] [PubMed]

41. Tuanyok, A.; Auerbach, R.K.; Brettin, T.S.; Bruce, D.C.; Munk, A.C.; Detter, J.C.; Pearson, T.; Hornstra, H.; Sermswan, R.W.; Wuthiekanun, V.; et al. A horizontal gene transfer event defines two distinct groups within *Burkholderia pseudomallei* that have dissimilar geographic distributions. *J. Bacteriol.* **2007**, *189*, 9044–9049. [CrossRef] [PubMed]

42. Sitthidet, C.; Korbsrisate, S.; Layton, A.N.; Field, T.R.; Stevens, M.P.; Stevens, J.M. Identification of motifs of *Burkholderia pseudomallei* BimA required for intracellular motility, actin binding, and actin polymerization. *J. Bacteriol.* **2011**, *193*, 1901–1910. [CrossRef] [PubMed]

43. Sarovich, D.S.; Price, E.P.; Webb, J.R.; Ward, L.M.; Voutsinos, M.Y. Variable virulence factors in *Burkholderia pseudomallei* (melioidosis) associated with human disease. *PLoS ONE* **2014**, *9*, e91682. [CrossRef] [PubMed]

44. Godoy, D.; Randle, G.; Simpson, A.J.; Aanensen, D.M.; Pitt, T.L.; Kinoshita, R.; Spratt, B.G. Multilocus sequence typing and evolutionary relationships among the causative agents of melioidosis and glanders, *Burkholderia pseudomallei* and *Burkholderia mallei*. *J. Clin. Microbiol.* **2003**, *41*, 2068–2079. [CrossRef] [PubMed]

45. Corea, E.M.; Merritt, A.J.; Ler, Y.-H.; Thevanesam, V.; Inglis, T.J.J. Sri Lankan national melioidosis surveillance program uncovers a nationwide distribution of invasive melioidosis. *Am. J. Trop. Med. Hyg.* **2016**, *94*, 292–298. [CrossRef] [PubMed]

46. Limmathurotsakul, D.; Dance, D.A.B.; Wuthiekanun, V.; Kaestli, M.; Mayo, M. Systematic review and consensus guidelines for environmental sampling of *Burkholderia pseudomallei*. *PLoS Negl. Trop. Dis.* **2013**, *7*, e2105. [CrossRef] [PubMed]

47. Nicholls, L. Melioidosis, with special reference to the dissociation of *Bacillus whitmori*. *Br. J. Exp. Pathol.* **1930**, *11*, 393–399.

48. Inglis, T.J.J. The treatment of melioidosis. *Pharmaceuticals* **2010**, *3*, 1296–1303. [CrossRef] [PubMed]

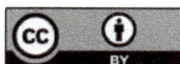

Tropical Medicine and Infectious Disease

MDPI

Review

Melioidosis in South Asia (India, Nepal, Pakistan, Bhutan and Afghanistan)

Chiranjay Mukhopadhyay [1,2,*], Tushar Shaw [1], George M. Varghese [3] and David A. B. Dance [4,5,6]

[1] Department of Microbiology, Kasturba Medical College, Manipal Academy of Higher Education, Manipal 576104, India; tusharshaw1990@gmail.com
[2] Center for Emerging and Tropical Diseases, Manipal Academy of Higher Education, Manipal 576104, India
[3] Department of Infectious Diseases, Christian Medical College, Vellore 632004, India; georgemvarghese@hotmail.com
[4] Lao-Oxford-Mahosot Hospital-Wellcome Trust Research Unit, Vientiane, Laos; David.d@tropmedres.ac
[5] Centre for Tropical Medicine and Global Health, University of Oxford, Oxford OX1 2JD, UK
[6] Faculty of Infectious and Tropical Diseases, London School of Hygiene and Tropical Medicine, London WC1E 7HT, UK
*   Correspondence: chiranjay.m@manipal.edu; Tel.: +91-082-0292-2717

Received: 12 March 2018; Accepted: 18 May 2018; Published: 22 May 2018

Abstract: Despite the fact that South Asia is predicted to have the highest number of cases worldwide, melioidosis is a little-known entity in South Asian countries. It has never been heard of by the majority of doctors and has as yet failed to gain the attention of national Ministries of Health and country offices of the World Health Organization (WHO). Although a few centers are diagnosing increasing numbers of cases, and the mortality documented from these institutions is relatively high (nearly 20%), the true burden of the disease remains unknown. In India, most cases have been reported from southwestern coastal Karnataka and northeastern Tamil Nadu, although this probably simply reflects the presence of centers of excellence and researchers with an interest in the disease. As elsewhere, the majority of cases have type 2 diabetes mellitus and occupational exposure to the environment. Most present with community-acquired pneumonia and/or bacteremia, especially during heavy rainfall. The high seropositivity rate (29%) in Karnataka and isolation of *B. pseudomallei* from the environment in Tamil Nadu and Kerala confirm India as melioidosis-endemic, although the full extent of the distribution of the organism across the country is unknown. There are limited molecular epidemiological data, but, thus far, the majority of Indian isolates have appeared distinct from those from South East Asia and Australia. Among other South Asian countries, Sri Lanka and Bangladesh are known to be melioidosis-endemic, but there are no cases that have conclusively proved to have been acquired in Nepal, Bhutan, Afghanistan or Pakistan. There are no surveillance systems in place for melioidosis in South Asian countries. However, over the past two years, researchers at the Center for Emerging and Tropical Diseases of Kasturba Medical College, University of Manipal, have established the Indian Melioidosis Research Forum (IMRF), held the first South Asian Melioidosis Congress, and have been working to connect researchers, microbiologists and physicians in India and elsewhere in South Asia to raise awareness through training initiatives, the media, workshops, and conferences, with the hope that more patients with melioidosis will be diagnosed and treated appropriately. However, much more work needs to be done before we will know the true burden and distribution of melioidosis across South Asia.

Keywords: *Burkholderia pseudomallei*; India; melioidosis; South Asia

1. Introduction

Melioidosis is a potentially fatal illness which is caused by the soil saprophyte and biothreat agent *Burkholderia pseudomallei*. It is known to be highly endemic in northeast Thailand and northern Australia, where annual incidence rates ranging from 4 to 41.7 cases per 100,000 population [1] have been reported. A recent modeling study predicted that as many as 165,000 people may be infected each year worldwide, with South Asia having the highest burden of the disease (44% of all cases) [2]. India is the largest country in South Asia and, having a suitable environment and an enormous diabetic population, might well be a 'hotspot' for the disease. However, the true melioidosis burden in India is unknown due to limited awareness and laboratory constraints throughout the country. Clinical diagnosis is exceptionally challenging due to the varied clinical presentations, especially as the disease can mimic other infections such as tuberculosis [3], which is highly endemic in resource-poor countries such as India.

The majority of the Indian population resides in rural settings and might readily acquire the infection through direct contact with soil and water. However, they have limited access to hospitals where there are well-equipped microbiology laboratories and well-trained professionals to diagnose the disease. The present-day situation in India is similar to that in Thailand in the mid-1980s when melioidosis started to be diagnosed increasingly as microbiology services improved. In countries such as India, limited awareness among clinicians and microbiologists about the disease has led to misdiagnosis and inappropriate treatment. Furthermore, the spectrum of disease manifestations ranges from the acute septicemic form to a chronic granulomatous form, and hence it mimics other endemic infections with which it may be confused. Although there has been a plethora of melioidosis case reports and short series published from India, there are no voluntary or mandatory surveillance systems to notify the cases, and so there has been limited evidence to encourage governments to formulate melioidosis-specific public health policies.

The challenges to the laboratory in diagnosing melioidosis are manifold. Wrinkled *B. pseudomallei* colonies are frequently thought to be aerobic spore bearing bacteria, which are relatively common environmental contaminants, and discarded. Any oxidase-positive Gram-negative, non-lactose fermenting bacillus is likely to be considered as a 'pseudomonad' or '*Pseudomonas* sp.', which is unlikely to be identified further to the species level. Even commercial identification kits and modern automated systems (e.g., API 20NE, VITEK 2, and MALDI-TOF) are not 100% reliable for identifying *B. pseudomallei*, especially in inexperienced hands [4]. However, awareness of the disease has recently been increasing in this subcontinent and it is being diagnosed more frequently, especially in India, Sri Lanka and Bangladesh. The current review aims to bring into focus a much neglected 'killer' disease from this region, focusing on India, Pakistan, Bhutan, Nepal, and Afghanistan, as Bangladesh and Sri Lanka are covered in separate reviews in this Special Issue.

2. History

Following the initial recognition of melioidosis by the British pathologist Alfred Whitmore and his Indian assistant, CS Krishnaswami, in Myanmar in 1911, the first case in South Asia was confirmed in Ceylon, now Sri Lanka, in 1927. The first case from India was not diagnosed until 1953, in a 40-year-old Scottish mining engineer suffering from prolonged fever, multiple abscesses and septicemia, who became infected while working in the central part of the country but was diagnosed post-mortem following his repatriation to Scotland [5]. Another fatal exported case was diagnosed in Switzerland in 1988 in a 40-year-old woman who had traveled extensively in India and Nepal [6]. It thus appeared likely that melioidosis was endemic within India.

The first indigenous case from India was detected in Mumbai in 1991 [7], which was followed by a long period of silence. Meanwhile, the epidemics thought to be the bubonic plague in Beed (Maharashtra) and pneumonic plague in Surat (Gujarat), which occurred in the mid-1990s, led to the suggestion that at least some of the cases may have been melioidosis [8], although this was questioned [9] and was never confirmed officially. This was followed by a series of publications from the Christian Medical College in Vellore, near the south-eastern coast of India, which raised the likelihood of melioidosis being endemic in the country and the probability of it being a silent killer due to incorrect diagnosis and treatment [10–14]. A small serosurvey carried out around the same time suggested that a proportion of the local rural population had evidence of exposure to *B. pseudomallei* [15].

3. Review of Melioidosis Cases and Presence of *B. pseudomallei* (Animal/Human/Environment)

We performed a PubMed search using the keywords '*melioidosis*', '*pseudomallei*', and '*India*', and reviewed the available references published between January 1991 and March 2018. Initially, titles and abstracts were screened and articles identified as possibly relevant were reviewed as full text. The reference lists of included articles were assessed for further relevant publications. A similar search strategy was applied for Nepal, Pakistan, Afghanistan, and Bhutan. In addition, cases reported from India were also identified from the website http://www.melioidosis.info. Duplicate cases were screened and removed manually. Additional cases were identified from the personal EndNote database of one of the authors (DABD), as many reports published in non-indexed journals were not available on PubMed. Further, more detailed information was obtained from our own laboratory database regarding cases diagnosed in Manipal since 2002, and Vellore since 2008.

3.1. India

The literature search revealed 190 articles (File S1) comprising case reports or series relating to 583 individual patients with melioidosis from different parts of India (Table 1 and Figure 1). The greatest number of cases were reported from Karnataka (306), followed by Tamil Nadu (146). Figure 1 shows clearly that these cases were predominantly diagnosed in coastal areas, probably reflecting the fact that the majority of the best-resourced hospitals are located in these regions. The ages ranged from 0 to 84 years, although many publications did not provide enough detail to calculate overall medians and interquartile ranges. A substantial majority of the patients were male, which may be attributable to men being more likely to be involved in occupations involving soil contact, but also to inequality in access to the health care between men and women. Diabetes was the most common predisposing factor reported (391/559, 70%). Ceftazidime was the most common antibiotic used in the intensive phase and cotrimoxazole for eradication therapy. The overall reported mortality was 95 (17%), although this may have been an underestimate as there were many cases in which the outcome was not reported (Table 1).

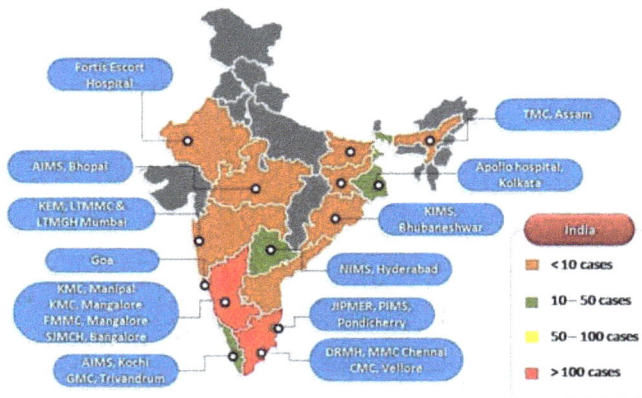

Figure 1. Cases reported from different parts of India and centers equipped to diagnose cases of melioidosis.

Trop. Med. Infect. Dis. **2018**, 3, 51

Table 1. Published cases of melioidosis reported from different states of India (1991–2018) (see Supplementary material for reference list).

State	Number of Cases	Age Range	Gender (Male: Female)	Diabetes n (%)	Intensive Treatment		Eradication Treatment		Mortality n (%)
					MER	CAZ	SXT	Others	
Karnataka	306	0–84	3:1	241 (79)	24	294	235	50	39 (13)
Tamil Nadu	146	4–65	3:1	75 (50)	3	82	80	2	37 (28)
Telangana	35	30–66	2:1	27 (77)	8	7	11	3	4 (11)
Kerala	34	9–66	5:1	24 (77)	3	15	14	2	5 (13)
Pondicherry	14	0–58	3:1	3 (21)	2	2	-	4	2 (14)
West Bengal	11	29–71	11:0	9 (82)	6	4	9	1	2 (18)
Maharashtra	9	10–72	7:1	5 (50)	0	4	4	0	4 (50)
Orissa	8	47–51	7:0	5 (63)	0	6	5	0	1 (12.5)
Assam	6	0–57	2:1	3 (50)	3	0	1	1	2 (33)
Goa	5	34–53	5:0	5 (100)	2	2	1	1	0
Bihar	4	50–65	4:0	4 (100)	2	1	2	1	0
Jharkhand	2	32–33	2:0	1 (50)	1	1	1	0	1 (50)
Rajasthan	1	49	1:0	0	1	0	1	0	0
Madhya Pradesh	1	56	1:0	1 (100)	0	1	0	0	0
Andhra Pradesh	1	23	1:0	1 (100)	0	0	0	0	1 (100)

Abbreviations: MER, meropenem; CAZ, ceftazidime; SXT, cotrimoxazole. Details are not given in many publications so denominators differ in each column.

3.2. Manipal

The tertiary care hospital of Kasturba Medical College in Manipal has more than 2000 beds and receives referred cases from primary and secondary health care centers. The hospital caters to the hilly regions and the plains of Udupi district, and other neighboring districts including Uttar Kannada, Shimoga, Davangere, Chikmagalur, Hassan, and Mangalore with many inpatient admissions (approximately 72,025/year) and outpatient visits (approximately 627,210/year). The greatest number of cases of melioidosis in any single center in India has been reported from Manipal since the first cases were recognized there in 2002 [16]. The incidence of melioidosis in Udupi district over the past three years was equivalent to 0.8/1000 hospital admissions and 1/100,000 population. The numbers have increased significantly since 2006 following the upgrading of laboratory facilities and the implementation of a program to raise awareness among doctors (Figure 2). However, being a tertiary referral center in the sparsely populated coastal Udupi district, most patients visiting this hospital are from middle and high socioeconomic backgrounds and may not have had as extensive exposure to the environment as daily laborers or tenant farmers, meaning that this experience may underestimate the true incidence of the disease in this district.

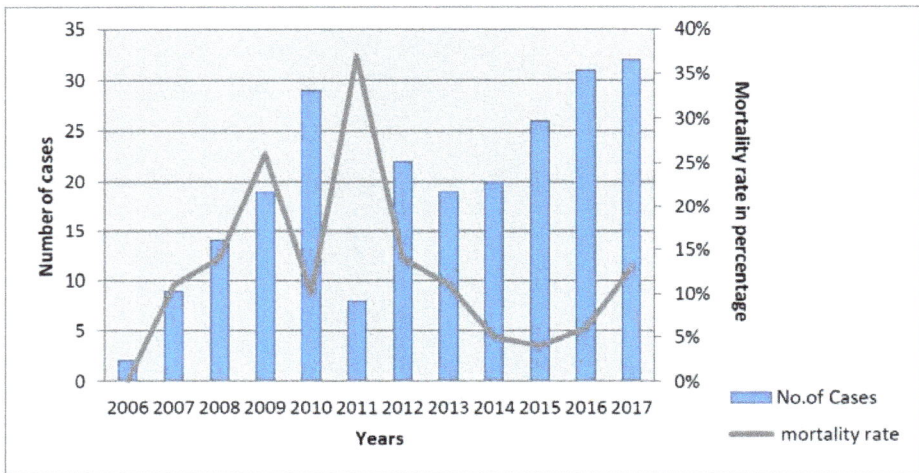

Figure 2. Annual numbers of melioidosis cases and mortality from Manipal.

Of the 231 patients with melioidosis diagnosed during 2006–2016 (which includes 82 cases included in the literature review described above), the majority (84, 36.3%) presented with pulmonary infection. Most patients presented during months of heavy rainfall (Figure 3). Organ failure was observed in 43 (19%). Diabetes mellitus was the most common co-morbidity (159, 69%). Overall, 48% of patients were bacteremic, and bacteremia (22/27; 81.4%) along with renal dysfunction (13/27, 48%) were significantly associated with mortality ($p = 0.004$). Mortality appears to have declined over the past decade (Figure 2) and at present the rate is surprisingly low (27, 12%) compared with that in Thailand (35%) [17], and equivalent to that in northern Australia (14%) [18]. In fact, melioidosis causes a relatively small proportion of all deaths attributable to infectious diseases in Manipal. There are no obvious links between changes in clinical management and this low mortality, although it is likely that there has been an increasing awareness over the years, which might have led to more accurate diagnosis and prompt treatment. The socioeconomic status of the patients seeking care at the tertiary center may also mean that they are in better general health than populations in some other settings. However, many patients are discharged against medical advice (DAMA) (mean 300/year over the past four years), mostly due to an inability to afford expensive medical treatment, and their outcome remains unknown. A point prevalence study conducted at Kasturba Hospital (unpublished data) showed that 60% of patients admitted to the hospital with suspected infection received empirical antibiotics that would have been expected to be effective against melioidosis, mainly carbapenems or beta-lactam/beta-lactamase inhibitor combinations. This could also be a cause of these patients remaining undiagnosed by culture as well as having low mortality. It is also likely that there are many patients who seek treatment in primary or secondary health care, private clinics, nursing homes or government hospitals, who remain undiagnosed or misdiagnosed and whose deaths would never be attributed to melioidosis.

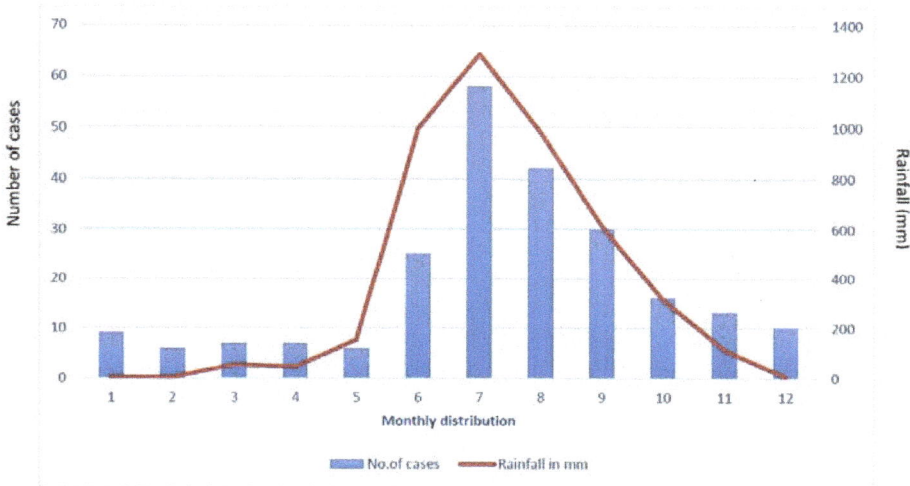

Month	Season
October–February	Post-monsoon
March–May	Summer
June–September	Monsoon

Figure 3. Average monthly rainfall and melioidosis cases in Manipal, 2006 to 2017.

3.3. Vellore

The Christian Medical College (CMC), Vellore, is a tertiary care teaching hospital with more than 2800 beds, which caters to a wide populace with substantial representation from most states in India, in addition to the patients referred from nearby districts in Tamil Nadu and Andhra Pradesh. The initial reports from CMC helped the recognition of the endemicity of melioidosis in India since 1996 [10]. The most recent retrospective analysis of 114 patients with culture-confirmed melioidosis at CMC between January 2008 and December 2014 reflects the current scenario [19]. Patients came from 15 states in India, but the greatest numbers were residents of West Bengal (26.3%), Jharkhand (22.8%) and Tamil Nadu (14.9%), predominantly from rural areas. As previous studies have shown, diabetes mellitus was found to be the most common risk factor (82.3%). Of the total cases, 41 (36%) presented with acute disease (<2 months duration) while 73 (64%) had chronic manifestations. Patients with acute septicemic melioidosis more frequently had bacteremia (80% vs. 41%; $p < 0.001$) and respiratory involvement (39% vs. 16.4%; $p = 0.007$). The mortality for acute septicemic melioidosis was 17% as opposed to 13.6% among those with chronic disease, with an overall case fatality rate of 14.9%. Respiratory involvement, bacteremia, septic arthritis and skin involvement more commonly occurred with acute melioidosis, while chronic melioidosis had splenic, genitourinary and bone involvement. Respiratory involvement and bacteremia were found to be independent predictors of mortality. Drug susceptibility to carbapenems and ceftazidime was 100%, while resistance to trimethoprim-sulfamethoxazole and doxycycline was found in 5.9% and 2.6%, respectively. Intensive therapy with ceftazidime or meropenem followed by eradication treatment with trimethoprim-sulfamethoxazole, with or without doxycycline, was administered in these patients. Relapse occurred in four (3.5%) patients after periods of 2–7 years. Since the patient population was representative of regions that are geographically distant, this is indicative of the widespread endemicity of the disease within India. However, the numbers are likely to be a substantial underestimate as the diagnosis was only made in patients who were managed at the tertiary care center and many cases are likely to have gone undetected in these regions due to inadequate diagnostic facilities and limited awareness.

3.4. Other Neighboring Countries

Only a single case of imported melioidosis has been reported to date from Nepal, in a 35-year-old patient returning from Malaysia [20]. There is some confusion in the literature about cases of melioidosis originating from Pakistan due to the previous designation of Bangladesh as 'East Pakistan' [21]. A case of pneumonia was diagnosed in the UK in a 60-year-old male described as being from Pakistan [22]. Inquiries of the author of this report by one of us (DABD) revealed some uncertainty about his true origin, and we have been unable to identify a single case of melioidosis that was unequivocally acquired in Pakistan. No cases were identified from Bhutan or Afghanistan. However, at this stage, it is unclear whether this reflects absence of the disease or simply lack of awareness and diagnostic capability in these countries, as Limmaturotsakul et al. predicted that it is likely that melioidosis exists undiagnosed in Nepal, Pakistan and Bhutan [2].

3.5. Serosurveillance

The only serosurveillance study undertaken in India since the 1990s was conducted among 711 healthy residents of Udupi Taluk. The study revealed an overall seropositivity rate (defined as a titer of $\geq$1:20 in the indirect hemagglutination (IHA) test) of 29% [23]. This suggests that exposure to *B. pseudomallei* is relatively common, although cross-reaction with closely-related organisms cannot be excluded [24].

3.6. Animals

There have been very few reports of animal melioidosis from any of the South Asian countries. A single case in a male rhesus monkey imported from India was reported from the USA in 1969 [25]. *B. pseudomallei* was also reported to have been associated with two cases of bovine abortion in India, although the antibiogram of the organisms isolated make it very unlikely that these were really *B. pseudomallei* [26].

3.7. Environmental Evidence

There have been very few studies attempting to isolate *B. pseudomallei* from the environment in India. One study in rice paddy along the southeast coast of Tamil Nadu confirmed four environmental isolates of *B. pseudomallei* [27]. Another study conducted along the Malabar coastal region of Kerala found that 22.7% of the *Burkholderia* spp. strains isolated were *B. pseudomallei* [28]. Both studies were conducted at a single time point and used culture followed by 16S rDNA sequencing rather than specific *B. pseudomallei* PCR. In addition, a study from the Lahore district in Pakistan reported the detection of *Burkholderia* spp. genomes in two (1.4%) environmental samples, although the method used could not distinguish between *B. pseudomallei* and *B. mallei* [29]. Until further studies are done in South Asia, the true distribution of *B. pseudomallei* in the environment will remain uncertain.

3.8. Molecular Epidemiology in South Asian Countries

The molecular epidemiology of South Asian isolates of *B. pseudomallei* has not been studied intensively. The first molecular typing of Indian strains revealed several novel sequence types, some of which were single locus variants (SLVs) of isolates from Thailand, Kenya, and China, suggesting the possibility of the spread of *B. pseudomallei* along historical trading routes [30]. A study using multi-locus sequence typing (MLST) of 32 clinical isolates from India found that the majority (93.7%) had novel allelic profiles, with ST 1368 as the most common sequence type [31]. The majority of the isolates were outliers in a population snapshot suggesting that Indian isolates are genetically distinct from Australian and Southeast Asian isolates. However, some of the Indian isolates were found to be single-locus variants of Sri Lankan isolates in the BURST analysis (Figure 4). This is perhaps not surprising, given that Sri Lanka is a neighboring country with which there has always been an active trade of goods and livestock. However, one of the sequence types (STs) reported from the northeastern region of India (ST1051) was similar to an Australian isolate, and homoplasy cannot be ruled out as a cause of such similarities without further molecular analysis such as whole genome sequencing [32].

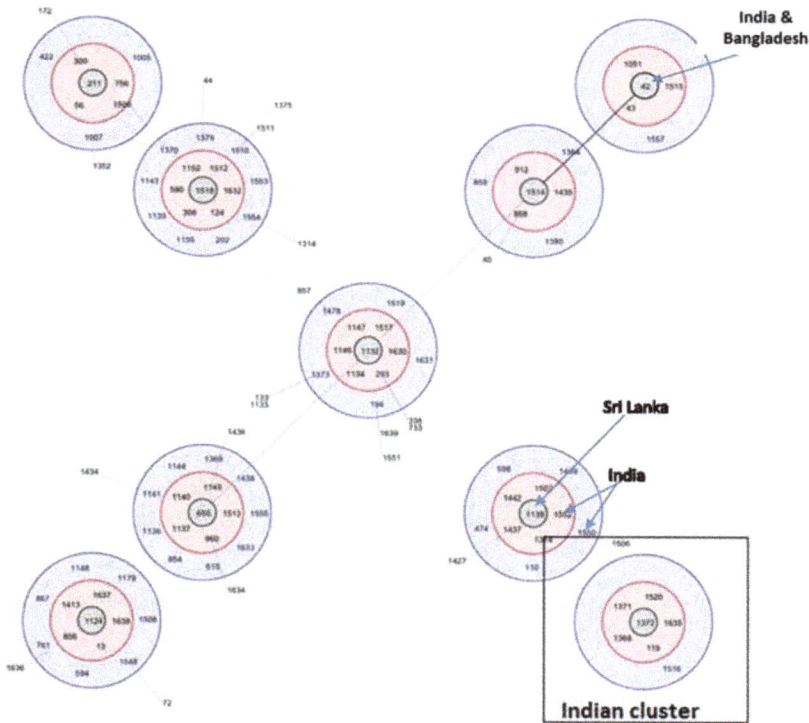

Figure 4. BURST cluster for South Asian countries with red shades depicting single locus variants and blue shades depict double locus variants linking the various STs. A group of Indian STs form a separate cluster not linked to other STs reported from other South Asian countries.

4. Current Recommendations and Availability of Measures against Melioidosis

It is well-established that melioidosis is associated with activities involving exposure to soil and water [33]. Although it is likely that the risk of disease can be reduced by simple measures such as the use of protective gear such as boots and consumption of boiled or bottled water [34], there are no current guidelines implemented in India or other South Asian countries for prevention of melioidosis. The need for enhanced surveillance is discussed below and it is hoped that, as the number of cases detected increases, state and national health authorities will develop and disseminate relevant guidance, particularly targeted at the areas and populations identified to be at greatest risk.

Surveillance Systems and Reporting

Melioidosis is not currently notifiable in any country in South Asia. In India, for example, diseases like tuberculosis, malaria, and dengue are highly endemic and are covered by specific guidelines and public health policies that have been promulgated by the government to both the public and health workers. The Integrated Disease Surveillance Program (IDSP) run by the Indian National Center for Disease Control (NCDC) encompasses the top 12 priority diseases for laboratory-based surveillance, which include dengue, chikungunya, Japanese encephalitis, meningococcal meningitis, typhoid fever, diphtheria, cholera, shigella dysentery, viral hepatitis (A and E), leptospirosis and malaria (http://idsp.nic.in/index1.php?lang=1&level=1&sublinkid=5985&lid=3925). An additional 22 syndromes are identified for 'presumptive' (i.e., clinically-based) surveillance. There are plans to integrate and decentralize surveillance activities at the grassroots level to combat these diseases, along with the development of human resource through training, upgrading of information and communication technology for collection, collation, compilation, analysis and dissemination of data, and strengthening of public health laboratories. However, melioidosis does not come under the surveillance program of NCDC. It has been predicted that the number of deaths from melioidosis globally is higher than that of dengue and leptospirosis [2], both of which are covered by IDSP. If so, the disease would warrant much greater attention. Nonetheless, it is unlikely that this will happen unless surveillance improves and greater numbers of cases are detected, an unfortunate 'Catch-22' situation. Currently, the only sources of hard data about melioidosis in South Asia are published case reports, which undoubtedly are still only the tip of the iceberg. It is thus down to South Asian researchers to provide evidence to local policymakers to raise melioidosis up their list of priorities with the ultimate aim of gaining a better understanding of the true burden of the disease through appropriate diagnosis and surveillance.

5. Diagnostic Facilities

The clinical features of melioidosis are not characteristic and may be confused with those of many other tropical diseases, especially tuberculosis. Diagnosis of melioidosis thus requires the facilities and expertise of the microbiology laboratory through isolation and identification of *B. pseudomallei*, which remains the 'gold standard' for diagnosis of the infection. Although the organism is classified as a 'Tier 1 Select Agent' in the USA (https://www.selectagents.gov/ohp-app1.html) and is worked on at biosafety level 3 in many countries, such facilities are generally not available in clinical laboratories in South Asian countries, and specimens are usually processed at biosafety level 2. Standard culture media are generally used, although it may take several days to grow the organism. Selective media such as Ashdown's agar and broth, which increase the yield of *B. pseudomallei* from non-sterile body sites, are rarely available outside a few specialist centers. In Manipal, for example, enrichment with 'CV-C50' broth for samples from non-sterile sites has improved the yield of culture [35]. Blood culture is the specimen most frequently received by laboratories for the investigation of melioidosis. Continuously monitored automated blood culture systems have largely replaced conventional blood culture broth or biphasic media in many settings, at least in most private tertiary care hospitals in India. In Manipal, the mean time to positivity for blood culture from patients with bacteremic melioidosis was 30.6 ± 14.2 h (unpublished data). Of 27 patients who died, the blood cultures became positive within 24 h in 21 (77.7%) and 6 (22.2%) within 48 h of the sample collection, results that probably reflect high levels of bacteremia, as has been shown in studies elsewhere [36].

Various methods are used to identify Gram-negative bacilli in South Asian laboratories. With the advent of automated identification systems, most laboratories use methods such as API 20NE and VITEK 2 for identification of the organisms. However, it is likely that many isolates are being dismissed as contaminants without being identified, or labeled, as *'Pseudomonas* sp.' or *'Burkholderia* sp.' *Burkholderia* spp. account for 1–9% of isolates from patients in various multicenter studies of bacteremia in India [37–39]. In Manipal, *Burkholderia* spp. were isolated from 1.6% (114/7100) of positive blood cultures over the past six years, of which 68.4% (78/114) were confirmed as *B. pseudomallei* by type III secretion system 1 (TTSS1) PCR. It is unlikely that Manipal is unique, which implies that many cases of melioidosis are probably being missed in places where such isolates are not being correctly identified to species level. In practice, any laboratory in South Asia could make a presumptive identification of an oxidase-positive Gram-negative rod as *B. pseudomallei* using a simple three-antibiotic disc test that was recently shown to be highly specific in Vietnam [40]. Such an approach might usefully be promoted.

New methods are needed to reduce the time to diagnosis and appropriate treatment. One such test, the Active Melioidosis Detect Lateral Flow Immunoassay (AMD-LFA) (InBios Inc., Seattle, WA, USA), has shown promising results as a 'point-of-care' (POC) test for early diagnosis of melioidosis [41]. The kit has been evaluated in Manipal on clinical samples from patients suspected of having melioidosis and had a sensitivity of 85.7% and specificity of 93.6% compared with enrichment culture [42]. However, the test gave some weak false-positive results on urine specimens and thus needs further development and evaluation before it can be recommended as a POC test in endemic regions like South Asia.

6. Antibiotic Susceptibility and Treatment

Although there are no national guidelines for treating melioidosis in India or other South Asian countries, physicians in centers where cases are regularly diagnosed generally follow international guidelines, i.e., ceftazidime during the acute phase and co-trimoxazole, which is cheap and widely available, for eradication therapy. Generally, the antimicrobial susceptibility of isolates of *B. pseudomallei* in South Asia mirrors that from other regions [43], although rare instances of ceftazidime resistance have been reported [44]. Clinical failure of treatment despite apparent in vitro susceptibility has also been described [45].

7. Awareness of Melioidosis

There is an overall lack of awareness of melioidosis in South Asian countries, as is even the case in countries where the disease is diagnosed more often, such as Thailand [46]. Although there have been no formal surveys of knowledge and understanding about the disease, our day-to-day observations reveal that most doctors outside a few specialist centers have never heard of it, the public is completely unaware of it, and it is not on the radar of policymakers, either at a state or a national level.

8. Establishing a Melioidosis Network

The Indian Melioidosis Research Forum (IMRF; www.melioidosisindia.com—Figure 5) was initiated in 2015 during the First South Asian Melioidosis Congress (1st SAMC) in Manipal as an interactive web portal intended to enhance communication between those in South Asia with an interest in melioidosis. Thus far, it has connected researchers from 12 states of India and encouraged research on melioidosis. An earlier workshop about laboratory processing and environmental sampling had been conducted in Manipal in collaboration with the University of Cambridge, UK, and Mahidol University, Thailand. Seven centers have already started detecting cases of melioidosis in their own states after becoming involved in the network and are in regular contact with IMRF regarding the diagnosis of the disease and confirmation of the isolates. IMRF is well connected with the International Melioidosis Network (www.melioidosis.info) and is in a position to act as a regional leader to connect enthusiastic researchers from South Asia with the international melioidosis community. The 'Center for Emerging and Tropical Diseases' in Manipal was established in 2017 and now acts as an informal reference laboratory for melioidosis. To date, it has confirmed 80 clinical isolates of *B. pseudomallei* from laboratories in different states of India, including Orissa, Hyderabad, Kerala, Pondicherry, and Assam (Table 2). The center is currently working with the Medical University of Graz, Austria (Indo-Austrian collaboration) and the Central Soil Salinity Research Institute (CSSRI), Haryana, on the ecology of *B. pseudomallei*, and the Defense Research and Development Organization (DRDO), Gwalior, on the molecular epidemiology of the pathogen. It has been instrumental in mentoring researchers and microbiologists around the country and encouraging them to share their expertise and collaborate in future projects.

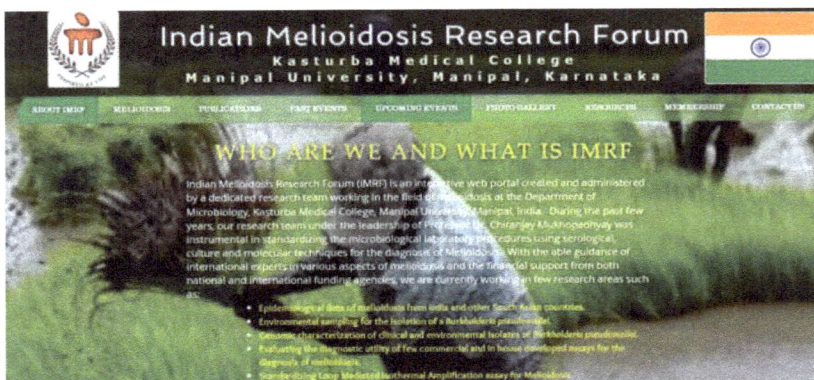

Figure 5. The Indian Melioidosis Research Forum (IMRF) has effectively brought researchers from all over India for research in melioidosis for the last two years.

Table 2. Isolates received by the Manipal Center for Emerging and Tropical Diseases for confirmation from various centers in India.

Institute (State)	Number of Isolates
Amritha Institute of Medical Sciences (Kerala)	34
Pondicherry Institute of Medical Sciences (Puducherry)	20
Nizams Institute of Medical Sciences (Hyderabad, Telangana)	12
Government Medical College (Tiruvanthapuram, Kerala)	7
Kalinga Institute of Medical Sciences (Orissa)	4
Government Medical College and Hospital (Mallapuram, Kerala)	2
Tripura Medical College (Assam)	1

9. Current and Future Challenges

Melioidosis is clearly an emerging disease in South Asia. The number of cases that have been microbiologically confirmed is still relatively small and it is too early to know whether the huge numbers of cases predicted to occur each year (more than 50,000 cases and 30,000 deaths in India alone) are anywhere near accurate. However, India faces an 'outbreak' of diabetes of enormous proportion. The prevalence of diabetes in India, according to the IDF Diabetes Atlas 2015 (http://www.diabetesatlas.org/across-the-globe.html), is reported to be 8.7% and, given the strong association between diabetes and melioidosis, it is likely that the latter will become more common as the former increases. Sadly, diagnostic microbiology services and laboratory-based surveillance across South Asia remain poorly developed, particularly those serving the rural poor, which is the very group that is at greatest risk of melioidosis.

The key challenges facing those with an interest in melioidosis in South Asia at this stage are as follows:

1. Collecting and collating better data on the number of cases of melioidosis occurring will require extensive communication with laboratories that are capable of identifying the organism.
2. Training more physicians and laboratory staff to recognize the clinical features of the disease and the characteristics of its causative organism (for example, through the use of the three-antibiotic disc test mentioned above) will require concerted efforts through universities and colleges and professional associations but will be difficult because of the fragmented nature of healthcare in the region.
3. Raising the profile of the disease with both policymakers and the general public at both local and national levels will inevitably have to be started locally, but, as the network of those with an interest grows, it should become easier to provide the necessary evidence that the morbidity and mortality of the disease warrant greater attention. One key objective would be to have melioidosis included in the list of diseases that are statutorily reportable by laboratories, which in turn would improve knowledge of the disease distribution and burden.

10. Conclusions

The burden of melioidosis in South Asia is predicted to be considerable, but as yet the evidence to support this is scant. However, given the huge population, the very high prevalence of underlying conditions predisposing to melioidosis such as diabetes mellitus, the shortcoming of diagnostic laboratory services, and the lack of awareness amongst health professionals, it remains possible that the predictions could indeed prove to be correct. There is evidence that interest in the disease is growing amongst healthcare workers and researchers, but the key challenge will be to coordinate efforts across this vast and diverse region. It is hoped that initiatives such as the IMRF and the SAMC (the second of which was held in Sri Lanka in 2017 and the next will take place in Bangladesh in 2020) will help to achieve this.

Supplementary Materials: They are available online at http://www.mdpi.com/2414-6366/3/2/51/s1.

Author Contributions: T.S. drafted the first version. C.M. reviewed and approved the final version. D.A.B.D. helped to revise and reorganize the review, supplied information about un-indexed reports, and corrected the English. G.M.V. supplied the data from Vellore and reviewed the final manuscript.

Conflicts of Interest: The authors declare no conflict of interest.

References

1. Cheng, A.C.; Currie, B.J. Melioidosis: Epidemiology, pathophysiology, and management. *Clin. Microbiol. Rev.* **2005**, *18*, 383–416. [CrossRef] [PubMed]
2. Limmathurotsakul, D.; Golding, N.; Dance, D.A.; Messina, J.P.; Pigott, D.M.; Moyes, C.L.; Rolim, D.B.; Bertherat, E.; Day, N.P.J.; Peacock, S.J.; et al. Predicted global distribution of *Burkholderia pseudomallei* and burden of melioidosis. *Nat. Microbiol.* **2016**, *1*, 15008. [CrossRef] [PubMed]
3. Vidyalakshmi, K.; Chakrapani, M.; Shrikala, B.; Damodar, S.; Lipika, S.; Vishal, S. Tuberculosis mimicked by melioidosis. *Int. J. Tuberc. Lung Dis.* **2008**, *12*, 1209–1215. [PubMed]
4. Lowe, P.; Engler, C.; Norton, R. Comparison of automated and nonautomated systems for identification of *Burkholderia pseudomallei. J. Clin. Microbiol.* **2002**, *40*, 4625–4627. [CrossRef] [PubMed]
5. Ives, J.; Thomson, T. Chronic melioidosis: The first report of a case infected in central India. *Glasgow Med. J.* **1953**, *34*, 61–67. [PubMed]
6. Thurnheer, U.; Novak, A.; Michel, M.; Ruchti, C.; Jutzi, H.; Weiss, M. Septic melioidosis following a visit to India. *Schweizerische Medizinische Wochenschrift* **1988**, *118*, 558–564. [PubMed]
7. Raghavan, K.; Shenoi, R.; Zaer, F.; Aiyer, R.; Ramamoorthy, P.; Mehta, M. Melioidosis in India. *Indian Pediatr.* **1991**, *28*, 184–188. [PubMed]
8. Bharadwaj, R.; Kagal, A.; Deshpandey, S.; Joshi, S.; Khare, P.; Junnarkar, A.; Phadke, M. Outbreak of plague-like illness caused by *Pseudomonas pseudomallei* in Maharashtra, India. *Lancet* **1994**, *344*, 1574. [CrossRef]

9. Dance, D.A.B.; Sanders, D.; Pitt, T.L.; Speller, D.C. *Burkholderia pseudomallei* and Indian plague-like illness. *Lancet* **1995**, *346*, 904–905. [CrossRef]

10. John, T.J.; Jesudason, M.V.; Lalitha, M.K.; Ganesh, A.; Mohandas, V.; Cherian, T.; Mathai, M.; Chandy, M.J. Melioidosis in India: The tip of the iceberg? *Indian J. Med. Res.* **1996**, *103*, 62–65. [PubMed]

11. Cherian, T.; John, T.J.; Ramakrishna, B.; Lalitha, M.K.; Raghupathy, P. Disseminated melioidosis. *Indian Pediatr.* **1996**, *33*, 403–406. [PubMed]

12. Murali, R.; Ganesh, A.; Jesudason, M.V.; Mathew, R.K.; Date, A. Surat '94: Was it melioidosis? Interesting observation from the first case of imported melioidosis in India. *J. Assoc. Phys. India* **1996**, *44*, 218–219.

13. Jesudason, M.V.; Shanthakumari, R.; John, T.J. *Burkholderia pseudomallei*—An emerging pathogen in India. *Indian J. Med. Microbiol.* **1997**, *15*, 1–2.

14. Jesudasom, M.V.; Anbarasu, A.; John, T.J. Septicaemic melioidosis in a tertiary care hospital in South India. *Indian J. Med. Res.* **2003**, *117*, 119–121.

15. Kang, G.; Rajan, D.P.; Ramakrishna, B.; Aucken, H.; Dance, D. Melioidosis in India. *Lancet* **1996**, *347*, 1565–1566. [CrossRef]

16. Rao, P.S.; Dhawan, R.; Shivananda, P. *Burkholderia pseudomallei* infections. *Trop. Dr.* **2002**, *32*, 174–175. [CrossRef] [PubMed]

17. Hinjoy, S.; Hantrakun, V.; Kongyu, S.; Kaewrakmuk, J.; Wangrangsimakul, T.; Jitsuronk, S.; Saengchun, W.; Bhengsri, S.; Akarachotpong, T.; Thamthitiwat, S.; et al. Melioidosis in Thailand: Present and future. *Trop. Med. Infect. Dis.* **2018**, *3*, 38. [CrossRef] [PubMed]

18. Currie, B.J.; Fisher, D.A.; Howard, D.M.; Burrow, J.N.; Lo, D.; Selva-Nayagam, S.; Anstey, N.M.; Huffam, S.E.; Snelling, P.L.; Marks, P.J.; et al. Endemic melioidosis in tropical northern Australia: A 10-year prospective study and review of the literature. *Clin. Infect. Dis.* **2000**, *31*, 981–986. [CrossRef] [PubMed]

19. Koshy, M.; Jagannati, M.; Ralph, R.; Punitha, J.V.; David, T.S.; Sathyendra, S.; Veeraraghavan, B.; Varghese, G.M. Clinical manifestations, susceptibility patterns and predictors of poor outcome of melioidosis in India. *Emerg. Infect. Dis.* **2018**. under review.

20. Shrestha, N.K.; Sharma, S.K.; Khanal, B.; Bhatta, N.; Dhakal, S.S. Melioidosis imported into Nepal. *Scand. J. Infect. Dis.* **2005**, *37*, 64–66. [CrossRef] [PubMed]

21. Stokes, K.J.; McCarthy, S. *Pseudomonas pseudomallei*: Isolation from a chronic sternal abscess. *J. Med. Lab. Technol.* **1969**, *26*, 199–201. [PubMed]

22. Sheppard, M.J.; Marriott, R.M.; Brown, T.J. Long latency pneumonia: A case of melioidosis. *J. Infect.* **1990**, *20*, 83–84. [CrossRef]

23. Vandana, K.E.; Mukhopadhyay, C.; Tellapragada, C.; Kamath, A.; Tipre, M.; Bhat, V.; Sathiakumar, N. Seroprevalence of *Burkholderia pseudomallei* among adults in coastal areas in southwestern India. *PLoS Negl. Trop. Dis.* **2016**, *10*, e0004610. [CrossRef] [PubMed]

24. Peacock, S.J.; Cheng, A.C.; Currie, B.J.; Dance, D.A. The use of positive serological tests as evidence of exposure to *Burkholderia pseudomallei*. *Am. J. Trop. Med. Hyg.* **2011**, *84*, 1021–1022. [CrossRef] [PubMed]

25. Moore, T.D.; Allen, A.M.; Palmer, A.E. Melioidosis—Maryland. *Morb. Mortal. Wkly. Rep.* **1969**, *18*, 278–279.

26. Das, A.M.; Paranjape, V.L. *Pseudomonas pseudomallei* associated with bovine abortion in India. *Vet. Med. Rev.* **1986**, *2*, 173–176.

27. Prakash, A.; Thavaselvam, D.; Kumar, A.; Kumar, A.; Arora, S.; Tiwari, S.; Barua, A.; Sathyaseelan, K. Isolation, identification and characterization of *Burkholderia pseudomallei* from soil of coastal region of India. *Springer Plus* **2014**, *3*, 438. [CrossRef] [PubMed]

28. Peddayelachagiri, B.V.; Paul, S.; Nagaraj, S.; Gogoi, M.; Sripathy, M.H.; Batra, H.V. Prevalence and identification of *Burkholderia pseudomallei* and near-neighbor species in the Malabar coastal region of India. *PLoS Negl. Trop. Dis.* **2016**, *10*, e0004956. [CrossRef] [PubMed]

29. Shabbir, M.Z.; Jamil, T.; Ali, A.A.; Ahmad, A.; Naeem, M.; Chaudhary, M.H.; Bilal, M.; Ali, M.A.; Muhammad, K.; Yaqub, T.; et al. Prevalence and distribution of soil-borne zoonotic pathogens in Lahore district of Pakistan. *Front. Microbiol.* **2015**, *6*, 917. [CrossRef] [PubMed]

30. Mukhopadhyay, C.; Kaestli, M.; Vandana, K.E.; Sushma, K.; Mayo, M.; Richardson, L.; Tuanyok, A.; Keim, P.; Godoy, D.; Spratt, B.G.; et al. Molecular characterization of clinical *Burkholderia pseudomallei* isolates from India. *Am. J. Trop. Med. Hyg.* **2011**, *85*, 121–123. [CrossRef] [PubMed]

31. Tellapragada, C.; Kamthan, A.; Shaw, T.; Vandana, K.; Kumar, S.; Bhat, V.; Mukhopadhyay, C. Unravelling the molecular epidemiology and genetic diversity among *Burkholderia pseudomallei* isolates from South India using multi-locus sequence typing. *PLoS ONE* **2016**, *11*, e0168331. [CrossRef] [PubMed]

32. De Smet, B.; Sarovich, D.S.; Price, E.P.; Mayo, M.; Theobald, V.; Kham, C.; Heng, S.; Thong, P.; Holden, M.T.; Parkhill, J.; et al. Whole-genome sequencing confirms that *Burkholderia pseudomallei* multilocus sequence types common to both Cambodia and Australia are due to homoplasy. *J. Clin. Microbiol.* **2015**, *53*, 323–326. [CrossRef] [PubMed]

33. Limmathurotsakul, D.; Kanoksil, M.; Wuthiekanun, V.; Kitphati, R.; Day, N.P.; Peacock, S.J. Activities of daily living associated with acquisition of melioidosis in northeast Thailand: A matched case-control study. *PLoS Negl. Trop. Dis.* **2013**, *7*, e2072. [CrossRef] [PubMed]

34. Suntornsut, P.; Wongsuwan, N.; Malasit, M.; Kitphati, R.; Michie, S.; Peacock, S.J.; Limmathurotsakul, D. Barriers and recommended interventions to prevent melioidosis in northeast Thailand: A focus group study using the behaviour change wheel. *PLoS Negl. Trop. Dis.* **2016**, *10*, e0004823. [CrossRef] [PubMed]

35. Tellapragada, C.; Shaw, T.; D'Souza, A.; Eshwara, V.K.; Mukhopadhyay, C. Improved detection of *Burkholderia pseudomallei* from non-blood clinical specimens using enrichment culture and PCR: Narrowing diagnostic gap in resource constrained settings. *Trop. Med. Int. Health* **2017**. [CrossRef] [PubMed]

36. Tiangpitayakorn, C.; Songsivilai, S.; Piyasangthong, N.; Dharakul, T. Speed of detection of *Burkholderia pseudomallei* in blood cultures and its correlation with the clinical outcome. *Am. J. Trop. Med. Hyg.* **1997**, *57*, 96–99. [CrossRef] [PubMed]

37. Mørch, K.; Manoharan, A.; Chandy, S.; Chacko, N.; Alvarez-Uria, G.; Patil, S.; Henry, A.; Nesaraj, J.; Kuriakose, C.; Singh, A.; et al. Acute undifferentiated fever in India: A multicentre study of aetiology and diagnostic accuracy. *BMC Infect. Dis.* **2017**, *17*, 665. [CrossRef] [PubMed]

38. Khan, I.D.; Sahni, A.K.; Bharadwaj, R.; Lall, M.; Jindal, A.K.; Sashindran, V.K. Emerging organisms in a tertiary healthcare set up. *Med. J. Armed Forces India* **2014**, *70*, 120–128. [CrossRef] [PubMed]

39. Gandra, S.; Mojica, N.; Klein, E.Y.; Ashok, A.; Nerurkar, V.; Kumari, M.; Ramesh, U.; Dey, S.; Vadwai, V.; Das, B.R.; et al. Trends in antibiotic resistance among major bacterial pathogens isolated from blood cultures tested at a large private laboratory network in India, 2008–2014. *Int. J. Infect. Dis.* **2016**, *50*, 75–82. [CrossRef] [PubMed]

40. Trinh, T.T.; Hoang, T.S.; Tran, D.A.; Trinh, V.T.; Gohler, A.; Nguyen, T.T.; Hoang, S.N.; Krumkamp, R.; Nguyen, L.T.N.; May, J.; et al. A simple laboratory algorithm for diagnosis of melioidosis in resource-constrained areas: A study from north-central Vietnam. *Clin. Microbiol. Infect.* **2018**, *24*, e1–e4. [CrossRef] [PubMed]

41. Houghton, R.L.; Reed, D.E.; Hubbard, M.A.; Dillon, M.J.; Chen, H.; Currie, B.J.; Mayo, M.; Sarovich, D.S.; Theobald, V.; Limmathurotsakul, D.; et al. Development of a prototype lateral flow immunoassay (LFI) for the rapid diagnosis of melioidosis. *PLoS Negl. Trop. Dis.* **2014**, *8*, e2727. [CrossRef] [PubMed]

42. Shaw, T.; Tellapragada, C.; Ke, V.; Au Coin, D.P.; Mukhopadhyay, C. Performance evaluation of Active Melioidosis Detect-Lateral Flow Assay (AMD-LFA) for diagnosis of melioidosis in endemic settings with limited resources. *PLoS ONE* **2018**, *13*, e0194595. [CrossRef] [PubMed]

43. Shaw, T.; Tellapragada, C.; Eshwara, V.K.; Bhat, H.V.; Mukhopadhyay, C. The antibiotics of choice for the treatment of melioidosis in Indian set up. *Indian J. Med. Microbiol.* **2016**, *34*, 353. [PubMed]

44. Behera, B.; Prasad Babu, T.L.; Kamalesh, A.; Reddy, G. Ceftazidime resistance in *Burkholderia pseudomallei*: First report from India. *Asian Pac. J. Trop. Med.* **2012**, *5*, 329–330. [CrossRef]

45. Pillai, M.P.; Faizal, B.P.; Urs, V.D. Emerging drug resistance in melioidosis. *Ann. Trop. Med. Public Health* **2014**, *7*, 263–265. [CrossRef]

46. Chansrichavala, P.; Wongsuwan, N.; Suddee, S.; Malasit, M.; Hongsuwan, M.; Wannapinij, P.; Kitphati, R.; Day, N.P.J.; Michie, S.; Peacock, S.J.; et al. Public awareness of melioidosis in Thailand and potential use of video clips as educational tools. *PLoS ONE* **2015**, *10*, e0121311. [CrossRef] [PubMed]

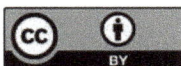

Tropical Medicine and
Infectious Disease

MDPI

Review

Transmission Modes of Melioidosis in Taiwan

Pei-Tan Hsueh [1], Wei-Tien Huang [2], Hsu-Kai Hsueh [2], Ya-Lei Chen [2,*,†] and Yao-Shen Chen [1,*,†]

[1]   Department of Internal Medicine, Kaohsiung Veterans General Hospital, Kaohsiung 813, Taiwan;
      mulberrymonster@gmail.com

[2]   Department of Biotechnology, National Kaohsiung Normal University, Kaohsiung 824, Taiwan;
      milo.huang1121@gmail.com (W.-T.H); cuprousion@yahoo.com.tw (H.-K.H.)

*   Correspondence: dan1001@ms31.hinet.net (Y.-L.C.); yschen@isca.vghks.gov.tw (Y.-S.C);
      Tel.: +886-7-717-2930 (Y.-L.C.); +886-7-342-2121 (Y.-S.C)

†   These authors contributed equally to this work.

Received: 29 January 2018; Accepted: 17 February 2018; Published: 28 February 2018

Abstract: In Taiwan, melioidosis is an emerging disease that suddenly increased in the Er-Ren River Basin, beginning in 2005 and in the Zoynan region during 2008–2012, following a typhoon. Additionally, the disease sporadically increased in a geography-dependent manner in 2016. Subcutaneous inoculation, ingestion, and the inhalation of soil or water contaminated with *Burkholderia pseudomallei* are recognized as the transmission modes of melioidosis. The appearance of environmental *B. pseudomallei* positivity in northern, central and southern Taiwan is associated with disease prevalence (cases/population: 0.03/100,000 in the northern region, 0.29/100,000 in the central region and 1.98/100,000 in the southern region). However, melioidosis-clustered areas are confined to 5 to 7.5 km^2 hot spots containing high-density populations, but *B. pseudomallei*-contaminated environments are located >5 km northwestern of the periphery of these hot spots. The observation that the concentration of *B. pseudomallei*-specific DNA in aerosols was positively correlated with the incidence of melioidosis and the appearance of a northwesterly wind in a hot spot indicated that airborne transmission had occurred in Taiwan. Moreover, the isolation rate in the superficial layers of a contaminated crop field in the northwest was correlated with PCR positivity in aerosols collected from the southeast over a two-year period. The genotype ST58 was identified by multilocus sequence typing in human and aerosol isolates. The genotype ST1001 has increased in prevalence but has been sporadically distributed elsewhere since 2016. These data indicate the transmission modes and environmental foci that support the dissemination of melioidosis are changing in Taiwan.

Keywords: melioidosis; *Burkholderia pseudomallei*; transmission modes

---

1. Introduction

Melioidosis is an emerging and fatally infectious disease that is endemic to Southeast Asia and northern Australia [1]. However, its incidence may be underestimated in many regions, such as India, South America, and Africa, because the disease is difficult to diagnose due to its very diverse clinical manifestations and the use of inadequate bacterial isolation and identification methods. Annual disease rates could be increasing worldwide as a result of transmission by travelers that were exposed to contaminants in melioidosis-endemic areas [2–4]. Overall, approximately 165,000 human melioidosis cases occur annually worldwide, and approximately 89,000 people die annually from this disease [5]. To date, no systematic international estimation of the clinical or sub-clinical incidence of melioidosis has been performed using a consistent, standardized, and quality-controlled method under the same health- or medically-controlled conditions. This makes it difficult to adequately compare the incidence of the disease among countries or regions and to predict the disseminated scope of melioidosis.

The pathogen underlying melioidosis is an environmental saprophyte and Gram-negative bacterium called *Burkholderia pseudomallei* that is usually found in the soil and surface water, and is sometimes seen in air particles [6,7]. People acquire melioidosis from directly contacting, ingesting or inhaling soil, water or dust contaminated with *B. pseudomallei* [8–10]. Nevertheless, melioidosis cases are usually clustered during the rainy season, particularly after the appearance of a heavy rainfall, cyclone, or typhoon [11–13]. The transmission modes of melioidosis probably differ because people's customs and lifestyles, as well as the geographical position of melioidosis case clusters differ. In this review, we focus on studies of the incidence of melioidosis in Taiwan that provide insight into the mechanism of melioidosis transmission.

2. Underestimated Period of Melioidosis in Taiwan (1984–2004)

The first reported case of melioidosis in Taiwan involved a patient who acquired melioidosis with multilobar pneumonia by drowning in the Philippines in 1984 [14]. Between 1984 and 2000, 12 pulmonary and two subcutaneous melioidosis cases and one melioidosis case with a mycotic aneurysm were reported [15]. Of those patients, 73.3% (11/15) had no overseas travel history. Because the symptoms of melioidosis are protean, melioidosis can go undetected. Its prevalence may therefore have been underestimated by physicians in Taiwan during the earlier years of its presence. Because *B. pseudomallei* is an uncertain airborne disease that belongs to a group of 'selected agents' that could be utilized to develop bacterial weapons for bioterrorism [16], melioidosis in Taiwan has been classified as a notifiable disease since 2000. This means that all of the culture-confirmed cases of melioidosis should be reported to the Centers for Disease Control (CDC) at the Department of Health in Taiwan. No case was reported from 2000 to 2002, five were reported in 2003, and 13 were reported in 2004. However, *B. pseudomallei* has consistently been isolated from soil at a depth of 30–60 cm in paddies in Taiwan and other countries [17,18]. In synthetic soil or water media, *B. pseudomallei* can survive for 150 days or more, indicating that affected Taiwanese individuals may have acquired melioidosis from indigenous bacteria, rather than by traveling to endemic areas [19]. To explore the potential for exposure to *B. pseudomallei* in Taiwan, an indirect ELISA (enzyme-linked immunosorbent assay) that targeted the truncated flagellin of the bacterium was developed [20]. Seropositive rates of approximately 4%, 2.8%, and 5% were detected in northern, central, and southern Taiwan, respectively [21]. Approximately 3% of the positive cases were patients with diabetes mellitus, which is a risk factor for melioidosis [22].

3. An Outbreak of Melioidosis in Taiwan (2005)

In 2005, after a typhoon event, melioidosis cases were clustered in the Er-Ren River Basin of Taiwan during a three-month period [23]. In 2005, while 0.3 cases/100,000 population were infected throughout the entire population of Taiwan, the incidence of melioidosis reached 122 cases/100,000 population in the area downstream of the Er-Ren River Basin. In the affected area, the incidence rates were higher than the 7.98–21.3 cases/100,000 population and 5.4–24.2 cases/100,000 population in Thailand and northern Australia, respectively [24–26]. Approximately 75% of these melioidosis patients had *B. pseudomallei* bacteremia, 50% had concomitant pleuropulmonary infections, and 20% died during hospitalization [27]. Pulsed-field gel electrophoresis (PFGE) typing revealed that two distinct genotypic clones appeared during this outbreak [27]. These two distinct types have been demonstrated to be ST58 and ST99 by the multilocus sequencing typing (MLST) method [28].

When compared with the seropositive rates of anti-*B. pseudomallei* flagellin antibodies of 2.8–5% in Taiwanese individuals before 2005, the rates were increased to as high as 36.6%, 21.6%, and 10.9% in the downstream, midstream, and upstream regions of the Er-Ren River, respectively. Those seropositive rates were associated with the incidence of melioidosis as follows: 120 cases/100,000 population in the downstream region, 68 cases/100,000 population in the midstream region and 36 cases/100,000 population in the upstream regions. However, *B. pseudomallei* was only isolated from the soil in the upstream region and never from the mid- or downstream regions, although PCR positivity to *B. pseudomallei*-specific amplicons was relatively higher in mid- and downstream regions than in upstream regions. People seemed to have acquired melioidosis through exposure to contaminated soil that had flowed down from the upstream river due to the heavy rain that was associated with the typhoon [26]. However, 70% (28/40) of the melioidosis patients in this outbreak denied recent contact with mud or dirty water before their illness [27]. Approximately 32.8–34.8% of the 105 adults who lived in the mid- and downstream areas of the Er-Ren River acknowledged having been flooded during this typhoon event [26].

After this outbreak, melioidosis was widely recognized as an indigenously emerging and fatally infectious disease in Taiwan. The CDC (Taiwan) reinforced the education and management of melioidosis using medical resources and improved the regulation of notifiable melioidosis in Taiwan. Thus, the numbers of melioidosis cases reported in the CDC database since this issue arose are more reliable than they previously were [29]. From 2005 to 2007, the average incidences of melioidosis were 0.03 cases/100,000 population in northern Taiwan, 0.29 cases/100,000 in central Taiwan and 1.98 cases/100,000 in southern Taiwan. The disease incidence was associated with PCR positivity for *B. pseudomallei*-specific amplicons, which was found in 1.3%, 10.1% and 19.4% of environmental samples in northern, central, and southern Taiwan, respectively. Viable *B. pseudomallei* was cultivated only from the soil in southern Taiwan (south of the Tropic of Cancer; isolation rate, 12.6%), and environmental isolates were never found in central and northern Taiwan (north of the Tropic of Cancer) [30]. *B. pseudomallei* is usually isolated from moist soil or water in tropical and subtropical countries, and is rarely found in temperate countries [1]. Although the favorable physical (pH and water content) and chemical (nutrients, salinity, organic, and inorganic compounds) conditions for the growth of *B. pseudomallei* are inconsistent in many soil studies [19,31–34], *B. pseudomallei* can thrive in rice fields when nutrients (e.g., fertilizer) are depleted during agriculture practices and rice field management [31]. After harvesting rice, the straw is frequently burned in the rice field in Taiwan. The presence or absence of *B. pseudomallei* related to rice field management in Taiwan is unknown. However, the soil, even if relatively dry, may act as a reservoir during the dry season, with an increase in the proliferation and potential for mobilization from soil into water in the wet season [35].

4. A Plateau in the Incidence of Melioidosis in Taiwan (2008–2012)

In 2008–2012, the annual incidence of melioidosis among the entire Taiwanese population increased to 0.19 cases/100,000 population as compared with 0.07 cases/100,000 population in 2007 [36]. Most of the cases were geographically clustered in the Er-Ren River Basin (size, 108 km^2; population, 79,790 people) and Zoynan region (size, 60 km^2; population, 127,438 people) in Taiwan [36,37]. The average incidences of melioidosis in both regions reached 16.7 cases/100,000 population (Er-Ren River Basin) and 10.9 cases/100,000 population, respectively, from 2008 to 2011 (Zoynan region). Approximately 62.5–67% of melioidosis patients were unemployed and had no recent travel history because most patients were elderly or had chronic diseases, such as diabetes, renal failure, or cancer [37,38]. Acute pulmonary melioidosis predominated (>70%). Furthermore, 88% of melioidosis cases were found during the rainy season, and 22% of the patients died [38]. Based on molecular tracing observations, ST99 (multilocus sequencing typing) was prevalent in the Er-Ren River Basin in 2005, but ST58 was found in the Zoynan region in 2008–2009, indicating that the epidemic strains of melioidosis were altered because the environmental foci contaminated with *B. pseudomallei* differed [28].

Two hot spots for melioidosis occurred 10.3 km apart, but the climatic conditions, including rainfall and wind strength, were different because the topographical characteristics differed, as described below. The Er-Ren River Basin is a plain, and the Zoynan Region is a hilly area. Rainfall that lasts for a period of 4–7 days is a trigger factor associated with an increase in melioidosis cases in both areas. However, rainfall lasting 6–8 days and wind with a speed >19 m/s (>17.2 m/s is defined as a typhoon) and a specific angle of wind direction (150°, 220°, or 280°) are associated with increases in the number of melioidosis cases in the flat Er-Ren River Basin. In the hilly Zoynan region, these wind speeds, when combined with rainfall lasing five days, was also associated the incidence of melioidosis [37]. In Taiwan, over 80% of melioidosis cases occurred in the rainy season when the typhoon appeared [13,26,27]. It is not surprising that the wind speed (>19 m/s) was associated with the occurrence of melioidosis in Taiwan. When considering the epidemiological survey described above, in the Er-Ren River Basin, *B. pseudomallei* was isolated from upstream areas, but melioidosis cases were increased in the mid- and downstream areas [26]. The direction of the sampled site contaminated with *B. pseudomallei* at the hot spot is from the southeast to northwest. Thus, the wind, with a 150° angle, as a vector could assist the transmission of *B. pseudomallei* to the patients if the airborne particles (aerosols) were generated from contaminated soil or water.

In contrast, in the Zoynan region, if a strong northwest wind originating from a counterclockwise cyclone occurred during the season the typhoon appeared, the incidence of melioidosis should be higher in the southeast districts, even though *B. pseudomallei* is isolated from environments in the northwestern region. In particular, the hills located south of the Zoynan region become a natural barrier to obstruct the transmission of aerosols contaminated with *B. pseudomallei*. Indeed, 96% (80/83) of melioidosis cases occurred north of the hilly Zoynan region, but rare cases occurred south of the Zoynan region [37]. To test this hypothesis, we first demonstrated that the concentration of *B. pseudomallei*-specific amplicons was increased in the rainy season when the typhoon appeared when compared with that in the dry season when the appearance of a typhoon is rare [39]. By sampling randomly but with an even distribution geographically as much as possible, several sites contaminated with *B. pseudomallei* in the northwestern wetted, cropped, or non-cropped soil of the hot spots were identified. The concentration of *B. pseudomallei*-specific amplicons in aerosols was positively correlated with the incidence of melioidosis and the appearance of a northwesterly wind. Moreover, the isolation rate in the superficial layers of the contaminated cropped field in the northwest was correlated with PCR positivity for aerosols that were collected from the southeast from 2011–2013. The genotype ST58 of *B. pseudomallei* was identified from soil, aerosol, and human isolates. The airborne transmission of melioidosis was demonstrated to move from contaminated soil to aerosols and/or to humans in the Zoynan region [6].

5. A New Hot Spot of Melioidosis in Taiwan (At the Present Time)

From 2000 to 2017, 516 melioidosis cases were reported in Taiwan. As melioidosis is a tropical disease, approximately 86% (444/516) of cases are geographically distributed south of the Tropic of Cancer in Taiwan (Figure 1A). Over 50% (223/444) of the cases were successively clustered in the Er-Ren River Basin in 2005 and in the Zoynan region in 2008–2012, and in Siaogang–Fengshan, more sporadic cases with subcutaneously localized infection have occurred since 2003 (Figure 1B). Usually, acute pulmonary melioidosis with bacteremia is clustered after extreme climate events, for example, heavy rainfall and typhoons, but melioidosis with localized infection can occur in dry seasons. For example, patients who were admitted with melioidosis 7–14 days after heavy monsoonal rainfall (188 mm) were more ill or were more likely to die (rainfall >211 mm) in Australia [40]. Over 1000 mm of rainfall during the wet season and a wind speed of >19 m/s (Er-Ren River Basin) were indicators for melioidosis occurrence in Taiwan [27,37,38]. The genotype ST1001 of *B. pseudomallei* was found in melioidosis patients dwelling in Siaogang–Fengshan in 2016. ST58 was prevalent in soil and human isolates during 2008–2012, while ST1001 has been sporadically found in humans and the environment. Both representative strains, vgh07 (ST58) and vgh16 (ST1001), have been sequenced. The vgh07 (ST58) strain contains 16 genomic islands, including a potential pathogenic island that harbors an invasive hemolytic gene, but vgh16 (ST1001) did not harbor any genomic island [41,42]. When the BALB/c mice were infected with the strains intravenously and the strains were re-isolated from liver extracts and used to re-infect the mice intravenously, repeatedly, the phenotypic levels of 3-hydroxytetradecanoic acid (an indicator of lipopolysaccharide of *B. pseudomallei*), biofilm formation and flagellar expression in both types were significantly increased when compared with those in the original parent strains. Moreover, the survival rates of the mice infected with both types that re-isolated from liver extracts were obviously decreased, indicating that the animals, as reservoirs, could increase the virulence of *B. pseudomallei* [43]. An environmental strain isolated from Pahang, Malaysia, was reported to show up-regulation of adhesins, virulence factors, and stress response-related proteins when the strain was injected intra-peritoneally into a mouse and re-isolated from the spleen [44]. If ST1001 persists in animals that serve as reservoirs for a long time, this strain can develop an increased virulence.

More research is needed to explore the molecular links among the environment, animals, and humans in Siaogang-Fengshan. However, since 2015, political considerations have resulted in a CDC (Taiwan) policy that involves tightly regulating the biosecurity and biosafety of *B. pseudomallei*. The ability to use a large panel of *B. pseudomallei* strains for molecular typing, as was previously possible, is now restricted. Only six strains, including ST1001, were identified in the soil ($n = 3$), animals ($n = 1$), and humans ($n = 2$) in Siaogang-Fengshan from 2015 to 2017. Their virulence in animals has not yet been determined.

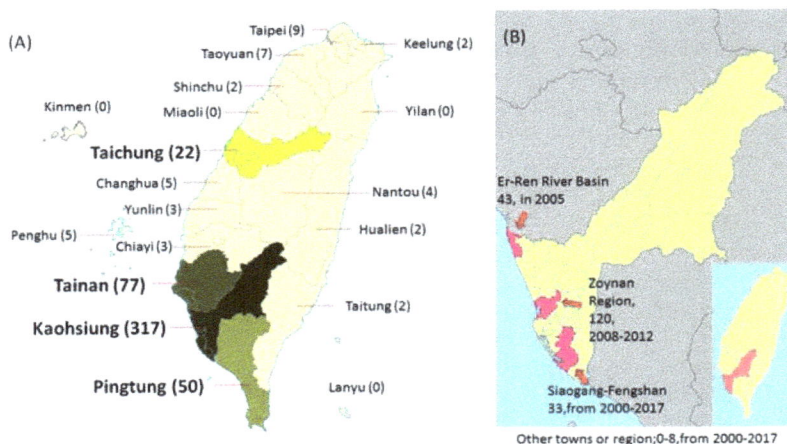

Figure 1. Geographical distribution of melioidosis in Taiwan. (**A**) In the entire island with the case number shown in brackets. (**B**) In Kaohsiung district. Two hot spots (Er-Ren River Basin and Zoynan Region) and Siagogan-Fengshan (location, case number, and year in which it occurred) are shown as red color.

6. Unresolved Problems Related to Melioidosis Dissemination in Taiwan

Melioidosis in Taiwan has successively clustered in certain areas, such as the Er-Ren River Basin, Zoynan regions, and Siaogang-Fengshan, consisting of small-sized regions with areas containing approximately 5–7.5 km^2, and has spread through different transmission modes or via exposure to different environmental foci [36]. As our insight into the geographical distribution of melioidosis cases and environmental foci improves, physicians will be able to increase alertness and awareness, leading to better control of the disease.

However, the pH value, solar strength, moisture, organic or inorganic content, temperature changes, and salinity of soil each affect the growth of *B. pseudomallei* in the environment [9,19,31–34]. To detect the presence of *B. pseudomallei* in the environment, the PCR detection rates are usually higher than those of microbiological cultures in our studies [6,26,30,36]. The presence of phages in *B. pseudomallei* strains has been reported to decrease their successful isolation from environmental samples [45]. Both *B. cenocepacia* and *B. multivorans*, which are antagonistic to *B. pseudomallei*, are widely distributed throughout the rice fields of Taiwan [46]. The secondary metabolites of *Bacillus amyloliquefaciens* isolated from soil can kill *B. pseudomallei* in vitro [47]. The amoeba *Paravahlkampfia ustiana* and some *Acanthamoeba* sp. are predators that graze on *B. pseudomallei*, while *Hartmannella* spp. and *Acanthamoeba astronyxis* may be reservoirs of *B. pseudomallei* in soil or water [48–50]. The physical or chemical parameters influencing the growth of *B. pseudomallei* in the environment are not completely understood in Taiwan. Although the geographical distribution of *B. pseudomallei* in the environment is very uneven, high isolation rates in soil or water are usually associated with a high incidence of melioidosis in surveys using a large area [26,30,36].

However, melioidosis-clustered cases are distributed within 5–7.5 km^2 of the hot spot regions with high-density populations, but an environment contaminated with *B. pseudomallei* was located

>5 km away from the periphery of the hot spot [6,36]. When most of the patients in a population are elderly or have diabetes and cannot participate in outdoor activities, a characterization of the vectors that carry contaminated *B. pseudomallei* should be performed [37,38]. The airborne transmission of infectious agents from aerosols to humans has been epidemiologically demonstrated using molecular linking and statistical methods. However, the finding that the isolation rates of *B. pseudomallei* in aerosols are very low contradicts the notion that the contaminated sources are contained in aerosols [6]. Additionally, in a rice paddy field in Ubon Ratchathani, northeast Thailand, *B. pseudomallei* was never isolated from air and rainwater samples during a 13-month prospective study [7]. In the absence of improved isolation techniques, it is uncertain whether environmental uncultivated *B. pseudomallei* can be considered an infective source.

Alternatively, it remains unclear how people become easily exposed to contaminated water or soil. In Taiwan, approximately 20% of water samples that were obtained in the Zoynan regions after 2012 appeared to contain *B. pseudomallei*-specific amplicons [36]. In contrast, the content of *B. pseudomallei* in samples obtained from rice field water is reportedly as high as 60% in Thailand [7]. The occupational risk of melioidosis is correlated with a farmer's exposure to contaminated soil through agricultural activity; approximately 86% of those diagnosed with melioidosis also lived near a river in Liao [1,51]. Spatial analysis revealed that, in northern Australia, melioidosis is particularly endemic in Townsville, north Queensland, where one set of melioidosis cases was clustered in the area of the old course of a major waterway [52]. In the Northern Territory of Australia, all of the *B. pseudomallei*-positive environmental sites (n = 104) were permanently waterlogged, or waterlogged during the wet season, or were irrigated [53]. Water serving as a transmission vehicle for *B. pseudomallei* has been suggested when melioidosis case clusters are associated with the water supply [54,55]. Ingestion of or contact with water contaminated with *B. pseudomallei* is probably the transmission mode. However, more importantly, Taiwanese individuals, especially the elderly or patients, drink boiled water or routinely avoid being in close proximity to rivers or waterlogged areas.

The *A. lenticulata* PT-14 strain was isolated from a well after a flood disaster caused by a typhoon and could become a host of the endosymbiont *Burkholderia* spp., as the 16S RNA genes of the bacterium were detected in the amoeba. *A. lenticulata* is widely distributed in aquatic and terrestrial environments and frequently contains various bacterial endosymbionts, such as *Mycobacterium* sp., *Legionella* sp., and *Burkholderia* sp. [56–58]. In an in vitro study, *A. lenticulata* PT-14 displayed endosymbiosis with *B. pseudomallei* vgh07 (ST58) and vgh16 (ST1001) (data not shown). The levels of *A. lenticulata* distributed in river or drinking water reservoirs differ according to season; specifically, certain 18S RNA genes of *A. lenticulata* are frequently detected during September to November [59,60], a period in which typhoon invasion usually occurs. Typhoons are an important environmental phenomenon that triggers the incidence of melioidosis case clusters and is associated with high detection rates of *B. pseudomallei*-specific amplicons in water [13,35,36]. The intracellular survival of bacteria in amoeba was not only evolutionarily designed to protect the bacteria from the harsh conditions of the environment, but also to enable the bacteria to develop a virulence that allows intracellular growth in mammals [61]. Thus, endosymbiotic *B. pseudomallei*, if they exist, not only interfere with microbiological cultures using filtered water, likely from sampling in Taiwan, but also become an alternative transmission mode of melioidosis from water to humans.

7. Conclusions

As an emerging and fatally infectious disease, melioidosis occurs because of exposure to soil or water contaminated with *B. pseudomallei*. Over 50% (223/444) of melioidosis cases were successively clustered in the Er-Ren River Basin in 2005 and in the Zoynan region in 2008–2012, and cases were also sporadically distributed throughout the Siaogang-Fengshan region in Taiwan. Subcutaneous inoculation, ingestion, and inhalation of contaminated soil or water are the main routes of melioidosis transmission. In 2005, individuals in the Taiwanese population acquired melioidosis seemingly through exposure to contaminated soil that flowed downstream from an upstream river area. While the upstream area had soil from which *B. pseudomallei* was isolated at high rates, the downstream region had a high incidence of melioidosis and high sero-prevalence for anti-*B. pseudomallei* antibodies. In 2008–2012, in the Zoynan region, melioidosis-clustered cases increased after typhoon events. In a prospective study, aerosols that contained *B. pseudomallei*-specific DNA were well distributed in the densely populated districts, but were rarely found in their surrounding areas. The concentration of specific DNA in aerosols was correlated with the melioidosis incidence and northwesterly wind in this endemic area. The isolation rate in the superficial layers of the contaminated crop field in the northwest was correlated with the PCR positivity of aerosols collected from the southeastern district over a two-year period. Because a strong northwest wind originating from a counterclockwise cyclone occurred during the wet season with a typhoon, the number of melioidosis cases was increased in a southeast district when *B. pseudomallei* was isolated from the northwestern region. Thus, melioidosis is airborne and was transmitted from contaminated soils to aerosols and/or to humans in Zoynan regions from 2008 to 2012. *B. pseudomallei* vgh07 (a representative strain of ST58) and its similar strain, which has a high virulence, have been prevalent in human and environmental isolates; however, the vgh16 strain (a representative strain of ST1001) and similar strains, with low virulence, were isolated from 2003 to 2016. If the ST1001 strain shows long-term persistence in animals or the environment as reservoirs, it could develop an increased virulence and potentially cause another outbreak in Taiwan. Although airborne transmission from aerosols to humans can occur in Taiwan, *B. pseudomallei* has a very low isolation rate in aerosols. Ingesting or coming into contact with water contaminated with *B. pseudomallei* is the likeliest mode of melioidosis transmission. However, more importantly, drinking boiling water and routinely avoiding proximity to rivers or waterlogged areas are common practices among the Taiwanese population. Most of the patients with melioidosis denied having contact with contaminated soil or water. Alternatively, the aim of endosymbiont *B. pseudomallei* to protect itself in harsh environments and develop a virulence to allow its intracellular growth in mammalian cells is likely another mode of melioidosis dissemination in Taiwan.

Acknowledgments: This project was supported by MOST (Ministry of Science and Technology, ROC) grants (MOST105-2320-B-017-003-MY3 [Y.-L.C.] and MOST106-2314-B-075B-009-MY3 [Y.-S.C.]).

Author Contributions: P.-T.H. collected and analyzed data, performed experiments and wrote the paper; W.-T.H. and H.-K.H. collected data; Y.-L.C. and Y.-S.C. analyzed the data, and wrote and led the manuscript. All authors have read and approved the final manuscript.

Conflicts of Interest: The authors declare no conflict of interest.

References

1. Cheng, A.C.; Currie, B.J. Melioidosis: Epidemiology, pathophysiology, and management. *Clin. Microbiol. Rev.* **2005**, *18*, 383–416. [CrossRef] [PubMed]
2. Doker, T.J.; Sharp, T.M.; Rivera-Garcia, B.; Perez-Padilla, J.; Benoit, T.J.; Ellis, E.M.; Elrod, M.G.; Gee, J.E.; Shieh, W.J.; Beesley, C.A.; et al. Contact investigation of melioidosis cases reveals regional endemicity in Puerto Rico. *Clin. Infect. Dis.* **2015**, *60*, 243–250. [CrossRef] [PubMed]
3. Birnie, E.; Wiersinga, W.J.; Limmathurotsakul, D.; Grobusch, M.P. Melioidosis in Africa: Should we be looking more closely? *Future Microbiol.* **2015**, *10*, 273–281. [CrossRef] [PubMed]
4. Vandana, K.E.; Mukhopadhyay, C.; Tellapragada, C.; Kamath, A.; Tipre, M.; Bhat, V.; Sathiakumar, N. Seroprevalence of *Burkholderia pseudomallei* among adults in coastal areas in southwestern India. *PLoS Negl. Trop. Dis.* **2016**, *10*, e0004610. [CrossRef] [PubMed]
5. Limmathurotsakul, D.; Golding, N.; Dance, D.A.; Messina, J.P.; Pigott, D.M.; Moyes, C.L.; Rolim, D.B.; Bertherat, E.; Day, N.P.J.; Peacock, S.J.; et al. Predicted global distribution of *Burkholderia pseudomallei* and burden of melioidosis. *Nat. Microbiol.* **2016**, *1*, 15008. [CrossRef] [PubMed]
6. Chen, P.S.; Chen, Y.S.; Lin, H.H.; Liu, P.J.; Ni, W.F.; Hsueh, P.T.; Liang, S.H.; Chen, C.; Chen, Y.L. Airborne transmission of melioidosis to humans from environmental aerosols contaminated with *B. pseudomallei*. *PLoS Negl. Trop. Dis.* **2015**, *9*, e0003834. [CrossRef] [PubMed]

7. Ong, C.E.L.; Wongsuvan, G.; Chew, J.S.W.; Kim, T.Y.; Teng, L.H.; Amornchai, P.; Wuthiekanun, V.; Day, N.P.J.; Peacock, S.J.; Cheng, T.Y.; et al. Presence of *Burkholderia pseudomallei* in soil and paddy rice water in a rice field in northeast Thailand, but not in air and rainwater. *Am. J. Trop. Med. Hyg.* **2017**, *97*, 1702–1705. [CrossRef] [PubMed]

8. Amadasi, S.; Dal Zoppo, S.; Bonomini, A.; Bussi, A.; Pedroni, P.; Balestrieri, G.; Signorini, L.; Castelli, F. A case of melioidosis probably acquired by inhalation of dusts during a helicopter flight in a healthy traveler returning from Singapore. *J. Travel Med.* **2015**, *22*, 57–60. [CrossRef] [PubMed]

9. Dance, D.A. Ecology of *Burkholderia pseudomallei* and the interactions between environmental *Burkholderia* spp. and human-animal hosts. *Acta Trop.* **2000**, *74*, 159–168. [CrossRef]

10. Mayo, M.; Kaesti, M.; Harrington, G.; Cheng, A.C.; Ward, L.; Karp, D.; Jolly, P.; Godoy, D.; Spratt, B.G.; Currie, B.J. *Burkholderia pseudomallei* in unchlorinated domestic bore water, tropical northern Australia. *Emerg. Infect. Dis.* **2011**, *17*, 1283–1285. [CrossRef] [PubMed]

11. Liu, X.; Pang, L.; Sim, S.H.; Goh, K.T.; Ravikumar, S.; Win, M.S.; Tan, G.; Cook, A.R.; Fisher, D.; Chai, L.Y.A. Association of melioidosis incidence with rainfall and humidity, Singapore, 2003–2012. *Emerg. Infect. Dis.* **2015**, *21*, 159–162. [CrossRef] [PubMed]

12. Merritt, A.J.; Inglis, T.J.J. The role of climate in the epidemiology of melioidosis. *Curr. Trop. Med. Rep.* **2017**, *4*, 185–191. [CrossRef] [PubMed]

13. Su, H.P.; Chan, T.C.; Chang, C.C. Typhoon-related leptospirosis and melioidosis, Taiwan, 2009. *Emerg. Infect. Dis.* **2011**, *17*, 1322–1324. [CrossRef] [PubMed]

14. Lee, N.; Wu, J.L.; Lee, C.H.; Tsai, W.C. *Pseudomonas pseudomallei* infection from drowning: The first reported case in Taiwan. *J. Clin. Microbiol.* **1985**, *22*, 352–354. [PubMed]

15. Hsueh, P.R.; Teng, L.J.; Lee, L.N.; Yu, C.J.; Yang, P.C.; Ho, S.W.; Luh, K.T. Melioidosis: An emerging infection in Taiwan? *Emerg. Infect. Dis.* **2001**, *7*, 428–433. [CrossRef] [PubMed]

16. Bossi, P.; Tegnell, A.; Baka, A.; van Loock, F.; Hendriks, J.; Werner, A.; Maidhof, H.; Gouvras, G. Bichat guidelines for the clinical management of glanders and melioidosis and bioterrorism-related glanders and melioidosis. *Euro Surveill.* **2004**, *9*, 35–36. [CrossRef] [PubMed]

17. Kao, C.M.; Chen, S.C.; Chen, Y.S.; Lin, H.M.; Chen, Y.L. Detection of *Burkholderia pseudomallei* in rice fields with PCR-based technique. *Folia Microbiol.* **2003**, *48*, 521–524. [CrossRef]

18. Manivanh, L.; Pierret, A.; Rattanavong, S.; Kounnavongsa, O.; Buisson, Y.; Elliott, I.; Maeght, J.L.; Xayyathip, K.; Silisouk, K.; Vongsouvath, M.; et al. *Burkholderia pseudomallei* in a lowland rice paddy: Seasonal changes and influence of soil depth and physico-chemical properties. *Sci. Rep.* **2017**, *7*, 3031. [CrossRef] [PubMed]

19. Chen, Y.S.; Chen, S.C.; Kao, C.M.; Chen, Y.L. Effects of soil pH, temperature and water content on the growth of *Burkholderia pseudomallei*. *Folia Microbiol.* **2003**, *48*, 253–256. [CrossRef]

20. Chen, Y.S.; Shiuan, D.; Chen, S.C.; Chye, S.M.; Chen, Y.L. Recombinant truncated flagellin of *Burkholderia pseudomallei* as a molecular probe for diagnosis of melioidosis. *Clin. Diagn. Lab. Immunol.* **2003**, *10*, 423–425. [CrossRef] [PubMed]

21. Chen, Y.S.; Chen, S.C.; Wu, T.R.; Kao, C.M.; Chen, Y.L. Seroprevalence of anti-flagellin antibody against *Burkholderia pseudomallei* in Taiwan. *Jpn. J. Inf. Dis.* **2004**, *57*, 224–225.

22. Chen, W.T.; Chen, Y.S.; Chye, S.M.; Wu, T.R.; Hong, W.G.; Lin, Y.N.; Bair, H.T.; Yang, S.C.; Chen, Y.L. Seroprevalence of melioidosis in diabetic patients in Taiwan. *J. Microbiol. Immunol. Infect.* **2005**, *38*, 267–270. [PubMed]

23. Su, H.P.; Chou, C.Y.; Tzeng, S.C.; Ferng, T.L.; Chen, Y.L.; Chen, Y.S.; Chung, T.C. Possible typhoon-related melioidosis epidemic, Taiwan, 2005. *Emerg. Infect. Dis.* **2007**, *13*, 1795–1797. [CrossRef] [PubMed]

24. Currie, B.J.; Jacups, S.P.; Cheng, A.C.; Fisher, D.A.; Anstey, N.M.; Huffam, S.E.; Krause, V.L. Melioidosis epidemiology and risk factors from a prospective whole-population study in northern Australia. *Trop. Med. Int. Health.* **2004**, *9*, 1167–1174. [CrossRef] [PubMed]

25. Limmathurotsakul, D.; Wongratanacheewin, S.; Teerawattanasook, N.; Wongsuvan, G.; Chaisuksant, S.; Chetchotisakd, P.; Chaowagul, W.; Day, N.P.J.; Peacock, S.J. Increasing incidence of human melioidosis in northeast Thailand. *Am. J. Trop. Med. Hyg.* **2010**, *82*, 1113–1117. [CrossRef] [PubMed]

26. Su, H.P.; Yang, H.W.; Chen, Y.L.; Ferng, T.L.; Chou, Y.L.; Chung, T.C.; Chen, C.H.; Chiang, C.S.; Kuan, M.M.; Lin, H.H.; et al. Prevalence of melioidosis in the Er-Ren River Basin, Taiwan: Implications for transmission. *J. Clin. Microbiol.* **2007**, *45*, 2599–2603. [CrossRef] [PubMed]

27. Ko, W.C.; Cheung, B.M.; Tang, H.J.; Shih, H.I.; Lau, Y.J.; Wang, L.R.; Chuang, Y.C. Melioidosis outbreak after typhoon, southern Taiwan. *Emerg. Infect. Dis.* **2007**, *13*, 896–898. [CrossRef] [PubMed]

28. Chen, Y.L.; Lin, Y.C.; Chen, Y.S.; Chen, S.C.; Liu, Y.M.; Tseng, I.L.; Chiang, C.S.; Lin, H.H.; Mu, J.J. Characterisation of predominant molecular patterns of *Burkholderia pseudomallei* in Taiwan. *Trans. R. Soc. Trop. Med. Hyg.* **2013**, *107*, 165–169. [CrossRef] [PubMed]

29. Centers for Disease and Control (Taiwan), Melioidosis Data Base. Available online: https://nidss.cdc.gov.tw/ch/SingleDisease.aspx?dc=1&dt=4&disease=025 (accessed on 15 February 2018).

30. Chen, Y.S.; Lin, H.H.; Mu, J.J.; Chiang, C.S.; Chen, C.H.; Buu, L.M.; Lin, Y.E.; Chen, Y.L. Distribution of melioidosis cases and viable *Burkholderia pseudomallei* in soil: Evidence for emerging melioidosis in Taiwan. *J. Clin. Microbiol.* **2010**, *48*, 1432–1434. [CrossRef] [PubMed]

31. Hantrakun, V.; Rongkard, P.; Oyuchua, M.; Amornchai, P.; Lim, C.; Wuthiekanun, V.; Day, N.P.J.; Peacock, S.J.; Limmathurotsakul, D. Soil nutrient depletion is associated with the presence of *Burkholderia pseudomallei*. *Appl. Environ. Microbiol.* **2016**, *82*, 7086–7092. [CrossRef] [PubMed]

32. Kaestli, M.; Mayo, M.; Harrington, G.; Ward, L.; Watt, F.; Hill, J.V.; Cheng, A.C.; Currie, B.J. Landscape changes influence the occurrence of the melioidosis bacterium *Burkholderia pseudomallei* in soil in northern Australia. *PLoS Negl. Trop. Dis.* **2009**, *3*, e364. [CrossRef] [PubMed]

33. Musa, H.I.; Hassan, L.; Shamsuddin, Z.H.; Panchadcharam, C.; Zakaria, Z.; Abdul Aziz, S. Physicochemical properties influencing presence of *Burkholderia pseudomallei* in soil from small ruminant farms in Peninsular Malaysia. *PLoS ONE* **2016**, *11*, e0162348. [CrossRef] [PubMed]

34. Wang-Ngarm, S.; Chareonsudjai, S.; Chareonsudjai, P. Physicochemical factors affecting the growth of *Burkholderia pseudomallei* in soil microcosm. *Am. J. Trop. Med. Hyg.* **2014**, *90*, 480–485. [CrossRef] [PubMed]

35. Larsen, E.; Smith, J.J.; Norton, R.; Corkeron, M. Survival, sublethal injury, and recovery of environmental *Burkholderia pseudomallei* in soil subjected to desiccation. *Appl. Environ. Microbiol.* **2013**, *79*, 2424–2427. [CrossRef] [PubMed]

36. Dai, D.; Chen, Y.S.; Chen, P.S.; Chen, Y.L. Case cluster shifting and contaminant source as determinants of melioidosis in Taiwan. *Trop. Med. Int. Health* **2012**, *17*, 1005–1013. [CrossRef] [PubMed]

37. Mu, J.J.; Cheng, P.Y.; Chen, Y.S.; Chen, P.S.; Chen, Y.L. The occurrence of melioidosis is related to different climatic conditions in distinct topographical areas of Taiwan. *Epidemiol. Infect.* **2014**, *142*, 415–423. [CrossRef] [PubMed]

38. Shih, H.I.; Chuang, Y.C.; Cheung, B.M.; Yan, J.J.; Chang, C.M.; Chang, K.; Chang, N.Y.; Lee, H.C.; Wu, C.J.; Chen, P.L.; et al. Sporadic and outbreak cases of melioidosis in southern Taiwan: Clinical features and antimicrobial susceptibility. *Infection* **2009**, *37*, 9–15. [CrossRef] [PubMed]

39. Chen, Y.L.; Yen, Y.C.; Yang, C.Y.; Lee, M.S.; Ho, C.K.; Mena, K.D.; Wang, P.Y.; Chen, P.S. The concentrations of ambient *Burkholderia pseudomallei* during typhoon season in endemic area of melioidosis in Taiwan. *PLoS Negl. Trop. Dis.* **2014**, *8*, e2877. [CrossRef] [PubMed]

40. Currie, B.J.; Jacups, S.P. Intensity of rainfall and severity of melioidosis, Australia. *Emerg. Infect. Dis.* **2003**, *9*, 1538–1542. [CrossRef] [PubMed]

41. Chen, Y.S.; Lin, H.H.; Hsueh, P.T.; Liu, P.J.; Ni, W.F.; Chung, W.C.; Lin, C.P.; Chen, Y.L. Whole-genome sequence of an epidemic strain of *Burkholderia pseudomallei* vgh07 in Taiwan. *Genome Announc.* **2015**, *3*, e00345-15. [CrossRef] [PubMed]

42. Hsueh, P.T.; Chen, Y.S.; Lin, H.H.; Liu, P.J.; Ni, W.F.; Liu, M.C.; Chen, Y.L. Comparison of whole-genome sequences from two colony morphovars of *Burkholderia pseudomallei*. *Genome Announc.* **2015**, *3*, e01194-15. [CrossRef] [PubMed]

43. Chen, Y.S.; Shieh, W.J.; Goldsmith, C.S.; Metcalfe, M.G.; Greer, P.W.; Zaki, S.R.; Chang, H.H.; Chan, H.; Chen, Y.L. Alteration of the phenotypic and pathogenic patterns of *Burkholderia pseudomallei* that persist in a soil environment. *Am. J. Trop. Med. Hyg.* **2014**, *90*, 469–479. [CrossRef] [PubMed]

44. Mariappan, V.; Vellasamy, K.M.; Vadivelu, J. Host-adaptation of *Burkholderia pseudomallei* alters metabolism and virulence: A global proteome analysis. *Sci. Rep.* **2017**, *7*, 9015. [CrossRef] [PubMed]

45. Withatanung, P.; Chantratita, N.; Muangsombut, V.; Saiprom, N.; Lertmemongkolchai, G.; Klumpp, J.; Clokie, M.R.J.; Galyov, E.E.; Korbsrisate, S. Analyses of the distribution patterns of *Burkholderia pseudomallei* and associated phages in soil samples in thailand suggest that phage presence reduces the frequency of bacterial isolation. *PLoS Negl. Trop. Dis.* **2016**, *10*, e0005005. [CrossRef] [PubMed]

46. Lin, H.H.; Chen, Y.S.; Li, Y.C.; Tseng, I.L.; Hsieh, T.H.; Buu, L.M.; Chen, Y.L. *Burkholderia multivorans* acts as an antagonist against the growth of *Burkholderia pseudomallei* in soil. *Microbiol. Immunol.* **2011**, *55*, 616–624. [CrossRef] [PubMed]

47. Boottanun, P.; Potisap, C.; Hurdle, J.G.; Sermswan, R.W. Secondary metabolites from *Bacillus amyloliquefaciens* isolated from soil can kill *Burkholderia pseudomallei*. *AMB Express* **2017**, *7*, 16. [CrossRef] [PubMed]

48. Howard, K.; Inglis, T.J. Disinfection of *Burkholderia pseudomallei* in potable water. *Water Res.* **2005**, *39*, 1085–1092. [CrossRef] [PubMed]

49. Inglis, T.J.; Foster, N.F.; Gal, D.; Powell, K.; Mayo, M.; Norton, R.; Currie, B.J. Preliminary report on the northern Australian melioidosis environmental surveillance project. *Epidemiol. Infect.* **2004**, *132*, 813–820. [CrossRef] [PubMed]

50. Noinarin, P.; Chareonsudjai, P.; Wangsomnuk, P.; Wongratanacheewin, S.; Chareonsudjai, S. Environmental free-living amoebae isolated from soil in Khon Kaen, Thailand, antagonize *Burkholderia pseudomallei*. *PLoS ONE* **2016**, *11*, e0167355. [CrossRef] [PubMed]

51. Rattanavong, S.; Wuthiekanun, V.; Langla, S.; Amornchai, P.; Sirisouk, J.; Phetsouvanh, R.; Moore, C.E.; Peacock, S.J.; Buisson, Y.; Newton, P.N. Randomized soil survey of the distribution of *Burkholderia pseudomallei* in rice fields in Laos. *Appl. Environ. Microbiol.* **2011**, *77*, 532–536. [CrossRef] [PubMed]

52. Corkeron, M.L.; Norton, R.; Nelson, P.N. Spatial analysis of melioidosis distribution in a suburban area. *Epidemiol. Infect.* **2010**, *138*, 1346–1352. [CrossRef] [PubMed]

53. Kaestli, M.; Mayo, M.; Harrington, G.; Watt, F.; Hill, J.; Gal, D.; Currie, B.J. Sensitive and specific molecular detection of *Burkholderia pseudomallei*, the causative agent of melioidosis, in the soil of tropical northern Australia. *Appl. Environ. Microbiol.* **2007**, *73*, 6891–6897. [CrossRef] [PubMed]

54. Currie, B.J.; Mayo, M.; Anstey, N.M.; Donohoe, P.; Haase, A.; Kemp, D.J. A cluster of melioidosis cases from an endemic region is clonal and is linked to the water supply using molecular typing of *Burkholderia pseudomallei* isolates. *Am. J. Trop. Med. Hyg.* **2001**, *65*, 177–179. [CrossRef] [PubMed]

55. Draper, A.D.; Mayo, M.; Harrington, G.; Karp, D.; Yinfoo, D.; Ward, L.; Haslem, A.; Currie, B.J.; Kaestli, M. Association of the melioidosis agent *Burkholderia pseudomallei* with water parameters in rural water supplies in Northern Australia. *Appl. Environ. Microbiol.* **2010**, *76*, 5305–5507. [CrossRef] [PubMed]

56. Michel, R.; Hauroder, B. Isolation of an *Acanthamoeba* strain with intracellular *Burkholderia pickettii* infection. *Zentralbl. Bakteriol.* **1997**, *285*, 541–557. [CrossRef]

57. Molmeret, M.; Jarraud, S.; Mori, J.P.; Pernin, P.; Forey, F.; Reyrolle, M.; Vandenesch, F.; Etienne, J.; Farge, P. Different growth rates in amoeba of genotypically related environmental and clinical *Legionella pneumophila* strains isolated from a thermal spa. *Epidemiol. Infect.* **2001**, *126*, 231–239. [CrossRef] [PubMed]

58. Ovrutsky, A.R.; Chan, E.D.; Kartalija, M.; Bai, X.; Jackson, M.; Gibbs, S.; Iii, J.O.F.; Iseman, M.D.; Reynolds, P.R.; Mcdonnell, G.; et al. Cooccurrence of free-living amoebae and nontuberculous *Mycobacteria* in hospital water networks, and preferential growth of *Mycobacterium avium* in *Acanthamoeba lenticulata*. *Appl. Environ. Microbiol.* **2013**, *79*, 3185–3192. [CrossRef] [PubMed]

59. Kao, P.M.; Chou, M.Y.; Tao, C.W.; Huang, W.C.; Hsu, B.M.; Shen, S.M.; Fan, C.W.; Chiu, Y.C. Diversity and seasonal impact of *Acanthamoeba* species in a subtropical rivershed. *Biomed. Res. Int.* **2013**, *2013*, 405794. [CrossRef] [PubMed]

60. Kao, P.M.; Hsu, B.M.; Hsu, T.K.; Liu, J.H.; Chang, H.Y.; Ji, W.T.; Tzeng, K.J.; Huang, S.W.; Huang, Y.L. Seasonal distribution of potentially pathogenic *Acanthamoeba* species from drinking water reservoirs in Taiwan. *Environ. Sci. Pollut. Res. Int.* **2015**, *22*, 3766–3773. [CrossRef] [PubMed]

61. Siddiqui, R.; Khan, N.A. Biology and pathogenesis of *Acanthamoeba*. *Parasit. Vectors* **2012**, *5*, 6. [CrossRef] [PubMed]

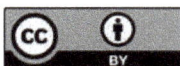

Tropical Medicine and Infectious Disease

MDPI

Review

Melioidosis in Thailand: Present and Future

Soawapak Hinjoy [1] [ID], Viriya Hantrakun [2] [ID], Somkid Kongyu [1], Jedsada Kaewrakmuk [3], Tri Wangrangsimakul [2,4] [ID], Siroj Jitsuronk [5], Weerawut Saengchun [6], Saithip Bhengsri [7], Thantapat Akarachotpong [7], Somsak Thamthitiwat [7], Ornuma Sangwichian [7], Siriluck Anunnatsiri [8], Rasana W Sermswan [8], Ganjana Lertmemongkolchai [9] [ID], Chayada Sitthidet Tharinjaroen [10], Kanya Preechasuth [10], Ratchadaporn Udpaun [10] [ID], Poomin Chuensombut [11], Nisarat Waranyasirikul [12], Chanihcha Anudit [13], Surapong Narenpitak [14], Yaowaruk Jutrakul [15], Prapit Teparrukkul [16], Nittaya Teerawattanasook [17], Kittisak Thanvisej [18], Alisa Suphan [19], Punchawee Sukbut [20], Kritchavat Ploddi [21], Poolsri Sirichotirat [22], Bongkoch Chiewchanyon [23], Kamolchanok Rukseree [24], Maliwan Hongsuwan [2], Gumphol Wongsuwan [2], Pornpan Sunthornsut [2], Vanaporn Wuthiekanun [2], Sandy Sachaphimukh [2], Prapass Wannapinij [2], Wirongrong Chierakul [2], Claire Chewapreecha [2], Janjira Thaipadungpanit [2], Narisara Chantratita [2,25], Sunee Korbsrisate [26], Apichai Taunyok [27], Susanna Dunachie [4] [ID], Prasit Palittapongarnpim [28,29], Stitaya Sirisinha [29], Rungrueng Kitphati [30], Sopon Iamsirithaworn [31], Wipada Chaowagul [16], Ploenchan Chetchotisak [8] [ID], Toni Whistler [7], Surasakdi Wongratanacheewin [8] and Direk Limmathurotsakul [2,4,*]

for Thailand Melioidosis Network

1. Bureau of Epidemiology, Department of Disease Control, Ministry of Public Health, Nonthaburi 11000, Thailand; soawapak@gmail.com (S.H.); skongyu@gmail.com (S.K.)
2. Mahidol-Oxford Tropical Medicine Research Unit, Faculty of Tropical Medicine, Mahidol University, Bangkok 10400, Thailand; viriya@tropmedres.ac (V.H.); tri@tropmedres.ac (T.W.); maliwan@tropmedres.ac (M.H.); gumphol@tropmedres.ac (G.W.); pornpan@tropmedres.ac (P.S.); lek@tropmedres.ac (V.W.); sandy@tropmedres.ac (S.S.); prapass@tropmedres.ac (P.W.); kae@tropmedres.ac (W.C.); cc12@sanger.ac.uk (C.C.); janjira@tropmedres.ac (J.T.); narisara@tropmedres.ac (N.C)
3. Faculty of Science, Prince of Songkla University, Songkla 90110, Thailand; jedsada.k@psu.ac.th
4. Centre for Tropical Medicine and Global Health, Nuffield Department of Medicine, University of Oxford, Oxford OX3 7FZ, UK; susie.dunachie@ndm.ox.ac.uk
5. Faculty of Medicine, Prince of Songkla University, Songkla 90110, Thailand; siroj.j@psu.ac.th
6. Department of Clinical Pathology, Chiang Rai Prachanukroh Hospital, Chiang Rai 57000, Thailand; mistermummy9@gmail.com
7. Division of Global Health Protection, Thailand Ministry of Public Health-US Centers for Disease Control and Prevention Collaboration, Nonthaburi 11000, Thailand; hpx4@cdc.gov (S.B.); hpt7@cdc.gov (T.A.); hpv2@cdc.gov (S.T.); xxc7@cdc.gov (O.S.); taw6@cdc.gov (T.W.)
8. Faculty of Medicine, Khon Kaen University, Khon Kaen 40002, Thailand; asiril@kku.ac.th (S.A.); rasanaw@gmail.com (R.W.S.); ploencha@kku.ac.th (P.C.); sura_wng@kku.ac.th (S.W.)
9. The Centre for Research & Development of Medical Diagnostic Laboratories, Faculty of Associated Medical Sciences, Khon Kaen University, Khon Kaen 40002, Thailand; g.lert@yahoo.co.uk
10. Division of Clinical Microbiology, Department of Medical Technology, Faculty of Associated Medical Sciences, Chiang Mai University, Chiang Mai 50200, Thailand; chayada.si@cmu.ac.th (C.S.T.); kanya.p@cmu.ac.th (K.P.); ratchadaudp@hotmail.com (R.U.)
11. Department of Clinical Pathology, Chiangkham Hospital, Phayao 56110, Thailand; chuensombut@hotmail.com
12. Department of Clinical Pathology, Somdejphrajaotaksin Maharaj Hospital, Tak 63000, Thailand; Nisarat_mt@hotmail.com
13. Department of Clinical Pathology, Uthai Thani Hospital, Uthai Thani 61000, Thailand; achanihcha@yahoo.com
14. Department of Internal Medicine, Udon Thani Hospital, Udon Thani 41000, Thailand; Suraponguth@hotmail.com

[15] Department of Clinical Pathology, Udon Thani Hospital, Udon Thani 41000, Thailand;
Yaowa_Ju@yahoo.co.th

[16] Department of Internal Medicine, Sunpasitthiprasong Hospital, Ubon Ratchathani 34000, Thailand;
prapith1@hotmail.com (P.T.); vipada_1@yahoo.com (W.C)

[17] Department of Clinical Pathology, Sunpasitthiprasong Hospital, Ubon Ratchathani 34000, Thailand;
nidteeraw@gmail.com

[18] Department of Internal Medicine, Nakhon Panom Hospital, Nakhon Panom 48000, Thailand;
kittisak97@gmail.com

[19] Ubon Ratchathani Provincial Public Health Office, Ubon Ratchathani 34000, Thailand; alisuphan@me.com

[20] Mukdahan Provincial Public Health Office, Mukdahan 49000, Thailand; mbdsmuk@yahoo.co.th

[21] The Office of Disease Prevention and Control 8, Udon Thani 41000, Thailand; dr.kritchavat@gmail.com

[22] The Office of Disease Prevention and Control 10, Ubon Ratchathani 34000, Thailand; bigtoii@yahoo.com

[23] The Office of Disease Prevention and Control 12, Songkla 90000, Thailand; b_chiewchanyon@yahoo.com

[24] Mahidol University Amnatcharoen Campus, Amnatcharoen 37000, Thailand;
kamolchanok.ruk@mahidol.ac.th

[25] Department of Microbiology and Immunology, Faculty of Tropical Medicine, Mahidol University,
Bangkok 10400, Thailand

[26] Department of Immunology, Faculty of Medicine Siriraj Hospital, Mahidol University,
Bangkok 10700, Thailand; Sunee.kor@mahidol.ac.th

[27] Department of Infectious Diseases & Immunology, Emerging Pathogens Institute, University of Florida,
Gainesville, FL 32611, USA; tuanyok@ufl.edu

[28] National Science and Technology Development Agency (NSTDA), Pathum Thani 12120, Thailand;
prasit@nstda.or.th

[29] Department of Microbiology, Faculty of Science, Mahidol University, Bangkok 10400, Thailand;
stitaya.sir@mahidol.ac.th

[30] Institute for Urban Disease Control and Prevention, Department of Disease Control, Ministry of Public Health,
Bangkok 10220, Thailand; drrungrueng@hotmail.com

[31] Bureau of General Communicable Diseases, Department of Disease Control, Ministry of Public Health,
Nonthaburi 11000, Thailand; sopon@ddc.mail.go.th

*   Correspondence: direk@tropmedres.ac; Tel.: +66-203-6333

Received: 31 January 2018; Accepted: 21 March 2018; Published: 8 April 2018

Abstract: A recent modelling study estimated that there are 2800 deaths due to melioidosis in Thailand yearly. The Thailand Melioidosis Network (formed in 2012) has been working closely with the Ministry of Public Health (MoPH) to investigate and reduce the burden of this disease. Based on updated data, the incidence of melioidosis is still high in Northeast Thailand. More than 2000 culture-confirmed cases of melioidosis are diagnosed in general hospitals with microbiology laboratories in this region each year. The mortality rate is around 35%. Melioidosis is endemic throughout Thailand, but it is still not uncommon that microbiological facilities misidentify *Burkholderia pseudomallei* as a contaminant or another organism. Disease awareness is low, and people in rural areas neither wear boots nor boil water before drinking to protect themselves from acquiring *B. pseudomallei*. Previously, about 10 melioidosis deaths were formally reported to the National Notifiable Disease Surveillance System (Report 506) each year, thus limiting priority setting by the MoPH. In 2015, the formally reported number of melioidosis deaths rose to 112, solely because Sunpasitthiprasong Hospital, Ubon Ratchathani province, reported its own data (*n* = 107). Melioidosis is truly an important cause of death in Thailand, and currently reported cases (Report 506) and cases diagnosed at research centers reflect the tip of the iceberg. Laboratory training and communication between clinicians and laboratory personnel are required to improve diagnosis and treatment of melioidosis countrywide. Implementation of rapid diagnostic tests, such as a lateral flow antigen detection assay, with high accuracy even in melioidosis-endemic countries such as Thailand, is critically needed. Reporting of all culture-confirmed melioidosis cases from every hospital with a microbiology laboratory, together with final outcome data, is mandated under the Communicable Diseases Act B.E.2558. By enforcing this legislation, the MoPH could raise the priority of this disease, and should consider implementing a campaign to raise awareness and melioidosis prevention countrywide.

Keywords: *Burkholderia pseudomallei*; melioidosis; Thailand; mortality; diagnosis; surveillance; awareness; treatment; prevention

---

1. Introduction

Indigenous melioidosis was first reported in Thailand by Chittivej et al. in 1955 [1]. The patient came from Saraburi Province, Central Thailand, presenting at Pramongkutklao Hospital, Bangkok, with lymphadenopathy. Pus collected from the patient was culture positive for *Burkholderia pseudomallei* [1]. In 1976, melioidosis was selected as the main discussion topic at the first meeting of the Infectious Disease Group of Thailand (now known as the Infectious Disease Association of Thailand) [2]. A total of 15 culture-confirmed melioidosis patients diagnosed in Bangkok up to 1976 was noted, and the clinical epidemiology of six fatal cases and two cases with unknown outcomes was discussed, raising the public health threat caused by melioidosis countrywide [2]. Subsequent workshops on melioidosis and interhospital case conferences organized by the Infectious Disease Group of Thailand and university hospitals increased the awareness of all physicians and laboratory staff of the need to look for melioidosis and *B. pseudomallei,* respectively, countrywide [3]. By 1985, 743 culture-confirmed cases of melioidosis had been reported from many provinces in Thailand; including Khon Kaen ($n = 386$; mortality 50%), Ubon Ratchathani ($n = 169$; mortality 61%), Bangkok ($n = 91$), Chiang Mai ($n = 61$), Nakhon Ratchasima ($n = 30$), Nonthaburi ($n = 11$), and Songkla ($n = 6$) [4].

In Thailand, underrecognition and misdiagnosis of melioidosis have been major obstacles to saving lives from this disease. Worldwide, untrained laboratory personnel commonly misidentify *B. pseudomallei* as a contaminant or other organism [5]. Leelarasamee et al. reported a total of 1165 isolates of *B. pseudomallei* identified in 46 hospitals from four regions of Thailand in 1995 (Northeast ($n = 19$), Central ($n = 11$), North ($n = 9$) and South ($n = 7$)) [6]. Nonetheless, the isolation rates were suspiciously low or absent in many hospitals when compared with adjacent hospitals that had reported very high numbers of melioidosis cases [6]. Focused training revealed that the microbiological laboratories in hospitals with unusually low numbers of melioidosis cases had misidentified the organisms, and the incidence rates of melioidosis in their areas were, in reality, also high [3].

From 1995 to 2015, melioidosis was heavily reported from Northeast Thailand [7,8] and rarely reported from the other regions. This led many clinicians and researchers to the misapprehension that melioidosis was not endemic in all regions of Thailand [9,10]. In this report, we review the latest information on melioidosis in Thailand and show that training in *B. pseudomalleii* identification for laboratory personnel is still needed countrywide.

The case fatality rate (CFR) of melioidosis in general hospitals in Thailand decreased markedly from 60–70% to 35–40% after the landmark study comparing ceftazidime with 'conventional' treatment was published in 1989 [11]. Unfortunately, in 2018—20 years later—the CFR of melioidosis in public hospitals is still around 30–35% [7,8]. Although the reported CFR is lower in university hospitals, at around 10–20% [9,12], most people in Thailand receive medical care in public hospitals, and university hospitals focus on tertiary care, providing service to less than 5% of the general population [13]. Generic ceftazidime is widely available, and the cost is covered by the universal coverage scheme; therefore, lack of effective antibiotics is not the issue in Thailand. To further reduce the CFR, it is likely that heavy investment in intensive care units, an increase in the ratio of nurses and doctors to patients, and an improvement in laboratory diagnostic capacity is needed. This has been done successfully in Australia, where the CFR of melioidosis is now approximately 10% [14–17]. For resource-limited countries such as Thailand, it might be better to invest in prevention campaigns and stop people from contracting melioidosis. However, the necessary developments leading to national prevention campaigns are impeded by the lack of disease awareness among lay people, lack of a national campaign by the MoPH to raise such awareness [18,19], and lack of official mortality data to support MoPH activities.

It is still unknown how many patients die of melioidosis in Thailand yearly. A recent modeling study estimated that there are 7572 human melioidosis cases per year in Thailand, of whom 2838 (37%) die [8]. This is strongly supported by publications showing high numbers of culture-confirmed melioidosis cases diagnosed annually at major public hospitals in Thailand. Approximately 400 cases are diagnosed at Sunpasitthiprasong Hospital, Ubon Ratchathani, each year, of which about 150 result in death [7,20]. At Nakhon Panom Hospital, about 100 cases are diagnosed each year with about 30 deaths [21,22]. Melioidosis is one of the 83 diseases notifiable by law under the National Communicable Disease Surveillance system in Thailand. However, only 15, 10, 13, 4, and 12 deaths caused by melioidosis were officially reported to the Thailand disease surveillance system (Report 506) in 2010, 2011, 2012, 2013, and 2014, respectively [23–27]. It has been advised by the Bureau of Epidemiology, MoPH, that the total number of deaths based on Report 506 should not be used to represent the burden of the disease. However, these numbers have been used periodically by policymakers to represent the burden of melioidosis in Thailand to the public via the mass media (including newspapers and television broadcasts) [28]. Stakeholders occasionally compare the reported number of deaths due to melioidosis (for example, 12 deaths in 2014) with that of dengue (49 deaths in 2014) and leptospirosis (24 deaths in 2014) [28], and regard melioidosis as less important. Therefore, the lack of official melioidosis death reports via Report 506 hampers initiatives to improve awareness, diagnosis, treatment, and prevention of melioidosis in Thailand.

The Thailand Melioidosis Network was formed in 2012, and has been working closely with the MoPH to investigate the burden, solve the problems of underreporting by Report 506, and develop initiatives on melioidosis. Here, we review the current guidelines for diagnosis, treatment and prevention of melioidosis in Thailand, explore how to improve the official data and increase awareness of melioidosis. We discuss the needs and future challenges to save lives from melioidosis in Thailand.

2. Melioidosis Cases and Presence of *B. pseudomallei* in Thailand

We reviewed evidence of melioidosis and presence of *B. pseudomallei* from 1910 to 2015 in Thailand (Figure 1). We searched PubMed for indigenous cases of melioidosis reported using the MeSH terms 'melioidosis' or '*pseudomallei*' and 'Thailand'. We also searched bibliographies from selected studies for secondary references. We included literature in English and Thai. Only culture-confirmed cases and cultures positive for *B. pseudomallei* from environmental samples were included. Clinically-suspected and serologically diagnosed melioidosis cases were excluded because of poor sensitivity and specificity of clinical manifestations and serological diagnostic tests for melioidosis [5]. We have described the evidence in each of six regions in Thailand: Northeast, North, East, West, South, and Central Thailand. This six-region division, developed by the National Geographic Committee in 1977, was used because it was set up for geographical and scientific purposes [29].

2.1. Northeast Thailand

Melioidosis is regarded as highly endemic in Northeast Thailand (Figure 1). It is the largest region of Thailand, and is divided into 20 provinces. This region is a plateau surrounded by mountain ranges, and much of the arable land consists of tropical sandy soil. Most of the published case reports and cohorts arise from four provinces: Khon Kaen, Nakhon Panom, Udon Thani, and Ubon Ratchathani. Srinagarind University, the Melioidosis Research Centre (MRC), Thailand MoPH–US Centers for Disease Control and Prevention Collaboration (TUC), and Mahidol Oxford Tropical Medicine Research Unit (MORU) have been collaboratively doing research with provincial hospitals in these four provinces for more than a decade. The published evidence demonstrates that melioidosis is highly endemic throughout the region. A study reported that 19 provincial hospital laboratories in Northeast Thailand diagnosed 1865 culture-confirmed cases of melioidosis in 2007 [7]. An environmental sampling study conducted in 2015 also found that *B. pseudomallei* is commonly present in six of the seven provinces evaluated, including Burirum, Chaiyaphum, Khon Kaen, Udon Thani, Nong Bua Lam Phu, and Loei, the exception being Nakhon Ratchasima [30]. We believe that the failure to detect *B. pseudomallei* in Nakhon Ratchasima is likely to be a false-negative result due to small sample size and poor sensitivity of the environmental sampling method [30], because *B. pseudomallei* is commonly found in clinical specimens in Nakhon Ratchasima Hospital [6]. The preliminary results of a large environmental study conducted by the Asia Partnership on Emerging Infectious Disease Research also found that *B. pseudomallei* was prevalent in fields on both sides of the main roads in Mukdahan province [31].

An increase in the total number of culture-confirmed cases diagnosed in Northeast Thailand, from 964 cases in 1994 (assuming one isolate per case) [6] to 1865 in 2007 [7], could be due to an increase in incidence rates of melioidosis, an increase in usage of bacterial culture as shown by the rise of the number of blood culture bottles used per year [32], and/or improved access to healthcare [33]. A genuine increase in incidence rates of melioidosis could be due to the rise in the prevalence of diabetes mellitus (an important risk factor for melioidosis) [34], the rising age of farmers in rural areas [35], increased land use for irrigated agriculture and rice farming [8], and/or depletion of soil nutrients caused by crop residue burning and poor farming practices [30]. The latter two points may also have led to an increase in presence of *B. pseudomallei* in the environment [8,30].

A number of captive zoo animals [36] and domestic animals [10,37] have been reported to have culture-confirmed melioidosis, both in Northeast Thailand and in all other regions in Thailand. A study by Kasantikul et al. on fatal culture-confirmed melioidosis in captive zoo animals in Thailand from 1997 to 2013 reported the highest incidence from the Northeast (*n* = 12) and South (*n* = 12) regions, followed by the East (*n* = 3), North (*n* = 1), and Central (*n* = 1) areas [36]. A descriptive study of culture-confirmed melioidosis in animals in Thailand from 2006–2015 by Kongkaew et al. also reported a total of 81 goats, 28 pigs, 18 cattle, 17 sheep, and 27 other livestock/pets at seven Veterinary Research and Development Center in six regions of Thailand [37].

2.2. North Thailand

North Thailand is composed of 9 provinces, some of which share a border with Myanmar and Laos. Its geography is comprised of several mountain ranges and the basins of four major rivers, which are tributaries of the Chao Phraya River in Central Thailand. Melioidosis has occasionally been reported from Chiang Mai, the largest province in the region [4,38,39]. From 2001 to 2003, 26 culture-confirmed cases were diagnosed at Maharaj Nakorn Chiang Mai Hospital, and 42% of them died [38]. A survey by Trakulsomboon et al. in 1999 reported that *B. pseudomallei* could be found in soil in North Thailand, but the details of locations were not reported, and an updated study has not been conducted [40].

In September 2017, a workshop organized by the MoPH, MRC, and Thailand Melioidosis Network was conducted at the Faculty of Associated Medical Sciences, Chiang Mai University, to provide information on melioidosis, the potential pitfalls in the identification of *B. pseudomallei* and diagnosis of melioidosis to laboratory staff from 17 hospitals in North Thailand and other regions. The immediate result was that Chiangkom Hospital, Phayao, North Thailand, diagnosed 20 culture-confirmed cases in 2017 [41]. During this workshop, we found that some provincial hospitals in North Thailand did not have high quality biochemical tests to identify *B. pseudomallei*, and misidentification as *Pseudomonas* spp. or contaminants was common. A recent study from Chiangrai Prachanukroh Hospital, Chiang Rai, also found that *B. pseudomallei* was commonly misidentified as *Acinetobacter* spp. [42]. Lack of laboratory staff training and the absence of an algorithm for identifying Gram-negative bacilli were likely to have been the main causes of the misidentification. In addition, the clinicians and laboratory staff were unaware that they were officially obliged to report culture-confirmed cases to the disease surveillance system (Report 506).

2.3. East Thailand

East Thailand is characterized by short mountain ranges alternating with alluvial plains. This region was historically not considered an endemic area for melioidosis; however, population-based surveillance activities by TUC in Sa Kaeo province, located on the Cambodian border about 200 kilometers from Bangkok, indicated otherwise [22]. Estimates from this project showed the average incidence of bacteremic melioidosis in Sa Kaeo from 2006–2008 to be 4.9 cases per 100,000 population (95% confidence interval (CI) = 3.9–6.1), with a population mortality rate of 1.9 per 100,000 (95% CI = 1.3–2.8) [22]. The annual incidence in Sa Kaeo was approximately 1/3 less than that determined for Nakhon Panom, an area considered highly endemic for *B. pseudomallei*, in this same study [22]. The CFR, however, was slightly higher in Sa Kaeo province at 44%, compared to Nakhon Panom province at 34% (*P* = 0.1) among patients with known outcomes from bacteremic melioidosis. These figures are likely to underestimate the true burden of *B. pseudomallei*, as the surveillance was focused on hospitalized cases. This study shows that the incidence of bacteremic melioidosis in Eastern Thailand is much higher than the figures reported to Report 506 of MoPH, Thailand suggest.

A descriptive study of animal melioidosis between 2006–2010 also reported a high number of culture-confirmed human melioidosis in two Eastern provinces, Chachoengsao (151 human cases and 2 goats), and Chonburi (76 human cases and 1 goat), where goat cases were diagnosed [10]. A recent environmental study also found *B. pseudomallei* to be highly prevalent in all six provinces (Sa Kaeo, Chachoengsao, Chonburi, Chanthaburi, Prachinburi, and Rayong) in East Thailand [30].

2.4. West Thailand

The geography of West Thailand is characterized by high mountains and steep river valleys along the border with Myanmar. Diagnosis of culture-confirmed melioidosis was rare within West Thailand until recently [10]. A descriptive study of melioidosis between 2006 and 2010 found a number of culture-confirmed human cases in two provinces, Ratchaburi (50 human cases and 16 goats) and Phetchaburi (8 human cases and 1 goat) [10]. A descriptive study of animal melioidosis by Kongkaew et al. also reported a high incidence of animal melioidosis in Ratchaburi, West Thailand, compared to all other provinces in the country [37].

During the workshop conducted at Chiang Mai University, North Thailand, in September 2017, laboratory staff from Somdejphrajaotaksin Maharaj Hospital, Tak, West Thailand, also participated. After the workshop, 3 culture-confirmed cases were diagnosed at the hospital that year [43]. TUC contacted Maesot General Hospital, Tak province, and noted that 15 bacteremic melioidosis patients had been diagnosed from 2013 to 2017. Finkelstein et al. also reported finding *B. pseudomallei* in soil samples collected from Prachuap Khiri Khan, West Thailand [44]. These results suggest that human melioidosis might have been misdiagnosed and underreported in West Thailand, which is on the border with Myanmar where melioidosis was first discovered in 1912 [45]. Training to improve diagnosis of melioidosis should include provincial hospitals in West Thailand.

2.5. South Thailand

South Thailand is famous for its beautiful beaches. The western part has steeper coastlines and is on the Andaman Sea, while the east side is mainly river plains and on the Gulf of Thailand. Melioidosis is increasingly recognized as endemic in South Thailand. One of the most striking phenomena was a number of culture-confirmed cases reported from tsunami survivors in 2004 in Phangnga [46–48], on the west coast of South Thailand. A foreign tourist was also suspected to have acquired melioidosis at Koh Samui, an island in Surat Thani on the east coast of South Thailand [49]. In 2012, an outbreak of 11 culture-confirmed cases (3 foreign tourists and 8 Thais) was observed in Koh Phangan, another island in Surat Thani on the east coast, and an environmental survey established that *B. pseudomallei* was widely found in water supplies on Koh Phangan [50]. Churangsuk et al. recently reported that, between 2002–2011, 134 culture-confirmed patients were diagnosed at Songklanagarind

Hospital, Hat Yai, South Thailand [9]. Overall, 50% had localized infection, 37% were blood culture positive, and the CFR was 7% [9]. The low CFR is likely to be due to the high proportion of patients with localized infection [9], compared to cohorts diagnosed in other regions. Finkelstein et al. also reported the finding of *B. pseudomallei* in all 14 provinces in South Thailand [44]. Therefore, it is possible that melioidosis is endemic in all provinces, and further studies are needed to reveal the true burden of melioidosis in South Thailand. A training workshop was organized by MRC, Prince Songkla University (PSU), and Thailand Melioidosis Network during 20–21 December 2017 at PSU. A standard operating procedure (SOP) for laboratory diagnosis was provided, and laboratory staff from 6 provinces participated. The preliminary unofficial report from the office of Disease Control in Songkla showed a significant number of melioidosis patients, with high mortality [51].

2.6. Central Thailand

Central Thailand is a large plain consisting of clay soil. It includes 21 provinces and the Greater Bangkok area, and all published evidence of culture-confirmed human cases come from university hospitals in this area (Figure 1a). Most published cases report a history of travelling to Northeast Thailand, leading to the general understanding that those cases acquired *B. pseudomallei* outside the region, and that melioidosis is not endemic in Central Thailand. However, recent evidence in 2014 showed the presence of culture-confirmed melioidosis in ten goats in Bangkok, suggesting that *B. pseudomallei* might be covertly present in the environment in the central region and in Bangkok (Figure 1b) [52]. In addition, an environmental study published in 2016 conducted in seven provinces in central Thailand also confirmed the presence of *B. pseudomallei* in Phitsanulok, Phetchabun, and Nakonnayok (Figure 1c) [30]. It is likely that melioidosis cases are occurring in those three provinces, but they are possibly misdiagnosed and not reported. A recent animal study also found that both captive animals in a zoo and domestic animals had died of culture-confirmed melioidosis in Central Thailand [36,37]. During the workshop conducted at Chiang Mai University, laboratory staff from Uthai Thani, Central Thailand, also participated. In 2017, after the workshop, a total of 35 culture-confirmed cases were diagnosed at Uthai Thani hospitals [53]. These findings all strongly suggest that the common statement, 'melioidosis is not endemic in Central Thailand', is incorrect.

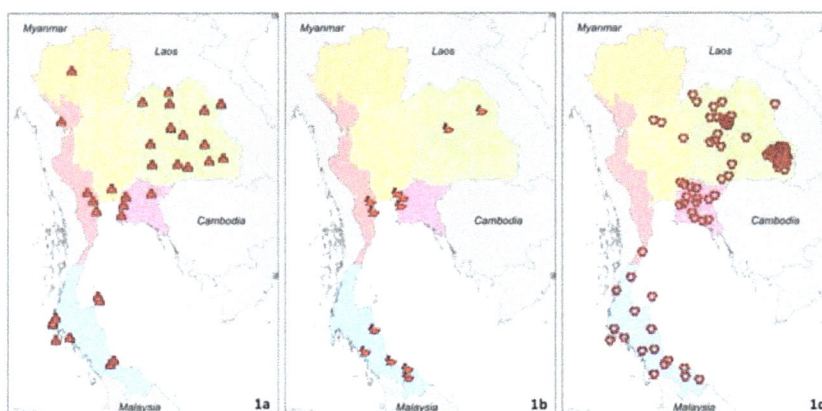

Figure 1. Evidence and distribution of melioidosis in Thailand from 1910 to 2015. Red icons represent geolocated records of culture-confirmed human cases (**1a**), culture-confirmed animal cases (**1b**) and presence of *B. pseudomallei* (**1c**). Green, orange, pink, rose, blue, and yellow colors represent Northeast, North, East, West, South, and Central Thailand, respectively. Interactive data are available online [54].

Geographically, melioidosis is likely to be endemic throughout Thailand. Action is needed to evaluate whether *B. pseudomallei* isolated from clinical samples in all regions can be accurately identified by laboratory personnel in hospitals, whether melioidosis cases are diagnosed and treated correctly, and whether all culture-confirmed melioidosis cases observed in each hospital, including university hospitals, are reported to Report 506 accurately.

3. Current Recommendations and Availability of Measures against Melioidosis

Currently there are no official, national guidelines for diagnosis, treatment and prevention of melioidosis in Thailand. In general, the international consensus guidelines for diagnosis [5] and treatment [55] are used.

Microbiological facilities are largely available in all provincial hospitals [32]. Following international sepsis campaigns [56], it is usual practice that doctors collect blood specimens for bacterial culture from every patient who presents at a provincial hospital and is prescribed parenteral antibiotics. In our experience, most Thai doctors do know about melioidosis and can diagnose and treat culture-confirmed cases of melioidosis appropriately if their laboratories can identify and report *B. pseudomallei* accurately.

However, there are no standard operating procedures (SOPs) or national guidelines for identification of *B. pseudomallei*. Most training and workshops are done ad hoc and do not include all microbiological laboratories in the country. The issue of misidentification of *B. pseudomallei* by many laboratories indicates that formal, national SOPs and training are critically needed to improve the identification of *B. pseudomallei*.

4. Surveillance Systems and Reporting of Melioidosis in Thailand

The National Communicable Disease Surveillance system (Report 506) was established in Thailand in 1968. Melioidosis has been one of the diseases for notification since 2002. However, until 2014, only about 10 fatal melioidosis cases per year were voluntarily reported in Report 506 [23–27]. The Thailand Melioidosis Network, together with the MoPH, has been investigating the issue of why provincial hospitals with microbiological facilities and fatal culture-confirmed melioidosis cases do not report them to the system. We found that many hospitals do not realize that they should report melioidosis cases, say that they are too busy to report them, or do not want to report a rapid increase of fatal melioidosis cases (for example, from 0 to 50 in a single province). We have been working through these issues since 2012, providing reassurance to hospitals that no negative consequences will result if the correct data are reported, that the MoPH is already aware of the situation, and that essential national action to reduce the deaths caused by melioidosis cannot be implemented if data are not reported. An improvement in reporting occurred in 2015. The number of melioidosis deaths formally reported rose to 112 in 2015 and 100 in 2016, solely because Sunpasithiprasong Hospital, Ubon Ratchathani province, began reporting (n = 107 and 87, respectively) [57?]. It is likely that if all hospitals with microbiological laboratories in Thailand were to report the outcomes of culture-confirmed cases, the total number of deaths caused by melioidosis could be higher than 1000 cases per year [7].

Since June 2016, reporting of culture-confirmed melioidosis cases from every hospital with a microbiology laboratory, together with final outcome, has been mandated under the Communicable Diseases Act B.E.2558 (A.D. 2015) [59]. Melioidosis is now one of the 57 diseases with a legal requirement for notification [59]. It is, therefore, important to educate and remind laboratory staff, clinicians, statisticians, and epidemiologists to comply with the requirements of the existing surveillance system by including every single case of melioidosis with cultures positive for *B. pseudomallei* in their Report 506. By enforcing this legislation, the MoPH could raise the priority of the disease, and should also consider implementing a large campaign to raise awareness and implement melioidosis-prevention measures countrywide.

We believe that the main cause for the discrepancy between the estimated number of fatal cases (n = 1000) and the model-predicted fatal cases (n = 2838) [8] is due to misdiagnosis and bacterial misidentification, which are still common outside Northeast Thailand.

In addition to the failure of reporting culture-confirmed cases, another important problem is the reporting of serologically diagnosed cases from community hospitals to the Report 506 system. Many of these cases are likely to be false positives, as it is well known that the indirect hemagglutination assay (IHA) should not be used to diagnose melioidosis in endemic countries due to the high background seropositivity [5]. This has led to a high number of false-positive melioidosis cases reported to Report 506, with few deaths, and therefore, reported CFRs are very low. For example, the CFR of melioidosis was officially reported as 0.5% (15/2902), 0.3% (10/3920), 0.2% (13/3711), 0.1% (4/2836), and 0.2% (12/2544) for Report 506 in 2010, 2011, 2012, 2013, and 2014, respectively [23–27]. These incorrect CFRs (ranging from 0.1 to 0.5%) have led to a false sense of security. People and policymakers mistakenly believe that melioidosis is not an important infectious disease in Thailand, as less than 1% of reported melioidosis cases were reported to have died. This is highly inaccurate, as the observed CFR of culture-confirmed cases in correctly designed studies in Thailand is between 30–35% [7,8].

The Thailand Melioidosis Network has proposed revising the reporting system to cover only culture-confirmed cases so that the true burden and true mortality (and CFR) could be demonstrated to the MoPH. Nonetheless, due to the problem of maintaining diagnostic capacity for melioidosis at community hospitals, the proposal was not accepted. The community hospitals require affordable rapid diagnostic tests (RDT) with high accuracy (particularly with high positive predictive value in melioidosis-endemic countries) to justify replacement of the IHA. Therefore, such an RDT is critically needed for Thailand.

Currently, the MoPH is working to rectify the underreporting of deaths caused by melioidosis in Report 506 by using (1) the hospital database known as '43 files reports' and (2) existing microbiological databases. The 43 file reports include International Statistical Classification of Diseases 10 (ICD-10). According to ICD-10, melioidosis is coded as A24. The MoPH is evaluating how many patients with the ICD-10 code of A24 were reported to Report 506, and how many of those died countrywide. Other work has used laboratory microbiological databases, and will evaluate how many patients with cultures positive for *B. pseudomallei* were reported to Report 506, and how many of those died countrywide. These activities will support the MoPH to improve understanding of the burden of melioidosis and the discrepancies between cases diagnosed by attending physicians, microbiologically-confirmed cases, and those reported to Report 506.

5. Awareness of Melioidosis in Thailand

Awareness of melioidosis in the general Thai population is very low. A recent study showed that 74% of lay adults had never heard of melioidosis, and 19% had heard of the disease, but had no further knowledge [18]. Information about melioidosis is rarely given to the public by the mass media, including television, newspapers, and radio stations. Basic information about the disease and its prevention is also not taught in schools in Thailand [18]. In contrast, public awareness of other common infections, such as HIV/AIDS, tuberculosis, malaria, leptospirosis, dengue, and influenza, are high, as these topics are taught in schools and are frequently mentioned by the national media [18].

A contributing factor to poor awareness of the disease is that many melioidosis patients die quickly before the microbiological results have been reported to the doctors caring for the patient. Even for culture-confirmed cases of melioidosis, doctors and healthcare workers are often too busy to explain to patients and their families what melioidosis is. This is because the relatives have usually never heard of this disease, and the explanation would take time. Most relatives in such scenarios are informed that the cause of death was sepsis, septic shock, or bacteremia, without explaining about melioidosis. They are also not informed about how to prevent other people in the family, or in the community, from acquiring the same disease. Although those who survive melioidosis are educated about the disease and receive oral eradicative treatment for up to 20 weeks, knowledge about the importance of the disease is not effectively shared with their relatives, friends, or communities. This is shown by the fact that most have never heard of the disease.

6. Major Changes and/or Achievements

The Thailand Melioidosis Network was formed during a meeting in March 2012 [60]. The meeting included scientists conducting melioidosis research and policymakers from across Thailand. The main purpose was to (1) provide updated information to participants, (2) form collaborations among research institutes and government authorities, and (3) discuss the important issues related to melioidosis in Thailand, including epidemiology, diagnosis, treatment, prevention, public awareness, and public engagement. The second meeting was held in September 2012 [61]. After the first two meetings, group email was used to communicate among the members.

The first international congress devoted to melioidosis held in Thailand, entitled 'International Congress on Melioidosis' with the theme 'State of the art discoveries and trends towards the 21st century', took place at the Siam City Hotel in Bangkok in 1998. The congress was organized by the Chulabhorn Research Institute and the chairperson was Prof. StitayaSirisinha. There were 150 delegates from Thailand and several other countries. The meeting was later referred to as 'The 2nd World Melioidosis Congress', which has since been held every three years and rotated through melioidosis-endemic countries. The international melioidosis meeting held in Kuala Lumpur, Malaysia in 1994 and chaired by Prof. Savithiri Puthucheary was regarded as the first World Melioidosis Congress (WMC). The 3rd and 4th WMC were held in 2001 in Perth, Australia, and 2004 in Singapore, respectively. In 2007, the 5th World Melioidosis Congress was again held in Thailand at Khon Kaen province and hosted by MRC, with Prof. Surasak Wongratanacheewin as chairperson [62], followed by the 6th WMC in Townsville, Australia. In 2013, over 300 delegates from 24 countries attended the 7th WMC in Bangkok [63]. It was hosted by MORU and the Faculty of Tropical Medicine, Mahidol University, with Dr. Wirongrong Chierakul as chairperson. The 8th WMC was hosted by University of Florida in Cebu, Philippines in 2016, with Asst. Prof. Apichai Tuanyok and Prof. Herbert Schweizer as chairpersons.

Hosting these meetings in Thailand has helped to raise the profile of melioidosis in the Thai medical, scientific, and political communities, as well as attracting media attention for the general public.

7. Current and Future Challenges

During the meetings of the Thailand Melioidosis Network in 2012, four priority areas were identified [61]. These included (1) to enhance the surveillance system, (2) to increase public awareness, (3) to improve diagnosis of melioidosis, and (4) to improve prevention of melioidosis.

First, the problem of underreporting by Report 506 must be solved. Although the rise in the reported number of deaths in 2015 occurred, more needs to be done. Only one provincial hospital (Sunpasitthiprasong Hospital) reported its melioidosis cases and their mortalities to Report 506. This was partially supported by the research unit in Sunpasitthiprasong Hospital. In future, the personnel who are responsible for the system might change jobs, and the system is not automated. Although a lot of discussion with many hospitals has taken place, the data from these hospitals have not yet been submitted to the national reporting system. An immediate need is educating and supporting all hospitals with microbiological facilities to report their culture-confirmed melioidosis cases and their mortalities to Report 506. A long-term solution is to automate the reporting system, similar to the systems in the Netherlands and China [64]. Another option is to have all admission and laboratory data from all hospitals in Thailand collected into one central data system. Then, formal analysis could be performed to identify the total number of cases for the Annual Epidemiological Surveillance Report of the MoPH [65], rather than using data from Report 506 alone.

Secondly, in order to raise public awareness of melioidosis, a large national campaign led by the MoPH is needed. Based on multiple studies in Thailand [18,19], lay people doubt that melioidosis is responsible for more than 1000 deaths of Thai people each year. They often ask, if that were true, "Why have I never heard or seen anything about this disease on television or in any campaign in hospitals?" Credible sources are a crucial component to provide information about the disease [18,19]. Thai people rely on doctors, nurses, healthcare workers, and the government to provide regular information about diseases and their prevention [18,19]. Therefore, information must come from the MoPH on a scale that is appropriate to a disease that kills more than 1000 people each year and is preventable. If people do not know about the disease and its true fatality rate, then prevention will be nearly impossible [18,19].

Third, the problem of misdiagnosis and bacterial misidentification in hospital microbiological laboratories outside Northeast Thailand has been described above. This is very likely due to the fact that (1) most laboratory technicians erroneously believe that melioidosis is endemic only in Northeast Thailand, (2) laboratory training around diagnostic testing is not adequate, (3) there is a lack of rapid bacterial identification tests, along with poor usage of *B. pseudomallei* selective culture media, and (4) a lack of RDTs for melioidosis diagnosis direct from clinical specimens, obviating the need for bacterial culture. Major university hospitals in Thailand could use instruments such as the Vitek 2 system (BioMerieux, Lombard, IL, USA) or matrix-assisted laser desorption ionization-time of flight mass spectrometry (MALDI-TOFMS), if the appropriate databases for *B. pseudomallei* are available [66]. However, it is crucial that all microbiology laboratory personnel in Thailand should be sufficiently familiar with *B. pseudomallei* to identify the organism within available resources, for example, using standard biochemistry and drug susceptibility tests. All technicians should be trained to recognize *B. pseudomallei* colonies, and not discard them as contaminants. All oxidase-positive Gram-negative bacilli should be tested to see whether they are *B. pseudomallei* [5]. Reports of *Pseudomonas* spp. should include a note that the organism was tested and confirmed not to be *B. pseudomallei*. A simple three-disc susceptibility testing method (demonstrating resistance to gentamicin and colistin but sensitivity to amoxicillin/clavulanic acid [67,68]) should be used in areas where resources are limited and secondary diagnostic tests (such as API 20NE and latex agglutination specific for *B. pseudomallei*) are not available. All uncertain isolates should be sent for confirmation to the Department of Medical Science, MoPH, Thailand, university hospital laboratories, or any research organizations in the area willing to receive bacterial isolates for confirmation of identity.

A latex agglutination assay using a monoclonal antibody specific for *B. pseudomallei* has been available in Thai research organizations for more than 17 years [69]. The test is useful for isolate confirmation, but cannot be used directly on clinical specimens. The Thailand Melioidosis Network strongly advocates for the latex agglutination assay to be one of the standard tests available to all microbiological laboratories in Thailand, together with the appropriate training. This should help to solve the problem of misidentification of *B. pseudomallei* countrywide [61].

A lateral flow immunoassay (LFI) using a similar monoclonal antibody to the latex agglutination assay has been developed by InBIOS (Seattle, WA, USA), and is currently being evaluated in several countries [70,71]. LFI can be used for rapid colony identification in a similar way to latex agglutination, and has the potential for application directly on clinical specimens [70,71]. Other advantages are lower cost when economy of scale is high, and longer shelf life. Currently, Prof. Wongratanacheewin at MRC is funded by the National Science and Technology Development Agency of Thailand, to develop a LFI for use in Thailand. The LFI could eventually replace latex agglutination as the production costs would likely be lower, and it should easily be manufactured at adequate levels to supply the whole country.

Fourth, recommendations for melioidosis prevention should be promoted thoroughly and intensively. Thailand is a hotspot for melioidosis, but only a small proportion of people in Thailand follow recommended behaviors that can prevent melioidosis [18,19]. These include using protective gear, such as rubber boots and gloves when in direct contact with soil and surface water, and consuming bottled or boiled water. However, changing behavior is typically complex, and providing information and boots alone is unlikely to be effective. This is shown by the fact that boots have been provided to Thai farmers for leptospirosis prevention since 2000 [72], yet many people still work in rice fields without using them [73]. Recent studies found that Thai people had no knowledge of melioidosis, believed that there was no need to adopt the recommended preventive behaviors, and were not inclined to use boots and gloves while working in muddy rice fields [18,19]. Practically, over-the-knee boots can be used in flooded rice fields without causing difficulty in walking, but they are still uncomfortable to wear in hot weather. Participants reported that input from numerous role models (physicians, diabetic clinics, friends, and families), and from the government via mass media, would be required for them to change their behavior. We strongly recommend that a multifaceted intervention at community and government levels is required to bring about the desired changes. It is still unknown how many melioidosis cases could be prevented by each recommended behavior. The size of the effect and cost-effectiveness of those preventive measures is being evaluated in a large behavioral change trial (NCT02089152). Nonetheless, the MoPH need not wait for the final results of this study (expected at the end of 2019) before launching a campaign, because the recommended preventive measures are simple and align with those for many other infectious diseases. The recommendations are supported by epidemiological studies [73,74], and are similar to prevention campaigns to raise awareness and reduce the number of cases and deaths due to melioidosis that have been conducted for several years in northern Australia [75].

In the long term, an effective vaccine against melioidosis, targeting at-risk groups, such as people with diabetes and agriculture workers, would be the ideal strategy for reducing the burden of disease and number of deaths from melioidosis in Thailand [76], and could be cost effective [77]. Ongoing research programs in Thailand [78] and internationally [79,80] to identify vaccine candidates are making progress, but vaccine development needs a long timeframe, and the case for ongoing funding of vaccine research relies on demonstrating the true extent of the disease burden in countries like Thailand.

In conclusion, we strongly believe that a prevention campaign should be undertaken now by the MoPH, together with enhancing disease surveillance systems, raising awareness of the disease and its true mortality, and improving the diagnosis of melioidosis. We believe that formal campaigns from the MoPH would enhance the usage of free boots that MoPH regularly provides to farmers. More lives could be saved, not only from leptospirosis, but also from melioidosis.

Acknowledgments: This work was funded by Department of Disease Control, Ministry of Public Health, Thailand. We thank all doctors, researchers and staff members in all participating hospitals and institutions in the Thailand Melioidosis Network. We thank Melioidosis Research Collaborative Network (RCN) and Cooperative Biological Engagement Program (CBEP), USA (HDTRA1-16-C-0017) for the support of open-access interactive map (www.melioidosis.info) and database of culture-confirmed melioidosis cases used. D.L. was funded by the Wellcome Trust (grant no. 101103). The laboratory network team for training and development of laboratory diagnosis was supported by National Science and Technology Development Agency (NSTDA), Thailand and Melioidosis Research Centre of KKU. The comments and conclusions in this article are those of the authors and do not necessarily represent the views of the organizations to which authors are affiliated.

Author Contributions: All authors are part of the Thailand Melioidosis Network. S.H., V.H., S.K. (Somkid Kongyu), S.T., S.A., R.W.S., G.L, P.T., N.T., V.W., N.C., S.D., P.P., S.S. (Stitaya Sirisinha), R.K., S.I., W.C. (Wipada Chaowagul), P.C. (Poomin Chuensombut), T.W.(Tri Wangrangsimakul), S.W. and D.L. conceived the study. V.H. and S.S. (Sandy Sachaphimukh) conducted the literature review. J.K., T.W. (Toni Whistler), S.J., W.S., S.B., T.A., O.S., C.S.T.,K.P.(Kanya Preechasuth), R.U., P.C. (Ploenchan Chetchotisa), N.W., C.A., S.N., Y.J., K.T., A.S., P.S. (Punchawee Sukbut), K.P.(Kritchavat Ploddi), P.S. (Poolsri Sirichotirat), B.C., K.R., M.H., G.W., P.S. (Pornpan Sunthornsut), P.W., W.C.(Wirongrong Chierakul), C.C., J.T., S.K. (Sunee Korbsrisate), A.T. contributed the data and assisted with the literature review. D.L. wrote the first draft. All authors contributed to the writing of the manuscript.

Conflicts of Interest: The authors declare no conflict of interest.

References

1. Chittivej, C.; Buspavanij, S.; Chaovanasai, A. Melioidosis with case report in a Thai. *R. Thai Army Med. J.* **1955**, *68*, 11–17.

2. Chayasirisobhon, S.; Intraprasit, S.; Jayanetsssra, P.; Punyagupta, S. Acute septicemic melioidosis. *J. Med. Assoc. Thai* **1976**, *59*, 375–379. [PubMed]

3. Leelarasamee, A. *Burkholderia pseudomallei:* The unbeatable foe? *Southeast Asian J. Trop. Med. Public Health* **1998**, *29*, 410–415. [PubMed]

4. Punyagupta, S.; Sirisanthana, T.; Stapatayavong, B. *Melioidosis;* Bangkok Medical Publisher: Bangkok, Thailand, 1989.

5. Hoffmaster, A.R.; AuCoin, D.; Baccam, P.; Baggett, H.C.; Baird, R.; Bhengsri, S.; Blaney, D.D.; Brett, P.J.; Brooks, T.J.; Brown, K.A.; et al. Melioidosis diagnostic workshop, 2013. *Emerg. Infect. Dis.* **2015**, *21*, e141045.
6. Leelarasamee, A.; Trakulsomboon, S.; Kusum, M.; Dejsirilert, S. Isolation rates of *Burkholderia pseudomallei* among the four regions in Thailand. *Southeast Asian J. Trop. Med. Public Health* **1997**, *28*, 107–113. [PubMed]
7. Limmathurotsakul, D.; Wongratanacheewin, S.; Teerawattanasook, N.; Wongsuvan, G.; Chaisuksant, S.; Chetchotisakd, P.; Chaowagul, W.; Day, N.P.; Peacock, S.J. Increasing incidence of human melioidosis in Northeast Thailand. *Am. J. Trop. Med. Hyg.* **2010**, *82*, 1113–1117. [CrossRef] [PubMed]
8. Limmathurotsakul, D.; Golding, N.; Dance, D.A.; Messina, J.P.; Pigott, D.M.; Moyes, C.L.; Rolim, D.B.; Bertherat, E.; Day, N.P.; Peacock, S.J.; et al. Predicted global distribution of *Burkholderia pseudomallei* and burden of melioidosis. *Nat. Microbiol.* **2016**, *1*, 15008. [CrossRef] [PubMed]
9. Churuangsuk, C.; Chusri, S.; Hortiwakul, T.; Charernmak, B.; Silpapojakul, K. Characteristics, clinical outcomes and factors influencing mortality of patients with melioidosis in Southern Thailand: A 10-year retrospective study. *Asian Pac. J. Trop. Med.* **2016**, *9*, 256–260. [CrossRef] [PubMed]
10. Limmathurotsakul, D.; Thammasart, S.; Warrasuth, N.; Thapanagulsak, P.; Jatapai, A.; Pengreungrojanachai, V.; Anun, S.; Joraka, W.; Thongkamkoon, P.; Saiyen, P.; et al. Melioidosis in animals, Thailand, 2006–2010. *Emerg. Infect. Dis.* **2012**, *18*, 325–327. [CrossRef] [PubMed]
11. White, N.J.; Dance, D.A.; Chaowagul, W.; Wattanagoon, Y.; Wuthiekanun, V.; Pitakwatchara, N. Halving of mortality of severe melioidosis by ceftazidime. *Lancet* **1989**, *2*, 697–701. [CrossRef]
12. Chetchotisakd, P.; Porramatikul, S.; Mootsikapun, P.; Anunnatsiri, S.; Thinkhamrop, B. Randomized, double-blind, controlled study of cefoperazone-sulbactam plus cotrimoxazole versus ceftazidime plus cotrimoxazole for the treatment of severe melioidosis. *Clin. Infect. Dis.* **2001**, *33*, 29–34. [CrossRef] [PubMed]
13. Limwattananon, S.; Tangcharoensathien, V.; Tisayaticom, K.; Boonyapaisarncharoen, T.; Prakongsai, P. Why has the universal coverage scheme in Thailand achieved a pro-poor public subsidy for health care? *BMC Public Health* **2012**, *12* (Suppl. 1), S6. [CrossRef] [PubMed]
14. Cheng, A.C.; Lowe, M.; Stephens, D.P.; Currie, B.J. Ethical problems of evaluating a new treatment for melioidosis. *BMJ* **2003**, *327*, 1280–1282. [CrossRef] [PubMed]
15. Stephens, D.P.; Thomas, J.H.; Higgins, A.; Bailey, M.; Anstey, N.M.; Currie, B.J.; Cheng, A.C. Randomized, double-blind, placebo-controlled trial of granulocyte colony-stimulating factor in patients with septic shock. *Crit. Care Med.* **2008**, *36*, 448–454. [CrossRef] [PubMed]
16. Currie, B.J.; Ward, L.; Cheng, A.C. The epidemiology and clinical spectrum of melioidosis: 540 cases from the 20-year Darwin prospective study. *PLoS Negl. Trop. Dis.* **2010**, *4*, e900. [CrossRef] [PubMed]
17. Stewart, J.D.; Smith, S.; Binotto, E.; McBride, W.J.; Currie, B.J.; Hanson, J. The epidemiology and clinical features of melioidosis in far North Queensland: Implications for patient management. *PLoS Negl. Trop. Dis.* **2017**, *11*, e0005411. [CrossRef] [PubMed]
18. Chansrichavala, P.; Wongsuwan, N.; Suddee, S.; Malasit, M.; Hongsuwan, M.; Wannapinij, P.; Kitphati, R.; Day, N.P.; Michie, S.; Peacock, S.J.; et al. Public awareness of melioidosis in Thailand and potential use of video clips as educational tools. *PLoS ONE* **2015**, *10*, e0121311. [CrossRef] [PubMed]
19. Suntornsut, P.; Wongsuwan, N.; Malasit, M.; Kitphati, R.; Michie, S.; Peacock, S.J.; Limmathurotsakul, D. Barriers and recommended interventions to prevent melioidosis in Northeast Thailand: A focus group study using the behaviour change wheel. *PLoS Negl. Trop. Dis.* **2016**, *10*, e0004823. [CrossRef] [PubMed]
20. Ong, C.E.L.; Wongsuvan, G.; Chew, J.S.W.; Kim, T.Y.; Teng, L.H.; Amornchai, P.; Wuthiekanun, V.; Day, N.P.J.; Peacock, S.J.; Cheng, T.Y.; et al. Presence of *Burkholderia pseudomallei* in soil and paddy rice water in a rice field in Northeast Thailand, but not in air and rainwater. *Am. J. Trop. Med. Hyg.* **2017**, *97*, 1702–1705. [CrossRef] [PubMed]
21. Bhengsri, S.; Lertiendumrong, J.; Baggett, H.C.; Thamthitiwat, S.; Chierakul, W.; Tisayaticom, K.; Tanwisaid, K.; Chantra, S.; Kaewkungwal, J. Economic burden of bacteremic melioidosis in Eastern and Northeastern Thailand. *Am. J. Trop. Med. Hyg.* **2013**, *89*, 369–373. [CrossRef] [PubMed]
22. Bhengsri, S.; Baggett, H.C.; Jorakate, P.; Kaewpan, A.; Prapasiri, P.; Naorat, S.; Thamthitiwat, S.; Tanwisaid, K.; Chantra, S.; Salika, P.; et al. Incidence of bacteremic melioidosis in Eastern and Northeastern Thailand. *Am. J. Trop. Med. Hyg.* **2011**, *85*, 117–120. [CrossRef] [PubMed]
23. Bureau of Epidemiology, Ministry of Public Health, Thailand. Annual Epidemiology Surveillance Report 2010; 2011. Available online: http://www.boe.moph.go.th/Annual/aesr2553/Open.html (accessed on 20 March 2018).

24. Bureau of Epidemiology, Ministry of Public Health, Thailand. Annual Epidemiology Surveillance Report 2011; 2012. Available online: http://www.boe.moph.go.th/Annual/AESR2011/main/AESR54_Part1/file4/2054_Melioidosis.pdf (accessed on 20 March 2018).

25. Bureau of Epidemiology, Ministry of Public Health, Thailand. Annual Epidemiology Surveillance Report 2012; 2013. Available online: http://www.boe.moph.go.th/Annual/AESR2012/main/AESR55_Part1/file4/2255_Melioidosis.pdf (accessed on 20 March 2018).

26. Bureau of Epidemiology, Ministry of Public Health, Thailand. Annual Epidemiology Surveillance Report 2013; 2014. Available online: http://www.boe.moph.go.th/Annual/AESR2013/annual/Melioidosis.pdf (accessed on 20 March 2018).

27. Bureau of Epidemiology, Ministry of Public Health, Thailand. Annual Epidemiology Surveillance Report 2014; 2015. Available online: http://www.boe.moph.go.th/Annual/AESR2014/aesr2557/Part1/1-4/melioidosis.pdf (accessed on 20 March 2018).

28. Farmers Warned of Disease Outbreak in Northeast Thailand. 25 August 2010.

29. Kashino, W.; Piyaphanee, W.; Kittitrakul, C.; Tangpukdee, N.; Sibunruang, S.; Lawpoolsri, S.; Yamashita, H.; Muangnoicharoen, S.; Silachamroon, U.; Tantawichien, T. Incidence of potential rabies exposure among Japanese expatriates and travelers in Thailand. *J. Travel Med.* **2014**, *21*, 240–247. [CrossRef] [PubMed]

30. Hantrakun, V.; Rongkard, P.; Oyuchua, M.; Amornchai, P.; Lim, C.; Wuthiekanun, V.; Day, N.P.; Peacock, S.J.; Limmathurotsakul, D. Soil nutrient depletion is associated with the presence of *Burkholderia pseudomallei*. *Appl. Environ. Microbiol.* **2016**, *82*, 7086–7092. [CrossRef] [PubMed]

31. Rukseree, K.; Mahidol University, Bangkok, Thailand; Palittapongarnpim, P.; National Science and Technology Development Agency, Bangkok, Thailand. Personal communication, 2017.

32. Teerawattanasook, N.; Tauran, P.M.; Teparrukkul, P.; Wuthiekanun, V.; Dance, D.A.B.; Arif, M.; Limmathurotsakul, D. Capacity and utilization of blood culture in two referral hospitals in Indonesia and Thailand. *Am. J. Trop. Med. Hyg.* **2017**, *97*, 1257–1261. [CrossRef] [PubMed]

33. Paek, S.C.; Meemon, N.; Wan, T.T. Thailand's universal coverage scheme and its impact on health-seeking behavior. *Springer Plus* **2016**, *5*, 1952. [CrossRef] [PubMed]

34. Shaw, J.E.; Sicree, R.A.; Zimmet, P.Z. Global estimates of the prevalence of diabetes for 2010 and 2030. *Diabetes Res. Clin. Pract.* **2010**, *87*, 4–14. [CrossRef] [PubMed]

35. The National Economic and Social Development Board, Thailand. Population Projections of Thailand 2000–2030. 2017. Available online: http://social.nesdb.go.th/social/Portals/0/Documents/pop_34.zip (accessed on 20 March 2018).

36. Kasantikul, T.; Sommanustweechai, A.; Polsrila, K.; Kongkham, W.; Chaisongkram, C.; Sanannu, S.; Kongmakee, P.; Narongwanichgarn, W.; Bush, M.; Sermswan, R.W.; et al. Retrospective study on fatal melioidosis in captive zoo animals in Thailand. *Transbound. Emerg. Dis.* **2016**, *63*, e389–e394. [CrossRef] [PubMed]

37. Kongkaew, W.; Thiptara, A.; Kaewkalong, S.; Hinjoy, S. Situation of melioidosis in Thailand, 2006–2015. *Thai-NIAH eJ.* **2017**, *12*, 80–102.

38. Chaiwarith, R.; Patiwetwitoon, P.; Supparatpinyo, K.; Sirisanthana, T. Melioidosis at Maharaj Nakorn Chiang Mai Hospital, Thailand. *J. Infect. Dis. Antimicrob. Agents* **2005**, *22*, 45–51.

39. Narata, R.; Wangkaew, S.; Kasitanon, N.; Louthrenoo, W. Community-acquired pneumonia in thai patients with systemic lupus erythematosus. *Southeast Asian J. Trop. Med. Public Health* **2007**, *38*, 528–536. [PubMed]

40. Trakulsomboon, S.; Vuddhakul, V.; Tharavichitkul, P.; Na-Gnam, N.; Suputtamongkol, Y.; Thamlikitkul, V. Epidemiology of arabinose assimilation in *Burkholderia pseudomallei* isolated from patients and soil in Thailand. *Southeast Asian J. Trop. Med. Public Health* **1999**, *30*, 756–759. [PubMed]

41. Sitthidet Tharinjaroen, C.; Chiang Mai University, Chiang Mai, Thailand; Preechasuth, K.; Chiang Mai University, Chiang Mai, Thailand; Chuensombut, v.; Chaingkham Hospital, Phayao, Thailand. Personal communication, 2017.

42. Wangrangsimakul, T.; Mahidol University, Bangkok, Thailand; Saengchun, W.; Chiang Rai Prachanukroh Hospital, Chiang Rai, Thailand. Personal communication, 2017.

43. Sitthidet Tharinjaroen, C.; Chiang Mai University, Chiang Mai, Thailand; Preechasuth, K.; Chiang Mai University, Chiang Mai, THailand; Waranyasirikul; Somdejphrajaotaksin Maharaj Hospital, Tak, Thailand. Personal communication, 2017.

44. Finkelstein, R.A.; Atthasampunna, P.; Chulasamaya, M. *Pseudomonas (burkholderia) pseudomallei* in Thailand, 1964–1967: Geographic distribution of the organism, attempts to identify cases of active infection, and presence of antibody in representative sera. *Am. J. Trop. Med. Hyg.* **2000**, *62*, 232–239. [CrossRef] [PubMed]

45. Whitmore, A. An account of a glanders-like disease occurring in Rangoon. *J. Hyg. (Lond.)* **1913**, *13*, 1–34. [CrossRef] [PubMed]

46. Chierakul, W.; Winothai, W.; Wattanawaitunechai, C.; Wuthiekanun, V.; Rugtaengan, T.; Rattanalertnavee, J.; Jitpratoom, P.; Chaowagul, W.; Singhasivanon, P.; White, N.J.; et al. Melioidosis in 6 tsunami survivors in Southern Thailand. *Clin. Infect. Dis.* **2005**, *41*, 982–990. [CrossRef] [PubMed]

47. Nieminen, T.; Vaara, M. *Burkholderia pseudomallei* infections in Finnish tourists injured by the December 2004 tsunami in Thailand. *Euro Surveill.* **2005**, *10*, E050303.4. [CrossRef] [PubMed]

48. Svensson, E.; Welinder-Olsson, C.; Claesson, B.A.; Studahl, M. Cutaneous melioidosis in a Swedish tourist after the tsunami in 2004. *Scand. J. Infect. Dis.* **2006**, *38*, 71–74. [CrossRef] [PubMed]

49. Rossi, B.; Epelboin, L.; Jaureguiberry, S.; Lecso, M.; Roos-Weil, D.; Gabarre, J.; Grenier, P.A.; Bricaire, F.; Caumes, E. Melioidosis and hairy cell leukemia in 2 travelers returning from Thailand. *Emerg. Infect. Dis.* **2013**, *19*, 503–505. [CrossRef] [PubMed]

50. Thaipadungpanit, J.; Chierakul, W.; Pattanaporkrattana, W.; Phoodaeng, A.; Wongsuvan, G.; Huntrakun, V.; Amornchai, P.; Chatchen, S.; Kitphati, R.; Wuthiekanun, V.; et al. *Burkholderia pseudomallei* in water supplies, Southern Thailand. *Emerg. Infect. Dis.* **2014**, *20*, 1947–1949. [CrossRef] [PubMed]

51. Kaewrakmuk, J.; Prince of Songkla University, Songkla, Thailand; Chiewchanyon, B.; The Office of Disease Prevention and Control 12, Songkla, Thailand. Personal communication, 2017.

52. Tonpitak, W.; Sornklien, C.; Chawanit, M.; Pavasutthipaisit, S.; Wuthiekanun, V.; Hantrakun, V.; Amornchai, P.; Thaipadungpanit, J.; Day, N.P.; Yingst, S.; et al. Fatal melioidosis in goats in Bangkok, Thailand. *Am. J. Trop. Med. Hyg.* **2014**, *91*, 287–290. [CrossRef] [PubMed]

53. Sitthidet Tharinjaroen, C.; Chiang Mai University, Chiang Mai, Thailand; Preechasuth, K.; Chiang Mai University, Chiang Mai, THailand; Anudit, C.; Uthai Thani Hospital, Uthai Thani, Thailand. Personal communication, 2017.

54. Melioidosis. Available online: www.melioidosis.info/map.aspx (accessed on 20 March 2018).

55. Lipsitz, R.; Garges, S.; Aurigemma, R.; Baccam, P.; Blaney, D.D.; Cheng, A.C.; Currie, B.J.; Dance, D.; Gee, J.E.; Larsen, J.; et al. Workshop on treatment of and postexposure prophylaxis for *Burkholderia pseudomallei* and *B. mallei* infection, 2010. *Emerg. Infect. Dis.* **2012**, *18*, e2. [CrossRef] [PubMed]

56. Dellinger, R.P.; Levy, M.M.; Rhodes, A.; Annane, D.; Gerlach, H.; Opal, S.M.; Sevransky, J.E.; Sprung, C.L.; Douglas, I.S.; Jaeschke, R.; et al. Surviving sepsis campaign: International guidelines for management of severe sepsis and septic shock: 2012. *Critical Care Med.* **2013**, *41*, 580–637. [CrossRef] [PubMed]

57. Bureau of Epidemiology, Ministry of Public Health, Thailand. Annual Epidemiology Surveillance Report 2015. 2016. Available online: http://www.boe.moph.go.th/Annual/AESR2015/aesr2558/Part1/04/melioidosis.pdf (accessed on 20 March 2018).

58. Bureau of Epidemiology, Ministry of Public Health, Thailand. Annual Epidemiology Surveillance Report 2016. 2017. Available online: http://203.157.15.110/annual/AESR2016/static/documents/sum-aesr/4/โรคเมลิออยโดสิส.pdf (accessed on 20 March 2018).

59. Department of Disease Control, Ministry of Public Health, Thailand. The Communicable Disease act B.E. 2558. 2015. Available online: http://www.ddc.moph.go.th/file/law/008.pdf (accessed on 20 March 2018).

60. Thailand Melioidosis Network. Minutes of the First Thailand Melioidosis Network Meeting, March 2012. Available online: http://www.melioidosis.info/download/20120515_102212%20tlmnm%2001%20meeting%20minute.pdf (accessed on 20 March 2018).

61. Thailand Melioidosis Network. Minutes of the Second Thailand Melioidosis Network Meeting, September 2012. Available online: http://www.melioidosis.info/download/20130207_084815%20tlmnm2%20minute%20eng%20ver1.pdf (accessed on 20 March 2018).

62. Proceedings from the 5th World Melioidosis Congress. Khon Kaen, Thailand. November 21–23, 2007. *Trans. R. Soc. Trop. Med. Hyg.* **2008**, *102* (Suppl. 1), S1–S156.

63. Schweizer, H.P.; Limmathurotsakul, D.; Peacock, S.J. New insights from the 7th World Melioidosis Congress 2013. *Emerg. Infect. Dis.* **2014**, *20*, e131737. [CrossRef] [PubMed]

64. Vlieg, W.L.; Fanoy, E.B.; van Asten, L.; Liu, X.; Yang, J.; Pilot, E.; Bijkerk, P.; van der Hoek, W.; Krafft, T.; van der Sande, M.A.; et al. Comparing national infectious disease surveillance systems: China and the Netherlands. *BMC Public Health* **2017**, *17*, 415. [CrossRef] [PubMed]

65. Coakley, M.F.; Leerkes, M.R.; Barnett, J.; Gabrielian, A.E.; Noble, K.; Weber, M.N.; Huyen, Y. Unlocking the power of big data at the national institutes of health. *Big Data* **2013**, *1*, 183–186. [CrossRef] [PubMed]

66. Suttisunhakul, V.; Pumpuang, A.; Ekchariyawat, P.; Wuthiekanun, V.; Elrod, M.G.; Turner, P.; Currie, B.J.; Phetsouvanh, R.; Dance, D.A.; Limmathurotsakul, D.; et al. Matrix-assisted laser desorption/ionization time-of-flight mass spectrometry for the identification of *Burkholderia pseudomallei* from Asia and Australia and differentiation between *Burkholderia* species. *PLoS ONE* **2017**, *12*, e0175294. [CrossRef] [PubMed]

67. Hodgson, K.; Engler, C.; Govan, B.; Ketheesan, N.; Norton, R. Comparison of routine bench and molecular diagnostic methods in identification of *Burkholderia pseudomallei*. *J. Clin. Microbiol.* **2009**, *47*, 1578–1580. [CrossRef] [PubMed]

68. Trinh, T.T.; Hoang, T.S.; Tran, D.A.; Trinh, V.T.; Gohler, A.; Nguyen, T.T.; Hoang, S.N.; Krumkamp, R.; Nguyen, L.T.N.; May, J.; et al. A simple laboratory algorithm for diagnosis of melioidosis in resource-constrained areas: A study from North-central Vietnam. *Clin. Microbiol. Infect.* **2017**, *24*, 84.e1–84.e4. [CrossRef] [PubMed]

69. Anuntagool, N.; Naigowit, P.; Petkanchanapong, V.; Aramsri, P.; Panichakul, T.; Sirisinha, S. Monoclonal antibody-based rapid identification of *Burkholderia pseudomallei* in blood culture fluid from patients with community-acquired septicaemia. *J. Med. Microbiol.* **2000**, *49*, 1075–1078. [CrossRef] [PubMed]

70. Robertson, G.; Sorenson, A.; Govan, B.; Ketheesan, N.; Houghton, R.; Chen, H.; AuCoin, D.; Dillon, M.; Norton, R. Rapid diagnostics for melioidosis: A comparative study of a novel lateral flow antigen detection assay. *J. Med. Microbiol.* **2015**, *64*, 845–848. [CrossRef] [PubMed]

71. Houghton, R.L.; Reed, D.E.; Hubbard, M.A.; Dillon, M.J.; Chen, H.; Currie, B.J.; Mayo, M.; Sarovich, D.S.; Theobald, V.; Limmathurotsakul, D.; et al. Development of a prototype lateral flow immunoassay (LFI) for the rapid diagnosis of melioidosis. *PLoS Negl. Trop. Dis.* **2014**, *8*, e2727. [CrossRef] [PubMed]

72. Phraisuwan, P.; Whitney, E.A.; Tharmaphornpilas, P.; Guharat, S.; Thongkamsamut, S.; Aresagig, S.; Liangphongphanthu, J.; Junthima, K.; Sokampang, A.; Ashford, D.A. Leptospirosis: skin wounds and control strategies, Thailand, 1999. *Emerg. Infect. Dis.* **2002**, *8*, 1455–1459. [CrossRef] [PubMed]

73. Limmathurotsakul, D.; Kanoksil, M.; Wuthiekanun, V.; Kitphati, R.; deStavola, B.; Day, N.P.; Peacock, S.J. Activities of daily living associated with acquisition of melioidosis in Northeast Thailand: A matched case-control study. *PLoS Negl. Trop. Dis.* **2013**, *7*, e2072. [CrossRef] [PubMed]

74. Limmathurotsakul, D.; Wongsuvan, G.; Aanensen, D.; Ngamwilai, S.; Saiprom, N.; Rongkard, P.; Thaipadungpanit, J.; Kanoksil, M.; Chantratita, N.; Day, N.P.; et al. Melioidosis caused by *Burkholderia pseudomallei* in drinking water, Thailand, 2012. *Emerg. Infect. Dis.* **2014**, *20*, 265–268. [CrossRef] [PubMed]

75. Boyd, R.; McGuinness, S.; Draper, A.; Neilson, M.; Krause, V. Melioidosis awareness campaign ....Don't get melioidosis.... *Northern Territ. Dis. Control Bull.* **2016**, *23*, 1–4.

76. Limmathurotsakul, D.; Funnell, S.G.; Torres, A.G.; Morici, L.A.; Brett, P.J.; Dunachie, S.; Atkins, T.; Altmann, D.M.; Bancroft, G.; Peacock, S.J.; et al. Consensus on the development of vaccines against naturally acquired melioidosis. *Emerg. Infect. Dis.* **2015**, *21*, e141480. [CrossRef] [PubMed]

77. Peacock, S.J.; Limmathurotsakul, D.; Lubell, Y.; Koh, G.C.; White, L.J.; Day, N.P.; Titball, R.W. Melioidosis vaccines: A systematic review and appraisal of the potential to exploit biodefense vaccines for public health purposes. *PLoS Negl. Trop. Dis.* **2012**, *6*, e1488. [CrossRef] [PubMed]

78. Dunachie, S.J.; Jenjaroen, K.; Reynssolds, C.J.; Quigley, K.J.; Sergeant, R.; Sumonwiriya, M.; Chaichana, P.; Chumseng, S.; Ariyaprasert, P.; Lassaux, P.; et al. Infection with *Burkholderia pseudomallei*—Immune correlates of survival in acute melioidosis. *Sci. Rep.* **2017**, *7*, 12143. [CrossRef] [PubMed]

79. Burtnick, M.N.; Shaffer, T.L.; Ross, B.N.; Muruato, L.A.; Sbrana, E.; DeShazer, D.; Torres, A.G.; Brett, P.J. Development of subunit vaccines that provide high level protection and sterilizing immunity against acute inhalational melioidosis. *Infect. Immun.* **2017**, *86*, e00724-17. [CrossRef] [PubMed]

80. Titball, R.W.; Burtnick, M.N.; Bancroft, G.J.; Brett, P. *Burkholderia pseudomallei* and *Burkholderia mallei* vaccines: Are we close to clinical trials? *Vaccine* **2017**, *35*, 5981–5989. [CrossRef] [PubMed]

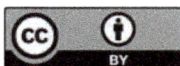

Tropical Medicine and Infectious Disease

MDPI

Review

Endemic Melioidosis in Southern China:
Past and Present

Xiao Zheng [1,2,*], Qianfeng Xia [3], Lianxu Xia [1] and Wei Li [1]

[1] State Key Laboratory for Infectious Disease Prevention and Control, Collaborative Innovation Center for Diagnosis and Treatment of Infectious Diseases, National Institute for Communicable Disease Control and Prevention, Chinese Center for Disease Control and Prevention, Beijing 102206, China; xialianxu@icdc.cn (L.X.); liwei@icdc.cn (W.L.)

[2] Chinese Field Epidemiology Training Program, Chinese Center for Disease Control and Prevention, Beijing 102206, China

[3] Laboratory of Tropical Biomedicine and Biotechnology, School of Tropical Medicine and Laboratory Medicine, Hainan Medical University, Haikou 571199, China; xiaqianfeng@sina.com

* Correspondence: zhengxiao@icdc.cn; Tel.: +86-010-6173-9444

Received: 16 November 2018; Accepted: 20 February 2019; Published: 25 February 2019

Abstract: Melioidosis is a severe tropical infectious disease caused by the soil-dwelling bacterium *Burkholderia pseudomallei*, predominantly endemic to Southeast Asia and northern Australia. Between the 1970s and the 1990s, the presence of *B. pseudomallei* causing melioidosis in humans and other animals was demonstrated in four coastal provinces in southern China: Hainan, Guangdong, Guangxi, and Fujian, although indigenous cases were rare and the disease failed to raise concern amongst local and national health authorities. In recent years, there has been a rise in the number of melioidosis cases witnessed in the region, particularly in Hainan. Meanwhile, although China has established and maintained an effective communicable disease surveillance system, it has not yet been utilized for melioidosis. Thus, the overall incidence, social burden and epidemiological features of the disease in China remain unclear. In this context, we present a comprehensive overview of both historical and current information on melioidosis in Southern China, highlighting the re-emergence of the disease in Hainan. Surveillance and management strategies for melioidosis should be promoted in mainland China, and more research should be conducted to provide further insights into the present situation.

Keywords: melioidosis; *Burkholderia pseudomallei*; epidemiology; China

1. Introduction

Melioidosis is a fatal infectious disease caused by *Burkholderia pseudomallei*, a saprophytic environmental bacterium that is endemic in many tropical regions of the world and affects both humans and animals [1,2]. In humans, although most organs of the body can be infected, acute pneumonia and septicaemia often represent the most common clinical manifestations, and are associated with a high mortality rate (10%–30%) for the disease [1,2]. Given the increase in the number of reported cases, as well as the extension of endemic regions in past decades, melioidosis is deemed to be a re-emerging infectious disease in many tropical countries [3], particularly in Southeast Asia and north Australia. More strikingly, a recent modeling study predicted that the true global burden of melioidosis was approximately 165,000 cases and 89,000 deaths a year [4], much higher than the total number of cases that are documented or reported. Although the true disease burden remains difficult to determine, it appears likely that there has been a dramatic underestimation of its scale in part due to misdiagnosis and underreporting in vast areas of the world appropriate for its endemicity. It is thus important to raise the profile of the disease across the tropical world.

Similar challenges have been encountered in mainland China. The environmental presence of *B. pseudomallei* was initially demonstrated in the 1970s and the first human case of melioidosis was identified in 1989 [5]; nonetheless, as only a few cases were identified at the time, attention soon declined and the disease was neglected for many years. However, with the rapid economic development and social transition over the past two decades, the situation has changed and there has been a substantial increase in the number of cases diagnosed in Hainan, with the occurrence of sporadic locally-acquired or imported cases in other areas throughout China. Clearly this shift requires a reconsideration of the current status and epidemiology of the disease within China. However, thanks to both preconceptions about the insignificance of the disease, and the fact that it has not been listed as a nationally notifiable infectious disease, studies of the epidemiology of melioidosis in China are few and far between and it is difficult to obtain resources to study it further.

Here, we provide an overview of the historical and current aspects of melioidosis in China by reviewing available data and information about human and animal melioidosis and *B. pseudomallei* in mainland China, with an emphasis on its resurgence in Hainan, including some publications that are only available in Chinese. We have excluded Hong Kong and Taiwan, which are both covered elsewhere in this issue. We hope that this review will help to inform clinicians and policy makers about the disease in southern China and lead to the formulation of plans to prevent and control it in the future.

2. History

The first event linking melioidosis to China occurred in France in the early 1970s when an outbreak of melioidosis at the Jardin des Plantes zoo was attributed to a giant panda from China [6]. Nevertheless, as pandas uniquely inhabit the high-altitude mountainous areas of Southwest China, where neither *B. pseudomallei* nor human or animal melioidosis has ever been reported, the panda might actually have been a victim of this outbreak rather than the source.

In mainland China, the discovery of environmental *B. pseudomallei* preceded the identification of the first human case of melioidosis by over 10 years. Since the early 1970s, horse farms and military establishments in Hainan and Guangdong had reported an increase of mallein test positive horses without any clinical features suggestive of glanders. A comprehensive environmental survey in the vicinity of mallein-positive stables was undertaken to investigate whether *B. pseudomallei* might be a potential cause of this phenomenon [7]. Between April and June 1975, Li and colleagues obtained 23 isolates of *B. pseudomallei* from 4.9% of pond waters sampled near these farms by inoculation in golden hamsters. Subsequent experiments showed that horses infected with *B. pseudomallei* gave positive mallein reactions [8]. From 1976 to 1979, the survey was extended to other southern provinces and another nine environmental isolates were obtained from Guangdong and Guangxi, two subtropical provinces close to Hainan, with no *B. pseudomallei* being cultured further north than this [8]. Subsequently, *B. pseudomallei* was isolated in 1985 from a paddy field in Putian, Fujian province, a subtropical region adjacent to Taiwan [9]. The first cases of culture-positive melioidosis were detected in 1982, when Lu isolated *B. pseudomallei* from slaughtered pigs in Hainan [10]. In 1981, Li found a prevalence of seropositivity (indirect hemagglutination (IHA) titer >1:40) ranging from 6.0% to 13.7% among people inhabiting the coastal areas of Hainan [8]. It thus appeared that exposure to *B. pseudomallei*, and therefore human melioidosis, was also likely to be present in this region.

Efforts to find cases of human melioidosis in Hainan continued throughout the 1980s, but most attempts were in vain. Eventually, the first human case of culture-positive melioidosis, presenting with an ulcer on his left leg, was identified in Sanya City in 1989 [11]. Two patients with fatal septicaemic melioidosis, both local farmers, were reported in 1990 from Zhanjiang City in Guangdong, which is located at the southernmost peninsula of mainland China opposite Hainan island [11]. Subsequently, Song et al. conducted a prospective survey looking for human cases at the largest provincial hospital on Hainan, Hainan People's Hospital, in 1995 [12]. Within a one-year period, a total of eight culture-confirmed cases were identified, four of whom had acute septicaemia and the others chronic forms with abscesses in different organs. As elsewhere, seasonal and occupational associations were seen, as all cases were farmers and most presented during the rainy season in Hainan (May to October). Based on these findings, it was concluded that animal and human melioidosis were rare in the region and few further studies were conducted on it during the 1990s.

3. Review of Melioidosis Cases and Resurgence of the Disease in Hainan

During the 21st century, particularly after the severe acute respiratory syndrome (SARS) outbreak in 2003, China's infectious disease surveillance, prevention and control systems expanded and improved considerably. Since then, the overall incidence of notifiable infectious diseases has been declining and some are even close to eradication [13]. By contrast, melioidosis has been one of the few infectious diseases whose incidence has increased in recent years, especially in the Hainan province. Clinical staff began to recognize increasing numbers of melioidosis cases in general hospitals in Hainan and their awareness of the infection grew [14,15]. For example, compared with a total of eight cases in 1996, approximately 20–30 cases were seen each year at Hainan People's Hospital during the 2010s [15,16]. As culture facilities and diagnostic guidelines were already well established in this institution, it is likely that this reflected a genuine increase in incidence.

This increased incidence drew the attention of local and national health authorities and so in 2011 the Institute for Communicable Disease Control and Prevention of China (ICDC) established a working group with the aim of identifying and monitoring the incidence and epidemiology of melioidosis throughout China. Following this, a preliminary sentinel network representing the major government and teaching hospitals within Hainan was established, resulting in the identification of a total of 396 culture-confirmed cases (392 from Hainan, three from Guangxi and one from Guangdong) between 2002 and 2016 (Figure 1). The available medical records of 289 cases (all from Hainan) were reviewed to establish information about the demographics, clinical features and outcomes. It was found that the patients were distributed around the periphery of Hainan Island with no cases originating from the two central mountainous prefectures (Wuzhishan and Qiong Zhong) as seen in Figure 2; three major port cities (Sanya, Haikou, and Dongfang) contributed to nearly half the cases (123, 42.6%). Of 289 patients for whom data were available, 245 were male and 44 were female; apart from one neonate (17 days), the other patients ranged from one year to 84 years old (median = 49.4 years), with the highest proportion in the 51–60 year age group (Figure 3). Cases were seen in each month, but the peak incidence occurred in August and September during the rainy season (from May to October) as seen in Figure 4. Of the 238 patients whose occupations were known, local farmers formed a large proportion (118, 49.6%). Among 277 cases with complete clinical information, septicaemia (153/277, 55.2%) and pneumonia (149/277, 53.8%) represented the two major clinical manifestations; other less common clinical features included musculo-skeletal or soft tissue abscesses (57/277, 20.6%), genitourinary or prostatic infection (18/277, 6.5%), brain infection (9/277, 3.3%), liver or splenic abscesses (8/277, 2.9%), pyogenic arthritis (5/277, 1.8%), upper gastrointestinal hemorrhage (4/277, 1.4%), neck abscess (4/277, 1.4%), suppurative parotitis (3/277, 1.1%), suppurative pharyngitis (3/277, 1.1%), and infected aortic aneurysm (3/277, 1.1%) as seen in Table 1. Death occurred in 64 cases, resulting in an overall mortality rate of 23.1% (64/277). The most common underlying co-morbidity was diabetes (131/277, 47.3%), followed by chronic liver disease (18/277, 6.5%), chronic lung disease (6/277, 2.2%), and chronic renal disease (5/277, 1.8%). During the survey period of 2011-2016, a notable peak in cases (*n* = 106) occurred in 2016, coinciding with record wet-season precipitation that year (Figure 2). This represented an annual incidence rate of 1.16 per 100,000 for this region, where the resident population was approximately 9,270,000 according to 2014 Census data. Even so, since this sentinel network did not include all the hospitals in the region and depended on voluntary surveillance rather than mandatory reporting, it is inevitable that a number of cases will have been missed and the true incidence would be higher.

Trop. Med. Infect. Dis. **2019**, *4*, 39

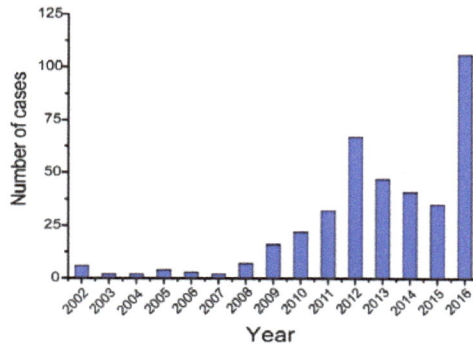

Figure 1. Number of melioidosis cases by year identified during surveillance, Hainan, China, 2002–2016.

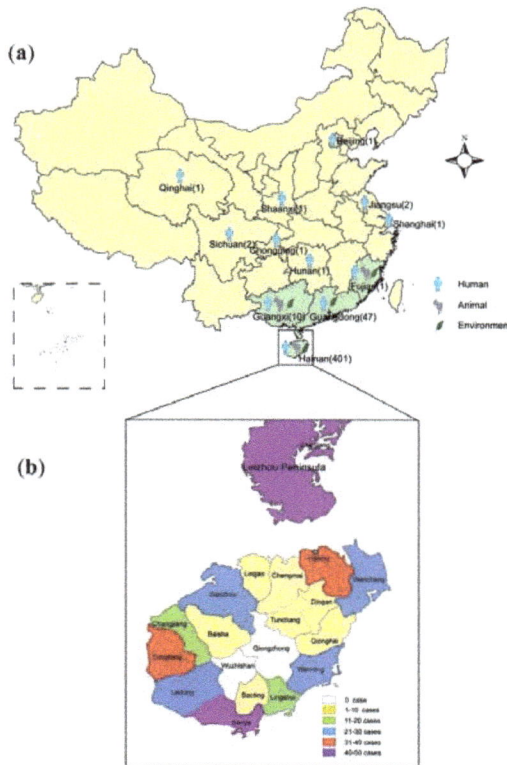

Figure 2. Location of *Burkholderia pseudomallei* and melioidosis cases in China. (**a**) The distribution of endemic areas (*n* = 4, with green shading) and melioidosis cases in mainland China, with locations of environmental isolation of *B. pseudomallei* and indigenous or imported human/animal cases of melioidosis indicated (The number of human cases for each province was indicated in parentheses. The patients outside the four endemic provinces all have a history of residence or travel to Hainan or overseas endemic areas and thus are deemed as imported cases); (**b**) The distribution of melioidosis cases according to different prefectures in Hainan (data only available for 289 of 401 cases) and in the Leizhou Peninsula (46 cases) of Guangdong, China.

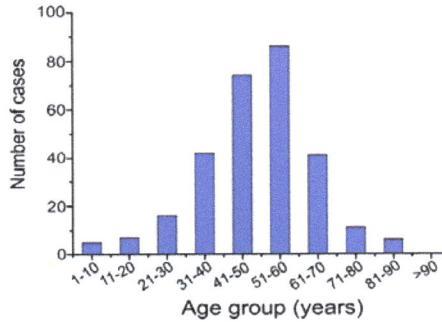

Figure 3. Age distribution of 288 human melioidosis patients from Hainan, China, 2002–2014.

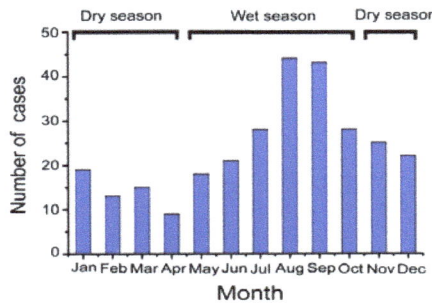

Figure 4. Monthly distribution of 289 melioidosis cases across 13 years (2002–2014) in Hainan, China.

Table 1. Summary of clinical presentation of 277 melioidosis cases from Hainan.

Presentation	Number of Cases	Percentage (%)
Septicaemia	153	55.2
Pneumonia	149	53.8
Musculoskeletal or soft tissue abscess	57	20.6
Genitourinary or prostatic infection	18	6.5
Brain infection	9	3.3
Internal organ (liver, kidney or splenic) abscess	8	2.9
Pyogenic arthritis	5	1.8
Upper gastrointestinal hemorrhage	4	1.4
Neck abscess	4	1.4
Suppurative parotitis	3	1.1
Infected aortic aneurysm	3	1.1
Orbital abscess	3	1.1
Suppurative pharyngitis	3	1.1

To search for additional records of melioidosis cases and *B. pseudomallei* isolates from mainland China, especially those occurring before the start of the ICDC surveillance (2011), we also consulted the international *B. pseudomallei* multi-locus sequence typing (MLST) database (https://pubmlst.org/bpseudomallei/) [17]. Up to the end of 2017, among over 5300 *B. pseudomallei* isolates deposited in this web accessible database, 205 were marked as originating from the Chinese mainland, comprising 195 human/animal isolates, five environmental isolates, and five isolates with unknown sources. The isolation dates spanned from 1975 to 2015, but strains prior to 2011 accounted for only a small proportion (66 isolates). As there were many duplicate cases between this dataset and our surveillance database, we excluded these and have only included records prior to 2002 (11 isolates) in this review.

4. Literature Review

Alongside this increase in the number of cases diagnosed, there has been a proliferation of publications on melioidosis in China, many of which have been published in Chinese and are thus not readily accessible to researchers in other countries. In order to undertake as comprehensive a review of the available literature as possible, we conducted a search of two domestic science databases (China Science Periodical Database, China Hospital Knowledge Database) and two international scientific databases (PubMed of the National Library of Medicine and Web of Science) to identify reports of documented human or animal cases of melioidosis from China. We used the key search terms "melioidosis", "*Burkholderia pseudomallei*" and "China". We identified 196 articles to the end of August 2018, which we reviewed for relevance based on whether they described melioidosis cases or *B. pseudomallei* isolates from mainland China. A total of 86 articles (from 1981 to 2018) were finally selected, of which only 31 were retrieved from international databases. Most of these documents dealt with endemic provinces, but there were also case reports from non-endemic areas of central and northern China, including Beijing [18], Shanghai [19], Jiangsu [20,21], Hunan [22], Qinghai [23], Chongqing [24], Shaanxi [25], and Sichuan [26] as seen in Figure 2. Except for the Hunan case for whom the residence/travel information was unavailable, each case occurring outside the known endemic provinces of Hainan, Fujian, Guangdong, and Guangxi had a history of residence or traveled to Hainan or overseas endemic regions before the onset of the disease, hence all of them should be considered imported cases.

It is notable that several series of melioidosis cases have been described in China (Table 2) over the past two decades. However, in most series, the individual case data have been omitted or summarized, making it difficult to identify duplications as well as to investigate clinical or epidemiological patterns on a larger scale. In a retrospective study, Fang et al. described the clinical and epidemiological features of 170 culture-confirmed cases hospitalized in three general hospitals in Hainan, between 2002 and 2014 [35]. As noted above, a steady increase in the numbers of melioidosis cases was seen; pneumonia (34.1%) was the most common manifestation, and people with diabetes and outdoor laborers were at greatest risk of contracting the disease. In a prospective survey, Zheng et al. characterized a cluster of 16 microbiologically confirmed cases occurring after Typhoon Rammasun hit northern Hainan on July 18th 2014 [36]. In a retrospective study undertaken by Chen et al., a total of 44 human cases were detected amongst 7786 febrile patients at the Affiliated Hospital of Guangdong Medical College in Zhanjiang City between 1990 and 2005, 25 of whom died (56.8%) [28]. Since all these cases came from surrounding counties/villages, it appears that the Leizhou Peninsula, which has contributed to the majority of documented cases from Guangdong, should also be considered a hotspot for melioidosis in southern China. Compared with Hainan and Guangdong, fewer melioidosis cases have been recognized in the provinces of Guangxi and Fujian, despite the fact that *B. pseudomallei* is known to be present in the environment [9,41]. However, a retrospective report was recently published, which describes seven culture-proven cases of melioidosis hospitalized in a teaching hospital in Nanning, the capital city of Guangxi, from October 2006 to March 2015 [40]. The clinical characteristics, drug susceptibility results and epidemiological features of these cases were similar to those in other known endemic regions. In parallel, although not documented in the published literature, an indigenous female patient from Fujian with severe melioidosis was reported online in November 2014 [42]. Interestingly, the patient was from Putian, where the environmental presence of *B. pseudomallei* had previously been identified in 1985. It is thus likely that Guangxi, and possibly Fujian, have been neglected as melioidosis-endemic, and improvements in awareness and diagnosis of the disease are needed to improve the understanding of its true prevalence in these provinces. In general, the range of clinical manifestations of melioidosis in China is similar to that seen elsewhere, with relatively rare clinical manifestations reported in the literature, including suppurative parotitis (one case) [43], osteomyelitis (three cases) [44] and pericarditis (one case) [45] from Hainan, as well as prostatic abscesses (two cases) [46] and co-infection with Japanese encephalitis (one case) [47] from Guangdong.

Table 2. Human melioidosis cases reported from Hainan, Guangdong, and Guangxi.

Year of Report	Location of Infection	Duration of Study	Number of Cases [1]	Outcome	Reference
1992	Hainan & Guangdong	1975–1992	3	1 Survived/2 Died	[8]
1998	Hainan	1995–1996	8	4 Survived/2 Died/2 Unknown	[12]
2005	Hainan	2002–2005	12	4 Survived/8 Died	[27]
2006	Guangdong	1990–2005	44	19 Survived/25 Died	[28]
2006	Hainan	1996–2005	32	21 Survived/3 Died/9 treatment withdrawn	[29]
2008	Hainan	2002–2006	19	12 Survived/7 Died	[30]
2008	Hainan	2000–2007	25	9 Survived/6 Died/10 treatment withdrawn	[31]
2009	Hainan	2000–2009	104	72 Survived/15 Died/17 treatment withdrawn	[32]
2011	Hainan	2002–2008	122	81 Survived/19 Died/22 treatment withdrawn	[14]
2013	Hainan	2007–2012	95	65 Survived/30 Died	[15]
2014	Hainan	2009–2012	40	34 Survived/6 Died	[33]
2014	Hainan	2010–2013	40	6 Survived /10 Died/24 Unknown	[34]
2015	Hainan	2002–2014	170	124 Survived/46 Died	[35]
2016	Hainan	2003–2014	60	32 Survived/26 Died/2 Unknown	[16]
2016	Hainan	Jul–Sep 2014	16	8 Survived/8 Died	[36]
2017	Hainan	2002–2015	7	5 Survived (4 had nervous system sequelae) /1 Died/1 treatment withdrawn	[37]
2017	Hainan	2000–2012	46	33 Survived/13 Died	[38]
2018	Hainan	2012–2017	35	26 Survived/7 Died/2 treatment withdrawn	[39]
2018	Guangxi	2006–2015	7	All Survived	[40]

[1] It was not possible to exclude duplicate reports and so there is overlap between these series.

In order to obtain a comprehensive dataset, we merged data from the three sources described above (ICDC, MLST database, and the literature review) to give an inclusive picture of the melioidosis distribution around mainland China (Supplementary Table S1), comprising 469 cases (401 from Hainan, 47 from Guangdong, 10 from Guangxi, one from Fujian and 10 cases imported into more northern provinces) identified in the present study. The distribution of these cases is shown in Figure 2.

5. Environmental and Molecular Investigations of *B. pseudomallei* in Hainan

5.1. Environmental Distribution of B. pseudomallei

The incidence of melioidosis is closely associated with the environmental density of *B. pseudomallei* in endemic areas. To estimate the abundance of the organism in soil and water and investigate its relationship with the recent increase in melioidosis cases, several environmental surveys have been conducted in Hainan over the past few years. In 2012, in a collaborative investigation by ICDC and Sanya People's Hospital, 70 soil and water samples were collected from 20 paddy fields scattered across southern Hainan Island. There was no *B. pseudomallei* found, but four isolates of *Burkholderia thailandensis*, a non-pathogenic species closely related to *B. pseudomallei*, were recovered from four different locations [48]. In 2014 and 2017, two further investigations were conducted by separate research groups [49,50], which were positive for *B. pseudomallei* by culture in 3 of 58 (5.2%) and 2 of 70 (2.9%) environmental samples, respectively. Comparison of clinical and environmental isolates using a combination of two discriminant genotyping techniques, multilocus sequence typing and multiple locus variable number tandem repeat analysis (MLST and MLVA), suggested an environmental origin for some of the cases. These studies were of limited scale, and could not determine the geographic distribution of *B. pseudomallei* all over the island, but from August to December 2016, Dong et al. conducted a more comprehensive environmental *B. pseudomallei* investigation, covering all 18 counties of Hainan Island [51]. Among 360 sampling sites, 48 (13.3%) were positive for the bacterium, and most of these were located in coastal counties (12/18), which corresponds with the distribution of clinical cases around the island. It is hoped that studies such as this will help to establish a risk map, which may assist in the prevention of the disease in Hainan.

5.2. Genetic Diversity of B. pseudomallei Isolates from Hainan

Latterly, molecular epidemiological studies of the increasing numbers of available isolates of *B. pseudomallei* have been a growing area of melioidosis research in Hainan. Using MLST, Fang et al. divided 102 isolates from three hospitals into 41 sequence types (STs), among which 11 STs were unique to Hainan and eight were novel [52]. In another recent study, 30 STs were found amongst 60 clinical isolates collected between 2003 and 2014, including six novel types [16]. It is clear from these studies that *B. pseudomallei* in Hainan are highly genetically diverse, with some major STs being shared with and linked to the subpopulations from other Southeast Asian endemic foci such as Thailand and Malaysia. This makes it likely that the introduction of *B. pseudomallei* into Hainan is not recent and that the island has probably been endemic for melioidosis for a long period. Interestingly, ST562 has been found in both Hainan and northern Australia [53]. On the basis of SNP-based phylogenetic analysis, Price et al. showed that Australian isolates of this clone belong to the Southeast Asian subpopulation, which appears to have spread to, and become established in, the Darwin region in recent years [54]. ST562 is also represented amongst the two genomes (BPC006 and 350105) of *B. pseudomallei* from China that have been sequenced and published [55,56]. Strain 350105 was obtained from Hainan in 1976 and represents the earliest known ST562 isolate, but precisely how and when this long-range transmission took place is unknown and would be worthy of further studies.

6. New Understanding of Melioidosis Epidemiology on Hainan

6.1. The Association between Typhoon and Case Clustering of Melioidosis

Climatic factors can exert a remarkable influence on the incidence of melioidosis, even causing outbreaks. However, despite the known endemic areas of southern China (Hainan, Guangdong, Guangxi, Fujian, and Hong Kong) being located in the typhoon-prone belt of the Western Pacific, it was only recently discovered that the potential impact of a typhoon strike on melioidosis incidence in the region was demonstrated when Typhoon Rammasun (a Category five super typhoon) struck Hainan in 2014 [36]. Within two months of the event, a cluster of 16 human cases of melioidosis concurred around the point at which the typhoon struck land. Moreover, the patients manifested severe clinical forms and a high mortality rate (50%), which had also been observed in typhoon-related melioidosis clusters in Taiwan [57]. A correlation between typhoons and the occurrence of melioidosis was also noted in a review of 15 confirmed cases (2002–2007) from a municipal hospital in Zhanjiang City, Guangdong [58]. Further studies are required to elucidate the mode and mechanism by which extreme weather events influence the incidence of melioidosis in southern China and how this may be affected by climate change.

6.2. Disease Burden and Risk Analysis

Defining the burden and risk factors for melioidosis is important to raise awareness of the disease in the public health community and develop preventive and control strategies for the disease [4]. However, although an increasing number of melioidosis cases have been witnessed in Hainan, our knowledge of its full magnitude and epidemiology are still lacking. It appears that the main disease burden is focused on the tropical coastal areas of southern China, especially those of Hainan Island, the Leizhou Peninsula, and southern Guangxi. Compared with inland regions, these coastal regions are characterized by higher population density, more abundant rainfall and more plentiful habitats for *B. pseudomallei* (such as paddy fields and artificial ponds), which would favor the occurrence of melioidosis. As with other endemic regions, diabetic and rural populations are at the highest risk of contracting the disease, and the incidence is associated with rainfall and extreme weather events. The rising incidence of melioidosis has been more evident in Hainan than in the other endemic provinces in recent years. The epidemiology of melioidosis represents the consequences of a complicated interaction between multiple natural and social factors, such as the physicochemical environment, climate, host population susceptibility and genetic variation of the pathogen [3], which is as yet poorly understood. The impact of climate change (such as a rise in precipitation or higher frequency of typhoon strikes) on the incidence of disease may be significant in Hainan. In addition, the booming real estate industry on the island, which is likely to cause considerable changes in land use and the ecological environment, together with the rapid growth of the diabetic population in Hainan [59] may also be implicated in the recently observed increased incidence. Thus, multiple factors have probably contributed to a genuine increase in the incidence of melioidosis in Hainan, and unless these factors are addressed, it is likely that the background incidence will continue to rise in Hainan and, under appropriate conditions, further clusters and outbreaks may occur.

7. Surveillance and Reporting of Melioidosis Cases in Mainland China

7.1. Human

Although a highly efficient nationwide reporting and monitoring network for infectious diseases has been established in China since 2004 [60], melioidosis is still not included, largely due to the lack of awareness and the fact that it is not listed as a statutorily notifiable infectious disease in the country. Given the evidence of increasing incidence, ICDC has prioritized surveillance work in Hainan through the establishment of the sentinel network described above. Between 2011 and 2017, this network has involved seven tertiary and 12 county-level hospitals. In addition, in order to improve the ability of medical and laboratory staff to recognize the disease, ICDC delivered training and workshops on melioidosis diagnosis and *B. pseudomallei* identification during 2016 and 2017 in Hainan. However, no such surveillance or training has yet been undertaken in the Leizhou Peninsula and southern Guangxi, despite the evidence that these are also melioidosis-endemic. It is therefore likely that underreporting cases remains a major issue in these regions. Even though melioidosis has not yet been incorporated into the national system for reportable infectious diseases, the disease should be added into the local infectious disease reporting systems of these regions in the future.

Molecular epidemiological surveillance, which is widely accepted as a powerful tool for the prevention and control of communicable diseases, has increasingly been implemented in China. With the recognition of melioidosis as an emerging threat to both endemic and non-endemic areas, since 2017 *B. pseudomallei* has been included in PulseNet China, a national monitoring platform for major bacterial pathogens led by ICDC. This should enhance nationwide surveillance and enable studies of the molecular epidemiology of the disease across China.

7.2. Animals

Melioidosis can affect a wide range of animal species, but its true incidence in wild and domestic animals is far from clear in almost all parts of China. Following the initial identification of *B. pseudomallei* from environmental samples in Hainan, Lu et al. carried out surveys on farm animals and succeeded in recovering *B. pseudomallei* from the viscera of pigs and goats collected in the slaughterhouses of Haikou and Nanning in 1982 [10]. In 1993, a rhesus monkey was confirmed as having died of melioidosis in a health research centre in Fuzhou, Fujian province [61]. In 2005, Chen isolated *B. pseudomallei* from dead dolphins at a marine park in Sanya City, Hainan [62]. Additionally, a melioidosis outbreak was reported at a livestock farm in Guangxi in October 2009, resulting in the death of 12 Boer goats [63]. Based on these accounts, we believe that animal melioidosis probably affects a variety of animal species in southern China, although the true range and economic loss it causes are yet unknown.

7.3. Guidelines

No standards or official guidelines for the diagnosis or management of melioidosis are available in mainland China. Although serological tests such as IHA and ELISA were established and used to diagnose melioidosis in some hospitals in Hainan and Guangdong in the 1990s [8], in our experience, culture and the identification of *B. pseudomallei* have now been accepted as the consensus standard and is what has now been adopted for the diagnosis and reporting of the disease at hospitals and institutes in endemic regions of China.

8. Diagnosis and Treatment

Accurate and efficient diagnosis of melioidosis cases is crucial, both for saving lives and for understanding the epidemiology of the disease. Unfortunately, owing to the lack of a consensus guideline and the scarcity of studies, the true situation as far as melioidosis diagnosis is concerned is largely unknown in mainland China. However, what is known from the literature does not give cause for optimism [32,33,39]. Due to a lack of laboratory capacity and a lack of familiarity with the clinical characteristics of the disease amongst clinicians, melioidosis patients are likely to be misdiagnosed in most ordinary hospitals [32,33]; even in good tertiary hospitals, the rate of initial misdiagnosis is high (80%–90%) [39]. Given the difficulty of clinical diagnosis of this protean disease, culture and identification of *B. pseudomallei* is accepted as the gold standard for the diagnosis of melioidosis countrywide [14,32,33,35,39]. However, as yet this capacity is restricted to a few general or teaching hospitals within endemic regions of China, where automated blood culture and commercial bacterial identification systems are deployed and microbiological investigations are routinely conducted. In addition to the use of commercial identification systems (e.g., VITEK, BD Phoenix, etc.), identification of *B. pseudomallei* commonly depends on laboratory staff recognizing the basic morphological and cultural characteristics of *B. pseudomallei* [15,38]. However, waiting for the results of cultures may lead to delays in initiating effective treatment. In a retrospective survey of 40 melioidosis cases in Hainan, the time from admission to diagnosis was 4–19 days (average 8.2 days) [33]. To improve efficiency and accuracy, molecular technologies (e.g., specific PCR, 16s rRNA sequencing, etc.) have been applied for the confirmation of the diagnosis by specialist centers in recent years; however, no proven rapid screening approaches for *B. pseudomallei* (such as the latex agglutination assay [64] or even the 'three disc test' for the characteristic antimicrobial susceptibility pattern [65]) are available in most hospitals in endemic areas of China. However, computed tomography (CT) scans, magnetic resonance imaging (MRI), and ultrasound have increasingly been used to identify internal abscesses in the liver, spleen, prostate and brain [37,39]. Clearly, the capability for melioidosis diagnostics need to be increased, and efficient rapid screening methods for detecting *B. pseudomallei* need to be introduced to Hainan and other endemic regions of mainland China.

As in other melioidosis-endemic regions of the world, lung or liver abscesses caused by *B. pseudomallei* are often mistaken for tumors or tuberculosis in Hainan, as the clinical and imaging features are difficult to distinguish [66]. In addition, although extremely rare, a case of human glanders was documented in China in 2004 [67]. A fatal human case of human *B. thailandensis* infection was also reported in 2017 [68], although the validity of this has been questioned [69].

With the rise of the incidence of melioidosis, the major general hospitals in Hainan have gradually gained experience and capability in providing effective diagnosis and treatment of melioidosis. Once the diagnosis has been made, the treatment regimens used are consistent with international consensus guidelines and consist of an initial intensive phase with intravenous antibiotics and a subsequent eradication phase with oral antibiotics [40]. Compared with that of over 20 years ago, the overall mortality rate of acute melioidosis cases has lowered from 50%–66% [27,28] to 15%–25% [34,38,39]. Recurrence has been observed, but only in a tiny proportion of cases that have received standardized treatment [32,39]. Improvements in patient outcomes are probably due to a combination of factors: advances in diagnostic techniques, availability of appropriate drugs (meropenem, imipenem and ceftazidime) and the regular performance of antibiotic susceptibility tests during therapy [40]. Nevertheless, the differences between hospitals and areas in their ability to diagnose and treat patients with melioidosis, remains a major concern. Based on our observations, most remote county-level hospitals in Hainan lack both the diagnostic capacity and access to appropriate antimicrobial drugs. Furthermore, it is worth noting that the economic burden of treatment on poor rural patients and their families is significant, and some even choose to withdraw from treatment [14,31,32].

Additionally, although the susceptibility of *B. pseudomallei* to carbapenems is almost universal, the emergence of ceftazidime resistance has been reported as a problem in some hospitals in Hainan in more recent years. Ceftazidime resistance was said to have risen from 0% to 20–30% of *B. pseudomallei* clinical isolates between 2002 and 2014 in one institution in Hainan [70]. This requires confirmation, and warrants our continued surveillance and concern.

9. Current and Future Challenges

Over 40 years has passed since the first identification of *B. pseudomallei* in southern China; nonetheless, our knowledge on this disease is still lacking and there are numerous challenges to revealing its true epidemiology. In particular, some crucial questions remain unanswered, including the ecology and distribution of *B. pseudomallei* in the environment within China, the true burden of the disease in local residents, and its incidence among domestic and wild animals. Therefore, institutions, hospitals and laboratories in this region and countrywide need to collaborate closely with each other and undertake more comprehensive epidemiological and ecological studies to enhance our knowledge and understanding of the disease within China.

Moreover, the main endemic area is the coastal zone (Hainan, Guangdong, Guangxi and Fujian), which has experienced rapid development and has become one of the major economic centers of China. In view of its proximity to Southeast Asia, the world's largest known melioidosis focus, and the booming economic and trade activities between them, close attention needs to be paid to the current and future trends of the disease in this area. In the meantime, under the national strategy of the Belt and Road Initiatives, Hainan has set the developmental goal of developing as a major international tourism island and seaborne trade centre in the next decade, with important progress towards these goals having already been made. In consequence, remarkable changes in the environment and population size can be anticipated for this region, which may increase the population at risk of infection with *B. pseudomallei* and pose greater challenges for the prevention and control of this disease in China and even regionally. Therefore, we recommend that melioidosis should be included in the national reportable diseases list, and that the sentinel surveillance network should be strengthened, which should lay a good foundation for risk assessment and the formulation of preventive strategies against this disease. Additionally, standard guidelines for the diagnosis and management of melioidosis need to be developed and distributed to all physicians and laboratory staff in both endemic and non-endemic areas of the country.

Although the national agency of disease control and prevention (ICDC) has set out to understand the current status through case and pathogen surveillance, the lack of awareness and attention of melioidosis amongst both government authorities and the general public is still a major challenge for the management and control of the disease in China. In a nationwide context, the public and the media hardly ever discuss this disease and threat it poses. Hence, we believe that a countrywide information campaign about melioidosis should be initiated in order to draw attention to this important disease.

10. Conclusions

In summary, this review presents a comprehensive account of the history, current status, and epidemiology of melioidosis in China. Surveillance data and a literature review clearly show that melioidosis has become more common in both endemic and non-endemic areas of mainland China, especially Hainan, in recent years, as in other parts of the world [71,72]. Surveillance and control strategies should be promoted to address this change, and further research should be conducted to provide new understanding and insights into the causes of this trend.

Supplementary Materials: The following are available online at http://www.mdpi.com/2414-6366/4/1/39/s1, Table S1: Summary of the number of human melioidosis cases from endemic and non-endemic provinces of mainland China identified from different sources.

Author Contributions: X.Z. conducted the data collection and wrote the first draft of the manuscript; Q.X. reviewed and revised the manuscript. L.X. and W.L. contributed to the writing of the manuscript.

Funding: This research was funded by National Natural Science Foundation of China (No. 81573208), National Science and Technology Major Project (No. 2018ZX10101003-001-009) and Natural Science Foundation of Hainan Province (No. 814389).

Acknowledgments: We thank Xiong Zhu, Hai Chen, Xuming Wang, Duorong Wu, Rushou Chen, Wenhui Mai, Zhicheng Wu, Xiaohua Zhang, Mei Xing and Ying Chen for assistance in case surveillance and data collection. We also thank David Dance for help with searching for the documented melioidosis cases from China and for editing the English.

Conflicts of Interest: The authors declare no conflict of interest.

References

1. Wiersinga, W.J.; Currie, B.J.; Peacock, S.J. Melioidosis. *N. Engl. J. Med.* **2012**, *367*, 1035–1044. [CrossRef] [PubMed]
2. Cheng, A.C.; Currie, B.J. Melioidosis: Epidemiology, pathophysiology, and management. *Clin. Microbiol. Rev.* **2005**, *18*, 383–416. [CrossRef] [PubMed]
3. Currie, B.J. Melioidosis: Evolving concepts in epidemiology, pathogenesis, and treatment. *Semin. Respir. Crit. Care Med.* **2015**, *36*, 111–125. [CrossRef] [PubMed]
4. Limmathurotsakul, D.; Golding, N.; Dance, D.A.; Messina, J.P.; Pigott, D.M.; Moyes, C.L.; Rolim, D.B.; Bertherat, E.; Day, N.P.; Peacock, S.J.; et al. Predicted global distribution of *Burkholderia pseudomallei* and burden of melioidosis. *Nat. Microbiol.* **2016**, *1*, 15008. [CrossRef] [PubMed]
5. Yang, S. Melioidosis research in China. *Acta Trop.* **2000**, *77*, 157–165. [CrossRef]
6. Mollaret, H.H. «L'affaire du jardin des plantes ou comment la mélioïdose fit son apparition en France. *Med. Maladies Infect.* **1988**, *18*, 643–654. (In French) [CrossRef]
7. Li, L. Survey on endemic foci of melioidosis. *Chin. J. Prev. Med.* **1981**, *15*, 1–5.
8. Li, L.; He, Y.W. *Pseudomonas pseudomallei* and melioidosis in China. *Chin. Med. J.* **1992**, *105*, 775–779. [PubMed]
9. Yang, S.; Tong, S.; Lu, Z. Geographical distribution of *Pseudomonas pseudomallei* in China. *Southeast Asian J. Trop. Med. Public Health* **1995**, *26*, 636–638. [PubMed]
10. Lu, Z.Z.; Zhang, W.D.; Mo, Z.S.; Wang, Y.X.; Fan, X.J.; Liang, J.Q.; Ouyang, X.M. Isolation of *Pseudomonas pseudomallei* from animals. *Chin. J. Vet. Med.* **1984**, *2*, 2–3.
11. Li, L.; Lu, Z.; Han, O. Epidemiology of melioidosis in China. *Chin. J. Epidemiol.* **1994**, *15*, 292–295.
12. Yang, S.; Tong, S.; Mo, C.; Jiang, Z.; Yang, S.; Ma, Y.; Lu, Z. Prevalence of human melioidosis on Hainan island in China. *Microbiol. Immunol.* **1998**, *42*, 651–654. [CrossRef] [PubMed]
13. Liu, Q.; Xu, W.; Lu, S.; Jiang, J.; Zhou, J.; Shao, Z.; Liu, X.; Xu, L.; Xiong, Y.; Zheng, H.; et al. Landscape of emerging and re-emerging infectious diseases in China: Impact of ecology, climate, and behavior. *Front. Med.* **2018**, *12*, 3–22. [CrossRef] [PubMed]
14. Lin, R.; Xie, C.; Chen, H.; Huang, Y. Clinical features and drug resistance analysis of melioidosis: 122 cases from Hainan. *Guangdong Med.* **2011**, *32*, 2303–2304.
15. Wu, H.; Wang, X.; Huang, D. Laboratory culture and identification on a collection of 95 *Burkholderia pseudomallei* strains. *Chin. J. Zoonoses* **2013**, *29*, 730–732.
16. Wang, X.M.; Zheng, X.; Wu, H.; Zhou, X.J.; Kuang, H.H.; Guo, H.L.; Xu, K.; Li, T.J.; Liu, L.L.; Li, W. Multilocus sequence typing of clinical isolates of *Burkholderia pseudomallei* collected in Hainan, a tropical island of southern China. *Am. J. Trop. Med. Hyg.* **2016**, *95*, 760–764. [CrossRef] [PubMed]
17. Godoy, D.; Randle, G.; Simpson, A.J.; Aanensen, D.M.; Pitt, T.L.; Kinoshita, R.; Spratt, B.G. Multilocus sequence typing and evolutionary relationships among the causative agents of melioidosis and glanders, *Burkholderia pseudomallei* and *Burkholderia mallei*. *J. Clin. Microbiol.* **2003**, *41*, 2068–2079. [CrossRef] [PubMed]

18. Tu, B.; Qin, E.; Zhao, M. A case of diabetes complicated with melioidosis septicemia. *J. Clin. Res.* **2011**, *28*, 2224.

19. Jin, H.; Chen, X.; Pan, Y.; Zhou, C.; Gao, X.; Hu, B.; He, L. Analysis and appraisal of difficult cases: No. 76, *Burkholderia pseudomallei* infection with fever, cough, swelling and pain of the right knee joint and bilateral pleural effusion with left hydropneumothorax. *Natl. Med. J. Chin.* **2005**, *85*, 1287–1289. [CrossRef]

20. Liu, Y.; Zhou, W.; Zhang, Z.; Si, J. One case of septicemia caused by *Burkholderia pseudomallei*. *Lab. Med. Clin.* **2016**, *13*, 575–576. [CrossRef]

21. Fang, Y.; Chen, J.; Zhu, Y.; Mao, X. Source tracking for an imported case of melioidosis. *J. Third Mil. Med. Univ.* **2016**, *38*, 1224–1225.

22. Li, Y.; Zhong, Y.; Liu, W.; Pu, Y.; Li, H.; Yan, Q.; Zou, M.; Guo, S. One death of sepsis caused by *Burkholderia pseudomallei*. *Chin. J. Infect. Control* **2013**, *12*, 475–476. [CrossRef]

23. Zhang, H. First imported and death case of melioidosis in Qinghai Province, China. *Int. J. Lab. Med.* **2015**, *36*, 1798–1799. [CrossRef]

24. Yang, L.; Lu, J. A case of cutaneous melioidosis infection misdiagnosed as rash over 10 years. *J. Third Mil. Med. Univ.* **2014**, *36*, 552.

25. Wang, Y. A case of melioidosis. *J. Clin. Dermatol.* **2014**, *43*, 163–164.

26. Li, L.; Wang, C.; Liu, J.; Gu, X.; Liang, R.; Sun, H. A case of *Burkholderia pseudomallei* septicemia associated with periorbit abscess. *Chin. J. Infect. Control* **2017**, *16*, 574–576. [CrossRef]

27. Lin, R.; Chen, H.; Yun, W. Clinical analysis of 12 cases of melioidosis in Hainan Province, 2002–2005. *Chin. J. Epidemiol.* **2005**, *26*, 824.

28. Chen, G.; Zeng, X.; Feng, X.; Liang, T.; Ke, S. Analysis of clinical feature and epidemiology investigation of melioidosis in Leizhou peninsula of Guangdong. *Chin. J. Infect. Dis.* **2006**, *24*, 406–409.

29. Cai, D.; Jia, J.; Wu, T.; Su, L. Clinical analysis of 32 *Pseudomonas pseudomallei* pneumonia patients. *Chin Trop. Med.* **2006**, *6*, 620–621.

30. Quan, H.; Fu, H.; Mo, C. Clinical analysis of 19 cases of type 2 diabetes mellitus complicated with septicemic melioidosis. *Chin. J. Endocrinol. Metab.* **2008**, *24*, 66–67. [CrossRef]

31. He, X.; Jia, J. Clinical analysis of 25 cases of septicemic melioidosis. *Chin. J. Modern Med.* **2008**, *18*, 956–958.

32. Cai, D.; Jia, J. Clinical features and drug resistance analysis of 104 melioidosis cases from Hainan. *Chongqing Med.* **2009**, *38*, 2362–2363.

33. Zhong, Y.; Lin, H. Clinical features and follow-up of melioidosis: 40 cases in Hainan island. *Chin. J. Lung Dis.* **2014**, *7*, 55–57.

34. Zhong, J.; Chen, R. Clinical analysis of 40 patients infected with *Burkholderia pseudomallei* in Sanya City. *Chin. Trop. Med.* **2014**, *14*, 1147–1149.

35. Fang, Y.; Chen, H.; Li, Y.L.; Li, Q.; Ye, Z.J.; Mao, X.H. Melioidosis in Hainan, China: A restrospective study. *Trans. R. Soc. Trop. Med. Hyg.* **2015**, *109*, 636–642. [CrossRef] [PubMed]

36. Zheng, X.; Wang, L.; Zhu, X.; Chen, H.; Wu, H.; Mai, W.; Li, W.; Xia, L. Preliminary study on incidence of melioidosis and molecular characteristics of clinical strains of *Burkholderia pseudomallei* after Typhoon Rammasun attack. *Dis. Surveill.* **2016**, *31*, 628–632. [CrossRef]

37. Zhan, Y.; Wu, Y.; Li, Q.; Yu, A. Neuromelioidosis: A series of seven cases in Hainan province, China. *J. Int. Med. Res.* **2017**, *45*, 856–867. [CrossRef] [PubMed]

38. Dong, S.; Lin, X.; Fu, S.; Wu, Q.; Xia, Q. Epidemiological features and clinical manifestations of melioidosis in 46 patients in Hainan. *J. Pathog. Biol.* **2017**, *12*, 579–582.

39. Zou, W.; Li, J.; Deng, C.; Liu, L.; Li, S. Clinical features of 35 cases of melioidosis. *Chin. J. Infect. Control* **2018**, *17*, 146–150.

40. Tang, Y.; Deng, J.; Zhang, J.; Zhong, X.; Qiu, Y.; Zhang, H.; Xu, H. Epidemiological and clinical features of melioidosis: A report of seven cases from southern inland China. *Am. J. Trop. Med. Hyg.* **2018**, *985*, 1296–1299. [CrossRef] [PubMed]

41. Ma, G.; Zheng, D.; Cai, Q.; Yuan, Z. Prevalence of *Burkholderia pseudomallei* in Guangxi, China. *Epidemiol. Infect.* **2010**, *138*, 37–39. [CrossRef] [PubMed]

42. One rare case of severe pneumonia caused by melioidosis infection in Putian. Sina Fujian, 27 November 2014. Available online: http://fj.sina.com.cn/news/s/2014-11-27/detail-iavxeafr5320356.shtml (accessed on 10 December 2018). (In Chinese)

43. Fu, Z.; Lin, Y.; Wu, Q.; Xia, Q. Pediatric suppurative parotitis caused by *Burkholderia pseudomallei*. *J. Venom. Anim. Toxins* **2016**, *22*, 31. [CrossRef] [PubMed]

44. Zou, W.; Jinghui, L.; Cao, Y.; Liu, F. Report of three cases of osteomyelitis caused by *Burkholderia pseudomallei* and literature review. *Chin. J. Infect. Chemo.* **2018**, *18*, 37–43. [CrossRef]

45. Cai, X.J.; Huang, Y.J.; Fu, Y.H. A case on acute *Burkholderia pseudomallei* pericarditis. *Chin. Med. J.* **2016**, *129*, 2256. [CrossRef] [PubMed]

46. Tan, G.; Li, J.; Chen, L.; Chen, X.; Zhang, S.; Ke, L.; Liu, J. Prostatic melioidosis rarely reported in China: Two cases report and literatures review. *Int. J. Clin. Exp. Med.* **2015**, *8*, 21830–21832. [PubMed]

47. Li, X.Y.; Ke, B.X.; Chen, C.N.; Xiao, H.L.; Liu, M.Z.; Xiong, Y.C.; Bai, R.; Chen, J.D.; Ke, C.W. First co-infection case of melioidosis and Japanese encephalitis in China. *BMC Infect. Dis.* **2018**, *18*, 452. [CrossRef] [PubMed]

48. Zheng, X.; Chen, H.; Zhu, X.; Cai, H.; Li, L.; Li, H.; You, X.; Ping, J.; Xia, L.; Li, W. Discovery of *Burkholderia thailandensis* isolated from melioidosis endemic areas of Hainan, China. *Chin. J. Epidemiol.* **2015**, *36*, 97–98.

49. Lin, Y.; Wu, Q.; Liu, X.; Dong, S.; Wu, L.; Pei, H.; Xu, K.; Xia, Q. Molecular tracking investigation of melioidosis cases reveals regional endemicity in Hainan, China. *Biomed. Rep.* **2016**, *5*, 766–770. [CrossRef] [PubMed]

50. Li, S.; Chen, H.; Li, H.; Li, W.; Xia, L.; Li, L.; Zheng, X.; Zhu, X. Molecular tracing investigation for one case of melioidosis in Hainan Island, China. *Chin. J. Zoonoses* **2018**, *34*, 673–676. [CrossRef]

51. Dong, S.; Wu, L.; Long, F.; Wu, Q.; Liu, X.; Pei, H.; Xu, K.; Lu, Y.; Wang, Y.; Lin, Y.; et al. The prevalence and distribution of *Burkholderia pseudomallei* in rice paddy within Hainan, China. *Acta Trop.* **2018**, *187*, 165–168. [CrossRef] [PubMed]

52. Fang, Y.; Zhu, P.; Li, Q.; Chen, H.; Li, Y.; Ren, C.; Hu, Y.; Tan, Z.; Gu, J.; Mao, X. Multilocus sequence typing of 102 *Burkholderia pseudomallei* strains isolated from China. *Epidemiol. Infect.* **2016**, *144*, 1917–1923. [CrossRef] [PubMed]

53. Chen, H.; Xia, L.; Zhu, X.; Li, W.; Du, X.; Wu, D.; Hai, R.; Shen, X.; Liang, Y.; Cai, H.; et al. *Burkholderia pseudomallei* sequence type 562 in China and Australia. *Emerg. Infect. Dis.* **2015**, *21*, 166–168. [CrossRef] [PubMed]

54. Price, E.P.; Sarovich, D.S.; Smith, E.J.; MacHunter, B.; Harrington, G.; Theobald, V.; Hall, C.M.; Hornstra, H.M.; McRobb, E.; Podin, Y.; et al. Unprecedented melioidosis cases in northern Australia caused by an Asian *Burkholderia pseudomallei* strain identified by using large-scale comparative genomics. *Appl. Environ. Microbiol.* **2016**, *82*, 954–963. [CrossRef] [PubMed]

55. Fang, Y.; Huang, Y.; Li, Q.; Chen, H.; Yao, Z.; Pan, J.; Gu, J.; Tang, B.; Wang, H.G.; Yu, B.; et al. First genome sequence of a *Burkholderia pseudomallei* isolate in China, strain BPC006, obtained from a melioidosis patient in Hainan. *J. Bacteriol.* **2012**, *194*, 6604–6605. [CrossRef] [PubMed]

56. Song, L.; Yu, Y.; Feng, L.; He, J.; Wang, T.; Zhu, H.; Duan, Q. Draft genome sequence of *Burkholderia pseudomallei* strain 350105, isolated in Hainan, China, in 1976. *Genome Announc.* **2015**, *3*. [CrossRef] [PubMed]

57. Chou, D.W.; Chung, K.M.; Chen, C.H.; Cheung, B.M. Bacteremic melioidosis in southern Taiwan: Clinical characteristics and outcome. *J. Formos. Med. Assoc.* **2007**, *106*, 1013–1022. [CrossRef]

58. Huang, Y.; Nie, X.; Huang, M.; Li, Y.; Chen, H.; Guo, X. Study on characteristics and epidemiology of *Burkholderia pseudomallei* in Zhanjiang area. *Chin. Infect. Control.* **2008**, *7*, 268–271.

59. Hu, C.; Jia, W. Diabetes in China: Epidemiology and genetic risk factors and their clinical utility in personalized medication. *Diabetes* **2018**, *67*, 3–11. [CrossRef] [PubMed]

60. Yang, S.; Wu, J.; Ding, C.; Cui, Y.; Zhou, Y.; Li, Y.; Deng, M.; Wang, C.; Xu, K.; Ren, J.; et al. Epidemiological features of and changes in incidence of infectious diseases in China in the first decade after the SARS outbreak: An observational trend study. *Lancet Infect. Dis.* **2017**, *17*, 716–725. [CrossRef]

61. Fan, C.; Li, Z.; Zhou, J.; Wen, W.; Chen, S.; Zhu, Y. Case report: A death of rhesus monkey caused by *Burkholderia pseudomallei* infection. *Chin. J. Zoonoses* **1994**, *10*, 64.

62. Chen, H.; Zhu, L. Separation of *Burkholderia pseudomallei* from dead dolphin. *Chin. J. Zoonoses* **2007**, *23*, 1269–1270.

63. Tao, L.; Peng, H.; Wei, Z.; Lan, M.; Li, J.; Qin, R.; Zhou, Y.; Chen, Z.; Yang, W. Diagnosis and treatment for *Burkholderia pseudomallei* infection in Boer Goats. *Chin. J. Zoonoses* **2011**, *47*, 39–40.

64. Anuntagool, N.; Naigowit, P.; Petkanchanapong, V.; Aramsri, P.; Panichakul, T.; Sirisinha, S. Monoclonal antibody-based rapid identification of *Burkholderia pseudomallei* in blood culture fluid from patients with community-acquired septicaemia. *J. Med. Microbiol.* **2000**, *49*, 1075–1078. [CrossRef] [PubMed]

65. Trinh, T.T.; Hoang, T.S.; Tran, D.A.; Trinh, V.T.; Gohler, A.; Nguyen, T.T.; Hoang, S.N.; Krumkamp, R.; Nguyen, L.T.N.; May, J.; et al. A simple laboratory algorithm for diagnosis of melioidosis in resource-constrained areas: A study from north-central Vietnam. *Clin. Microbiol. Infect.* **2018**, *24*, e81–e84. [CrossRef] [PubMed]

66. Cai, D.; Jia, J.; Wu, T.; Su, L. Analysis of 15 cases of melioidosis misdiagnosed as pulmonary tuberculosis. *Chin. J. Misdiagn.* **2006**, *6*, 2135–2136.

67. Lu, L.; Zhao, C.; Sun, Q. Misdiagnosis of a case of human glanders. *Chin. J. Mult Organ. Dis Eld.* **2004**, *3*, 184.

68. Kai, C.; Jie, L.; Huan, X.; Min, L.; Fengling, Z.; Jin, L.; Dayong, G.; Shaoli, D.; Ming, C.; Weiping, L. Human infection with *Burkholderia thailandensis*, China, 2013. *Emerg. Infect. Dis.* **2017**, *23*, 1416–1418.

69. Dance, D.A.B.; Sarovich, D.; Price, E.P.; Limmathurotsakul, D.; Currie, B.J. Human infection with *Burkholderia thailandensis*, China, 2013. *Emerg. Infect. Dis.* **2018**, *24*, 953–954. [CrossRef] [PubMed]

70. Chenyang, J.; Hu, C.; Fang, Y.; Mao, X. Drug resistance spectrum of clinical *Burkholderia pseudomallei* strains in China and related mechanism. *J. Third Mil. Med. Univ.* **2016**, *38*, 1220–1223. [CrossRef]

71. Hinjoy, S.; Hantrakun, V.; Kongyu, S.; Kaewrakmuk, J.; Wangrangsimakul, T.; Jitsuronk, S.; Saengchun, W.; Bhengsri, S.; Akarachotpong, T.; Thamthitiwat, S.; et al. Melioidosis in Thailand: Present and future. *Trop. Med. Infect. Dis.* **2018**, *3*, 38. [CrossRef] [PubMed]

72. Trinh, T.T.; Nguyen, L.D.N.; Nguyen, T.V.; Tran, C.X.; Le, A.V.; Nguyen, H.V.; Assig, K.; Lichtenegger, S.; Wagner, G.E.; Do, C.D.; et al. Melioidosis in Vietnam: Recently improved recognition but still an uncertain disease burden after almost a century of reporting. *Trop. Med. Infect. Dis.* **2018**, *3*, 39. [CrossRef] [PubMed]

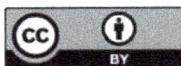

MDPI

St. Alban-Anlage 66

4052 Basel

Switzerland

Tel. +41 61 683 77 34

Fax +41 61 302 89 18

www.mdpi.com

Tropical Medicine and Infectious Disease Editorial Office

E-mail: tropicalmed@mdpi.com

www.mdpi.com/journal/tropicalmed

www.ingramcontent.com/pod-product-compliance
Lightning Source LLC
Chambersburg PA
CBHW051723210326
41597CB00032B/5584